HANDBOOK ON
PERSONALIZED MEDICINE

Handbook on Personalized Medicine

Zen Obi
Kwesi Crow

Kruger Brentt
Publishers

2026

Kruger Brentt Publishers UK. LTD.
Company Number 9728962

Regd. Office: 68 St Margarets Road, Edgware, Middlesex HA8 9UU

ISBN: 978-1-78715-615-9

Disclaimer:

Every possible effort has been made to ensure that the information contained in this book is accurate at the time of going to press, and the publisher and author cannot accept responsibility for any errors or omissions, however caused. No responsibility for loss or damage occasioned to any person acting, or refraining from action, as a result of the material in this publication can be accepted by the editor, the publisher or the author. The Publisher is not associated with any product or vendor mentioned in the book. The contents of this work are intended to further general scientific research, understanding and discussion only. Readers should consult with a specialist where appropriate.

Every effort has been made to trace the owners of copyright material used in this book, if any. The author and the publisher will be grateful for any omission brought to their notice for acknowledgement in the future editions of the book.

For information on all our publications visit our website at http://krugerbrentt.com/

PREFACE

Personalized medicine represents a transformative approach to healthcare, moving away from the traditional "one-size-fits-all" model toward treatments tailored to individual patients based on their genetic, environmental, and lifestyle factors. Advances in genomics, bioinformatics, molecular diagnostics, and data analytics have made it possible to design more precise, effective, and safer therapeutic strategies. Personalized medicine holds the promise of improving patient outcomes, reducing adverse drug reactions, and optimizing healthcare delivery on a global scale.

This book, Handbook on Personalized Medicine, provides a comprehensive overview of the principles, technologies, and applications of personalized healthcare. It is designed for medical professionals, researchers, students, and healthcare policymakers seeking an in-depth understanding of how individualized approaches are reshaping modern medicine.

The book begins with an introduction to the foundational concepts of personalized medicine, including genomics, proteomics, metabolomics, and pharmacogenomics. Subsequent chapters explore diagnostic technologies, biomarker identification, and molecular profiling techniques that enable clinicians to make informed decisions about disease prevention, diagnosis, and treatment.

Special emphasis is placed on the application of personalized medicine across major therapeutic areas, including oncology, cardiology, neurology, and rare genetic disorders. The book also discusses the integration of big data, artificial intelligence, and machine learning in analyzing patient-specific information to guide therapy and predict outcomes. Ethical, regulatory, and social considerations related to personalized medicine, such as data privacy, equity, and accessibility, are thoroughly addressed.

Real-world case studies illustrate how personalized medicine is applied in clinical settings, highlighting successes, challenges, and ongoing research. By combining scientific rigor with practical insights, the book equips readers with the knowledge necessary to understand, implement, and advance personalized approaches in healthcare.

Handbook on Personalized Medicine serves as an essential resource for anyone involved in modern healthcare, from clinicians and researchers to educators and policymakers. By integrating cutting-edge science with clinical applications, this book provides a roadmap for delivering more precise, effective, and patient-centered care.

Zen Obi

Kwesi Crow

CONTENTS

1 Chapter INTRODUCTION TO PERSONALIZED MEDICINE

1.0 INTRODUCTION: AN OVERVIEW

The field of medicine is undergoing a transformative shift from a generalized, population-based approach toward a more precise, individualized strategy known as Personalized Medicine. This emerging model of healthcare aims to tailor medical treatment to the unique characteristics of each patient by integrating genetic, molecular, environmental, and lifestyle information. Rather than relying on the traditional "one-size-fits-all" model—where patients with the same condition receive the same treatment—personalized medicine seeks to provide the right treatment to the right patient at the right time. At its core, personalized medicine recognizes that individuals vary in their susceptibility to disease, in the biology of their conditions, and in their responses to treatment. These differences often have a genetic basis. Advances in genomics, proteomics, metabolomics, and bioinformatics have made it possible to explore these variations more precisely than ever before. The Human Genome Project, completed in 2003, laid the foundation by decoding the entire human genetic blueprint. Since then, a new era of precision diagnostics and targeted therapies has emerged, revolutionizing how we predict, prevent, diagnose, and treat diseases. In oncology, for example, personalized medicine is already yielding significant results. Biomarker testing and genomic profiling can identify mutations that drive tumour growth, allowing clinicians to match patients with targeted therapies that directly address those mutations. This has led to improved treatment outcomes, reduced side effects, and better quality of life for many cancer patients. Similar approaches are being developed in cardiology, neurology, psychiatry, infectious diseases, and rare genetic disorders.

One of the key components of personalized medicine is pharmacogenomics, the study of how genes affect a person's response to drugs. Genetic testing can reveal variations in drug metabolism, enabling physicians to avoid adverse drug reactions and to select medications and dosages that are more likely to be effective. For instance, variations in the CYP450 enzymes can determine how patients metabolize drugs like warfarin, clopidogrel, or antidepressants, guiding more precise prescriptions.

Another important pillar is predictive and preventive medicine. Genetic and molecular data allow clinicians to assess an individual's risk for developing certain diseases—such as breast cancer, Alzheimer's, or Type 2 diabetes—before symptoms appear. This proactive approach empowers individuals to adopt lifestyle changes, undergo early screening, or consider preventive treatments, shifting the focus from disease treatment to health maintenance and risk reduction.

Personalized medicine also plays a crucial role in rare and undiagnosed diseases. Whole-genome and exome sequencing have helped uncover the genetic basis of many conditions that had previously eluded diagnosis, offering hope to patients and families after years of uncertainty. These discoveries often pave the way for targeted interventions and greater understanding of the biological pathways involved. The digital revolution has accelerated the growth of personalized medicine. Wearable devices, electronic health records, artificial intelligence, and machine learning enable the integration and analysis of massive amounts of patient data. These technologies help identify subtle patterns, optimize treatment pathways, and support evidence-based clinical decision-making. Moreover, the convergence of biotechnology, data science, and cloud computing is fostering more dynamic, real-time, and continuous health monitoring (Fig. 1).

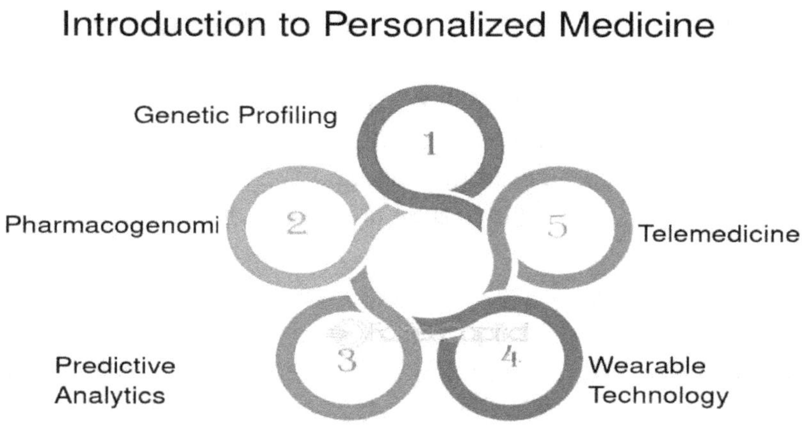

Fig. 1 Introduction to Personalized Medicine

Despite its promise, personalized medicine also raises ethical, social, and economic challenges. Issues such as data privacy, genetic discrimination, health equity, and informed consent are central to public trust and responsible implementation. Furthermore, disparities in access to advanced diagnostics and targeted therapies remain a concern, particularly in low-resource settings. The cost-effectiveness of personalized interventions also needs rigorous evaluation to ensure sustainable healthcare systems. In education and training, personalized medicine demands a new generation of clinicians, researchers, and health professionals skilled in genomics, data interpretation, and interdisciplinary collaboration. Medical curricula must evolve to incorporate these competencies and foster a deeper understanding of patient diversity and individuality. Personalized medicine represents a paradigm shift—from reactive to proactive, from generalized to individualized, and from treatment-focused to prevention-centered care. It holds the potential to redefine modern medicine, offering more precise, predictive, and participatory approaches that benefit patients, providers, and society alike. While challenges remain, the integration of scientific innovation, clinical insight, and ethical responsibility will be key to unlocking the full promise of this transformative field.

1.1 DEFINITION AND CORE CONCEPTS

Personalized Medicine, also known as precision medicine, is a medical model that customizes healthcare—decisions, practices, and treatments—to the individual characteristics of each patient. It integrates information about a person's genetic makeup, molecular profile, environment, and lifestyle to tailor prevention, diagnosis, and therapy strategies. Rather than applying uniform treatments to all patients with the same disease, personalized medicine recognizes and responds to the biological uniqueness of each individual. In summary, personalized medicine integrates modern biology, technology, and patient data to move beyond generalized approaches and toward highly individualized healthcare. It holds the potential to significantly improve outcomes by offering more precise, predictive, preventive, and participatory medical care.

Core Concepts of Personalized Medicine: Personalized medicine represents a transformative approach to healthcare that emphasizes the uniqueness of each individual. Unlike traditional models that treat patients based on population averages, personalized medicine leverages advanced tools in genomics, molecular biology, and data science to understand the intricate biological differences among individuals. At the heart of this medical paradigm are several foundational concepts that guide its application—from genomic profiling and biomarker discovery to targeted therapies and pharmacogenomics. These concepts enable clinicians to predict disease risks, diagnose conditions more accurately, and tailor treatments that align with each patient's genetic and physiological profile. Personalized medicine also integrates real-time health monitoring, wearable technologies, and artificial intelligence to refine decisions and optimize outcomes. It fosters a shift from reactive care to proactive prevention, ensuring interventions are timely, effective, and minimally invasive. The multi-omics approach—encompassing genomics, proteomics, metabolomics, and more—offers a holistic view of health at the molecular level. Central to this field is patient empowerment and shared decision-making, emphasizing individualized care and respect for personal values. Furthermore, personalized medicine underscores the ethical use of sensitive health data, equity in access to innovations, and ongoing education for both providers and patients (Fig. 2).

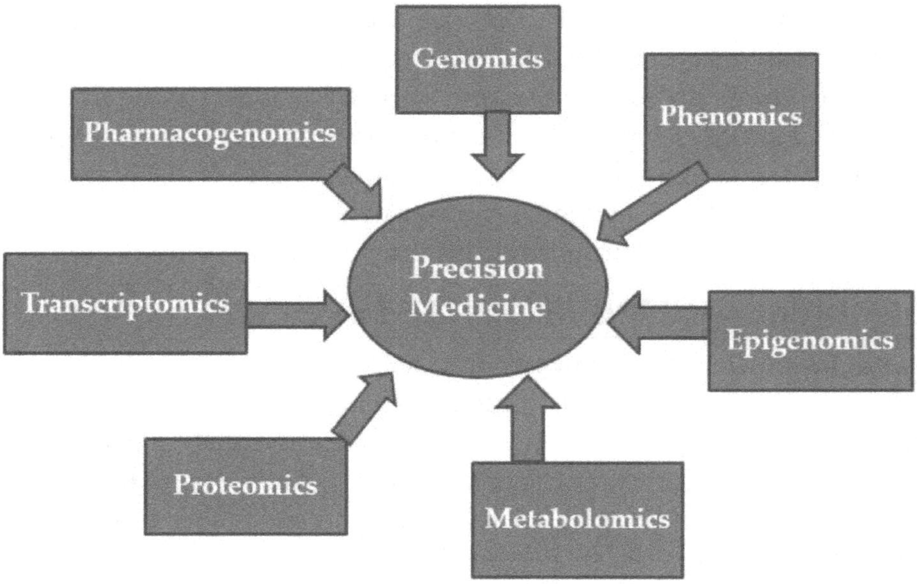

Fig. 2 Revolutionizing Personalized Medicine

These core concepts collectively define the framework that is reshaping the future of modern medicine (Table-1).

- **Genomic Profiling:** Central to personalized medicine is the analysis of an individual's DNA to detect genetic variations, mutations, or polymorphisms that influence disease susceptibility, progression, and response to treatment. For instance, mutations in the BRCA1/2 genes increase the risk of breast and ovarian cancers.
- **Biomarkers:** Biological markers (biomarkers) are measurable indicators of a biological condition or response. They help in disease detection, risk assessment, and therapy selection. For example, HER2 protein expression guides treatment in breast cancer.
- **Pharmacogenomics:** This is the study of how genes affect a person's response to drugs. It enables the optimization of drug therapy—maximizing effectiveness and minimizing toxicity—based on an individual's genetic makeup. Drugs like warfarin and tamoxifen are prescribed more effectively with pharmacogenomic data.
- **Risk Stratification:** Personalized medicine uses genetic and molecular tools to categorize individuals into different risk groups. This allows for early intervention, focused monitoring, or preventive measures tailored to the individual's risk profile.
- **Targeted Therapies:** These are treatments developed to specifically target molecular pathways or mutations responsible for disease. Unlike

conventional therapies that affect both healthy and diseased cells, targeted therapies aim for precision with fewer side effects.

- **Data Integration and AI:** Personalized medicine requires the integration of large-scale data—genomic, clinical, lifestyle, and environmental. AI and machine learning tools are used to analyze complex datasets and generate individualized treatment plans.
- **Preventive Medicine:** By understanding genetic predispositions and lifestyle factors, physicians can develop personalized preventive strategies to reduce disease risk, such as dietary changes, prophylactic treatments, or enhanced screening schedules.
- **Patient-Centered Care:** Personalized medicine emphasizes the active participation of patients in their healthcare decisions. It values the individual's preferences, beliefs, and values, promoting a shared decision-making model.
- **Molecular Diagnostics:** These advanced diagnostic tests detect disease at a molecular level, often before symptoms appear. They are crucial in identifying the most effective treatment or determining whether treatment is necessary.
- **Multi-Omics Approach:** Personalized medicine uses data from genomics (DNA), transcriptomics (RNA), proteomics (proteins), and metabolomics (metabolites) to gain a holistic understanding of an individual's health status.
- **Real-Time Monitoring and Wearables:** Digital health technologies such as wearable devices collect continuous health data (e.g., heart rate, glucose levels) to monitor patient conditions in real time, enabling dynamic personalization of treatment.
- **Ethical and Legal Considerations:** The use of genetic and personal health data brings challenges around privacy, consent, data sharing, and potential misuse. Personalized medicine must operate within a framework of ethical standards and regulations.
- **Health Equity:** A core principle is ensuring that advancements in personalized medicine are accessible and affordable to diverse populations, not limited by socioeconomic or geographic disparities.

Table 1 Summary of the Core Concepts of Personalized Medicine

Core Concept	Description	Example / Application
Genomic Profiling	Analysis of DNA to detect genetic variations that affect disease risk and treatment response.	BRCA1/2 gene mutations and breast/ovarian cancer risk.

Biomarkers	Measurable biological indicators used in disease diagnosis, risk assessment, and therapy selection.	HER2 protein expression in breast cancer.
Pharmacogenomics	Study of how genes influence drug response to ensure optimal drug selection and dosage.	Warfarin or tamoxifen dosage based on CYP gene variants.
Risk Stratification	Categorizing individuals into risk groups using genetic and molecular tools for early intervention.	Genetic screening for heart disease or diabetes risk.
Targeted Therapies	Drugs or treatments designed to specifically target disease-causing molecular pathways or mutations.	EGFR inhibitors in lung cancer.
Data Integration & AI	Combining large-scale clinical, genomic, and lifestyle data analyzed using AI for personalized treatment plans.	AI predicting cancer treatment responses.
Preventive Medicine	Using personal risk data to design strategies that prevent disease before symptoms appear.	Prophylactic mastectomy for BRCA mutation carriers.
Patient-Centered Care	Emphasizing shared decision-making and individual values in treatment planning.	Customizing care plans based on patient preferences.
Molecular Diagnostics	Early detection of disease at the molecular level using specialized tests.	Liquid biopsies for early cancer detection.
Multi-Omics Approach	Integrating genomics, proteomics, transcriptomics, and metabolomics for a comprehensive understanding of health.	Systems biology models of disease.
Real-Time Monitoring	Use of wearables and digital devices to continuously collect and analyze health data.	Continuous glucose monitors for diabetics.
Ethical & Legal Issues	Ensuring privacy, informed consent, and data security in handling genetic and health data.	Regulations like HIPAA and GDPR.
Health Equity	Striving for equitable access to personalized medicine technologies and therapies across populations.	Subsidizing genomic tests in low-income communities.

1.2 HISTORICAL EVOLUTION: FROM ONE-SIZE-FITS-ALL TO TAILORED THERAPIES

The journey from generalized medicine to personalized healthcare is marked by key scientific discoveries, technological advancements, and paradigm shifts in medical philosophy. Below is a detailed, headwise explanation of the historical evolution of personalized medicine:

1.2.1. Ancient and Pre-Modern Practices

Early Individualization (Before 19th Century): Long before the advent of modern science and molecular medicine, ancient healing traditions practiced forms of individualized care based on holistic principles. In traditional systems such as Ayurveda (India), Traditional Chinese Medicine (China), and Unani and Greek Medicine (Middle East and Europe), physicians emphasized the uniqueness of each individual. Rather than adopting a uniform treatment for all patients, these traditions focused on temperament, body constitution, age, environment, diet, and emotional state. For example, in Ayurveda, a person's constitution—known as prakriti—was categorized into three doshas: Vata, Pitta, and Kapha, each representing different physiological and psychological tendencies. Treatment plans in Ayurveda were tailored according to the balance or imbalance among these doshas, including personalized regimens of herbs, diet, physical activity, and meditation. Similarly, Traditional Chinese Medicine (TCM) recognized the interplay of yin and yang, the five elements, and vital energy or qi in determining the health profile of an individual. Diagnosis in TCM was based on detailed patient observation, pulse reading, and tongue inspection, leading to highly personalized herbal, dietary, and acupuncture-based therapies. Greek physician Hippocrates, often called the father of Western medicine, also emphasized individualized care. His theory of the four humors—blood, phlegm, yellow bile, and black bile—was used to explain disease as a result of imbalance. Treatments included lifestyle changes, diet modifications, and bloodletting, depending on the person's specific humoral composition. While these systems lacked the molecular understanding of disease, they operated on the principle that no two individuals are exactly alike, and health is a balance between internal and external factors unique to each person. This early form of "personalization" in healthcare, although based on observation and philosophy rather than scientific evidence, demonstrates humanity's long-standing awareness of individual variability in disease manifestation and response to treatment. These practices were empirical and intuitive, derived from centuries of accumulated knowledge, clinical observation, and experience rather than controlled experiments. There were no tools to measure DNA, proteins, or metabolic profiles, yet the practitioners of these ancient systems understood that treating the whole person, rather than just the disease, was key to effective healing. Despite the limitations of their time, these systems laid the philosophical and clinical groundwork for what would eventually evolve into modern personalized medicine. In many parts of the world, especially in Asia and Africa, such traditional systems are still used in parallel with modern medicine. Modern research is now revisiting these age-old traditions through the lens of science, exploring whether ancient classifications like prakriti have genetic or metabolic correlates. While ancient and pre-modern practices lacked the molecular and technological sophistication of today's personalized medicine, they strongly embraced individual-centered care. They understood health as a dynamic equilibrium shaped by personal constitution, environment, and lifestyle. Their legacy continues to influence integrative medicine today, reinforcing the notion that personalization in healthcare is not a new idea—but rather a deep-rooted principle that has evolved alongside human civilization.

1.2.2 The Rise of Modern Medicine

One-Size-Fits-All Begins (19th–20th Century): The 19th and 20th centuries witnessed a profound transformation in medicine, characterized by the emergence of a more standardized, scientific, and population-based approach to diagnosis and treatment. This era, marked by monumental discoveries such as the germ theory of disease by Louis Pasteur and Robert Koch, brought clarity to the causes of many infectious illnesses. With the understanding that microorganisms were responsible for diseases like tuberculosis, cholera, and anthrax, medical interventions became more targeted and universally applied. Alongside this scientific advancement, the development of anesthesia and antiseptics, led by pioneers like William Morton and Joseph Lister, revolutionized surgical practices by reducing pain, infection, and mortality, allowing safer and more consistent procedures. Another groundbreaking development was the discovery and mass production of antibiotics, most notably penicillin in the 1920s and 1940s. Antibiotics drastically reduced the death toll from bacterial infections and reinforced the model of uniform treatment for specific diseases, regardless of patient variability. Medical education and clinical practice became increasingly rooted in symptomatology and population norms, leading to the birth of the "one-size-fits-all" paradigm. Diseases were diagnosed through observable signs and symptoms, and treatments were prescribed based on what worked on the average patient, as determined by population-wide studies. The mid-20th century introduced another major milestone: the Randomized Controlled Trial (RCT). RCTs, first popularized by Sir Austin Bradford Hill, became the gold standard in clinical research, enabling scientists to determine the safety and efficacy of new drugs and therapies in a statistically rigorous manner. While RCTs greatly improved medical reliability and eliminated bias, they were designed to measure average treatment effects rather than account for individual differences. As a result, patients who deviated from the average in terms of genetics, metabolism, or comorbidities were often excluded or underrepresented in both studies and treatment guidelines. This era also marked the rise of evidence-based medicine (EBM), which emphasized decision-making rooted in empirical data from clinical trials and meta-analyses. EBM was a major step forward in ensuring that healthcare was grounded in proven effectiveness. However, it came at the cost of individualized nuance, as guidelines and protocols were generalized to large populations. Personal factors such as genetic predisposition, metabolic rate, or immune response were not yet measurable or understood, so they were largely ignored in mainstream treatment approaches.

In essence, while the 19th and 20th centuries laid the scientific and institutional foundations of modern medicine, they also entrenched a model that prioritized universality over individuality. The progress achieved in controlling infectious diseases, reducing surgical mortality, and introducing mass drug therapies was remarkable. Yet, this progress also fostered a reliance on standardization, assuming that what worked for the majority would work for all. This assumption, though efficient in many cases, overlooked the complex biological variability among individuals, which would only come to light with the advent of genetics and molecular medicine in the 21st century. Thus, the rise of modern medicine brought remarkable advances in public health and medical practice, but it also marked a period where the individual patient was often overshadowed by statistical averages. It was a time when medicine moved toward precision in tools and procedures, but not yet toward precision in personalization. The eventual shift toward personalized medicine in the late 20th and early 21st centuries would emerge as a necessary response to the limitations of this generalized, population-focused medical model

1.2.3 Discovery of DNA and the Genetic Basis of Disease (1950s–1970s)

The period from the 1950s to the 1970s marked a pivotal chapter in the history of medical science with the emergence of molecular biology and genetics as core disciplines. A major breakthrough occurred in 1953, when James Watson and Francis Crick, building on the work of Rosalind Franklin and Maurice Wilkins, unveiled the double-helix structure of DNA. This discovery revolutionized our understanding of heredity, establishing that DNA is the molecule that carries genetic information and directs the formation of proteins in all living organisms. It not only launched the molecular era in biology but also laid the foundational framework for modern genetics and personalized medicine. Following this, scientists began decoding the genetic code, identifying how sequences of DNA nucleotides determine the sequence of amino acids in proteins. This set the stage for understanding how gene mutations could lead to disease. During this period, Mendelian genetics—based on Gregor Mendel's 19th-century work—gained renewed attention. Researchers began to correlate specific gene mutations with monogenic (single-gene) diseases, such as sickle-cell anemia, cystic fibrosis, hemophilia, and Huntington's disease. These diseases followed predictable inheritance patterns (dominant or recessive), enabling doctors and genetic counselors to trace familial risk and offer early diagnosis or reproductive guidance. However, the scope of genetic medicine during this time was relatively limited. The tools for sequencing DNA were still rudimentary, and there was little understanding of complex, polygenic diseases like heart disease, diabetes, cancer, or schizophrenia. These conditions involved interactions between multiple genes and environmental factors, making them difficult to decipher using the available techniques. Furthermore, the idea of using genetic information to personalize treatment was still a theoretical concept, far from clinical application.

Despite these limitations, the 1950s–1970s era was crucial in reshaping medical thought. It marked the transition from observational medicine to molecular explanation, shifting focus from treating symptoms to investigating underlying biological mechanisms. It also fostered the early development of molecular diagnostics, such as karyotyping and enzyme assays, which could detect chromosomal abnormalities and inherited metabolic disorders. These innovations, though primitive by today's standards, signaled the beginning of genotype-based disease understanding. Research institutions worldwide began investing in molecular biology, and genetics was increasingly integrated into medical education and research. The growing body of genetic knowledge also raised new ethical questions about privacy, reproductive decisions, and genetic discrimination—questions that would become more prominent in the coming decades. Importantly, this period ignited a scientific momentum that would eventually culminate in large-scale projects like the Human Genome Project.

The discovery of DNA's structure and the identification of the genetic basis for certain diseases in the 1950s–1970s laid a conceptual foundation for personalized medicine. It marked the first time diseases were understood not merely as external invasions or organ dysfunctions, but as molecular disruptions at the genetic level. Although still limited to a small subset of diseases, this understanding planted the seeds for the future revolution in individualized healthcare, where genetic information would become central to prediction, diagnosis, and treatment.

1.2.4 The Human Genome Project (1990–2003): The Genomic Revolution

The Human Genome Project (HGP) stands as one of the most ambitious and transformative scientific undertakings in modern history. Launched in 1990 and successfully completed in 2003, this international, collaborative effort aimed to map and sequence the entire human genome, comprising over 3 billion DNA base pairs. Spearheaded by the U.S. National Institutes of Health (NIH) and the Department of Energy, along with global partners from the UK, Japan, France, Germany, and China, the HGP sought to identify and understand all the approximately 20,000–25,000 human genes encoded within our DNA. The completion of the project marked a historic milestone—a genomic blueprint of humanity was finally revealed. The significance of the HGP extended far beyond sequencing DNA. It marked a turning point in biomedical science, opening a new era of genomic medicine where the relationship between genes and disease could be systematically studied. Researchers could now investigate how genetic variations, such as single nucleotide polymorphisms (SNPs), contribute to disease susceptibility, progression, and drug response. This knowledge began to reshape our understanding of a wide range of diseases—from monogenic disorders like cystic fibrosis to complex, multifactorial conditions such as cancer, diabetes, cardiovascular diseases, and Alzheimer's. The project provided scientists with tools to identify disease-causing genes, understand gene-environment interactions, and develop new diagnostic and therapeutic strategies.

Perhaps most importantly, the HGP catalyzed the birth of personalized and precision medicine. By understanding the genetic basis of disease, clinicians could begin tailoring treatments to the molecular profile of each patient, rather than relying solely on symptom-based, generalized approaches. For example, recognizing specific mutations in cancer-related genes allowed for the design of targeted therapies, such as HER2 inhibitors in breast cancer or EGFR inhibitors in lung cancer. Moreover, the availability of the human genome sequence fueled advancements in pharmacogenomics, helping predict how individuals would respond to certain medications based on their genetic makeup. The Human Genome Project also revolutionized research methods and data analysis in biology. It led to the development of high-throughput DNA sequencing technologies, powerful bioinformatics tools, and massive genomic databases that could store and analyze vast amounts of genetic information. These innovations drastically reduced the time and cost of sequencing—from billions of dollars per genome to just a few hundred today—making genetic testing more accessible for clinical and research use. Beyond the science, the HGP raised important ethical, legal, and social issues (ELSI), such as genetic privacy, potential discrimination, and informed consent. These concerns were addressed through dedicated ELSI programs integrated into the project, setting precedents for future genomic research. It also spurred public dialogue about the implications of knowing one's genetic risk and how such information should be handled in medicine, insurance, and employment. The Human Genome Project served as the genomic revolution's launching pad, redefining how we study, understand, and treat disease. It turned the vision of personalized medicine from theory into possibility. With the entire genetic code of Homo sapiens mapped, medicine was no longer confined to observable symptoms but could now delve into the molecular architecture of life itself. The legacy of the HGP continues to shape contemporary research, clinical practice, and healthcare policy, anchoring a future where treatment is informed by the patient's genome, not just their condition.

1.2.5 Rise of Genomic Technologies and Bioinformatics (2000s–2010s)

The decade following the completion of the Human Genome Project saw an unprecedented acceleration in genomic technologies and computational biology, transforming how scientists and clinicians explored the human genome. In the 2000s to 2010s, new and powerful tools such as microarrays, next-generation sequencing (NGS), and CRISPR-Cas9 gene editing revolutionized genomic research and clinical applications. These technologies enabled the rapid, high-throughput, and cost-effective analysis of DNA, RNA, and epigenetic modifications, making genetic profiling faster, cheaper, and more accurate than ever before. Microarrays allowed researchers to study thousands of genes simultaneously, while NGS enabled complete genome or exome sequencing within days, a task that once took years. Simultaneously, the rise of CRISPR-Cas9 in the early 2010s introduced a groundbreaking method for precise genome editing, giving scientists the ability to modify DNA at specific locations with unprecedented ease and accuracy. This opened new frontiers in studying gene function, correcting genetic mutations, and developing novel gene-based therapies. These innovations drastically expanded the scope and scale of genomic medicine, turning once-theoretical possibilities into clinical realities.

1.2.6 Emergence of Pharmacogenomics and Targeted Therapies

The early 21st century witnessed a major shift in medical treatment strategies with the emergence of pharmacogenomics and the rise of targeted therapies, both of which formed the clinical backbone of personalized medicine. Pharmacogenomics, a fusion of pharmacology and genomics, focuses on understanding how genetic variations influence an individual's response to drugs. This field gained momentum as researchers discovered that certain gene mutations and polymorphisms significantly affect how drugs are metabolized, absorbed, or transported in the body. These genetic differences can determine whether a medication will be effective, ineffective, or even harmful to a particular patient. With this understanding, treatment began to evolve from a trial-and-error process to a more predictable and tailored approach, improving outcomes and reducing adverse effects. A landmark development in this era was the introduction of targeted cancer therapies that were designed to interfere with specific molecular pathways involved in tumor growth. For example, trastuzumab (Herceptin) was developed to treat breast cancer patients whose tumors overexpress the HER2 protein, a condition found in approximately 20–25% of cases. This drug marked one of the first clinically successful examples of using a molecular biomarker to guide therapy, demonstrating how precision targeting could significantly improve patient survival. Similarly, imatinib (Gleevec) transformed the treatment of chronic myeloid leukemia (CML) by targeting the BCR-ABL fusion gene, the genetic abnormality responsible for the disease. Imatinib not only provided a highly effective treatment but also became a model for how understanding disease at the molecular level could lead to revolutionary breakthroughs in therapy.

Pharmacogenomics further influenced the safe and effective prescription of common medications. For instance, variations in the CYP450 family of liver enzymes, especially CYP2D6 and CYP2C19, affect the metabolism of a wide range of drugs, including antidepressants, antiepileptics, beta-blockers, and anticoagulants like warfarin. By genotyping these enzymes before prescribing, clinicians could now adjust dosages or choose alternative medications to minimize toxicity and enhance efficacy, reducing the risk of life-threatening complications. This era also expanded the relevance of companion diagnostics, which are laboratory tests used to determine whether a patient will benefit from a specific drug based on their genetic or molecular profile. The co-development of therapies and diagnostics became a cornerstone of precision medicine, especially in oncology, where biomarkers such as EGFR mutations in lung cancer or KRAS mutations in colorectal cancer were used to guide targeted interventions. Beyond cancer, pharmacogenomics began influencing other fields, including cardiology, psychiatry, infectious diseases, and pain management. For example, genetic testing could predict hypersensitivity reactions to the HIV drug abacavir, or inform dosing of painkillers like codeine based on how well a patient metabolizes opioids. As evidence accumulated, pharmacogenomic guidelines were developed by organizations like CPIC (Clinical Pharmacogenetics Implementation Consortium) to help integrate genetic information into routine clinical practice. The emergence of pharmacogenomics and targeted therapies marked the transition from theory to application in personalized medicine. It demonstrated that tailoring treatments to a patient's molecular and genetic profile could lead to safer, more effective care. These advances not only improved individual outcomes but also introduced new standards for drug development, regulatory approval, and clinical practice, setting the stage for a future where every prescription could be personalized.

1.2.7 Multi-Omics and Systems Biology (2010s–Present)

The 2010s marked a pivotal evolution in personalized medicine with the emergence of multi-omics and systems biology, offering an integrative framework to study human health in its full molecular complexity. While genomics laid the foundation by decoding DNA, it became increasingly evident that DNA alone could not explain the dynamic behaviour of cells, tissues, and organs. This realization led to the incorporation of multiple omics layers—genomics, transcriptomics, proteomics, metabolomics, and epigenomics—each contributing a unique dimension to understanding disease and physiology. By examining these data collectively, researchers began to view health not as the product of a single gene or mutation, but as the result of complex, interrelated networks operating across biological systems.

Genomics provided the blueprint of genetic code; transcriptomics examined gene expression patterns that change in response to internal and external stimuli. Proteomics explored the functional proteins that carry out biological processes, while metabolomics profiled the small molecules involved in cellular metabolism. Epigenomics, meanwhile, revealed how environmental factors and life experiences can switch genes on or off without altering the DNA sequence itself. Collectively, these omics approaches helped unravel how genetic predispositions interact with lifestyle, nutrition, medication, and the environment to influence health outcomes. Another crucial layer is the microbiome, the trillions of microbes residing in the human body, which are now understood to play essential roles in digestion, immunity, brain function, and even drug metabolism. Differences in microbiome composition between individuals have been linked to conditions like obesity, diabetes, and autoimmune diseases, and are being explored as targets for personalized therapies and dietary interventions.

Systems biology uses computational modeling and data integration techniques to synthesize information from these diverse omics sources, constructing network models that simulate how various pathways and biological entities interact. This holistic approach enables clinicians and researchers to move beyond reductionist methods—where a single gene or protein is studied in isolation—toward a comprehensive understanding of how entire systems behave in health and disease. The clinical implications of this shift are profound. In oncology, multi-omic profiling of tumors allows for the identification of molecular subtypes and resistance mechanisms, guiding combination therapies tailored to each patient's cancer biology. In cardiovascular disease, metabolomic signatures can predict risk with higher precision than traditional biomarkers. Neurodegenerative diseases like Alzheimer's are now being studied through the lens of integrated omics, revealing patterns of dysregulation across genes, proteins, and metabolites long before clinical symptoms emerge. Moreover, AI and machine learning are essential tools in processing and interpreting the vast data generated by multi-omics platforms. These technologies can uncover hidden patterns, build predictive models, and assist in clinical decision-making—turning complex molecular data into actionable insights. Personalized nutrition, pharmacometabolomics (tailoring drugs based on metabolic profile), and predictive diagnostics are just a few applications emerging from this systems-oriented paradigm. In essence, multi-omics and systems biology have propelled personalized medicine into a new era of precision and contextualization, where treatment and prevention strategies are informed not just by static genes, but by dynamic biological processes. As these technologies mature and become more accessible, they promise to refine the way clinicians approach complex and chronic diseases, enabling care that is not only more targeted but also deeply responsive to the ever-changing molecular landscape of each individual.

1.2.8 Real-Time Personalization: Wearables, AI, and Digital Health

The advent of real-time personalization marks a significant leap in the evolution of personalized medicine, fueled by the convergence of wearable technology, artificial intelligence (AI), and digital health platforms. This new paradigm shifts healthcare from episodic, clinic-based visits to continuous, dynamic, and context-aware care. With the widespread adoption of wearable devices—such as smartwatches, fitness trackers, ECG patches, glucose monitors, and even smart clothing—patients' physiological parameters can now be monitored 24/7. These devices capture an array of data points including heart rate, sleep quality, physical activity, respiratory rate, glucose levels, and more, providing a detailed and ongoing picture of a person's health. This real-time data is often transmitted to cloud-based platforms where AI and machine learning algorithms process and analyze it in real time. By detecting patterns, trends, and deviations, these intelligent systems can predict health risks, detect early signs of disease exacerbation, and offer personalized alerts or interventions. For example, a wearable may detect subtle heart rate variability indicating atrial fibrillation long before symptoms appear, or a continuous glucose monitor may signal an approaching hypoglycemic event and alert the patient instantly. This level of proactive care enables early intervention, improves adherence to treatment, and significantly reduces hospitalizations and emergency visits. In chronic disease management, real-time personalization has been particularly transformative. For people with diabetes, continuous glucose monitors (CGMs) combined with insulin pumps and AI-driven insulin dosing algorithms allow for automated, real-time glycemic control. In cardiovascular health, wearables can monitor blood pressure, detect arrhythmias, and offer personalized fitness or diet recommendations. In mental health, apps that track sleep, mood, voice patterns, and activity can detect early warning signs of anxiety, depression, or bipolar disorder, prompting timely psychological or pharmacological support. Moreover, digital health platforms provide a two-way communication channel between patients and healthcare providers. Patients can share data in real time with clinicians, who can then adjust treatment plans dynamically based on ongoing feedback. This ensures that care is adaptive and individualized, reflecting the patient's actual, day-to-day health rather than periodic snapshots. It also empowers patients to take a more active role in managing their health, enhancing self-awareness and health literacy. The integration of electronic health records (EHRs) with wearable and app data further enriches the personal health profile, allowing a comprehensive view that includes genetic, lifestyle, environmental, and behavioral factors. AI systems can aggregate and synthesize this complex data landscape to create predictive models that guide therapy choices, dosage adjustments, and lifestyle interventions with high precision.

Another frontier in real-time personalization is just-in-time adaptive interventions (JITAIs), where AI delivers personalized support at the moment it is most needed—for instance, sending a motivational prompt when the user is sedentary for too long, or adjusting a diet recommendation after detecting poor sleep quality. These micro-interventions create a responsive health ecosystem that adapts to the user's evolving needs, behaviours, and environmental contexts. However, the real-time personalization era also raises challenges around data privacy, device accuracy, digital literacy, and regulatory oversight. Ensuring that the data generated is secure, the insights are clinically validated, and the technologies are equitably accessible remains a critical focus as this field matures. Real-time personalization, powered by wearables, AI, and digital platforms, is revolutionizing the way healthcare is delivered. It transforms static diagnostics and fixed treatment plans into fluid, responsive, and personalized care pathways, enabling better outcomes, improved quality of life, and a more proactive, participatory model of medicine.

1.2.9 Precision Medicine Initiative and Global Support

The launch of the Precision Medicine Initiative (PMI) by the United States government in 2015 marked a watershed moment in the evolution of personalized medicine, formally aligning national health policy with genomic and data-driven care. Announced by President Barack Obama during his State of the Union Address, the PMI aimed to revolutionize the way diseases are understood and treated by incorporating individual variability in genes, environment, and lifestyle. It represented a bold investment in a long-term vision where health care is not only reactive but also predictive, preventive, and precisely tailored to each individual. One of the major components of this initiative was the development of a large-scale research cohort—now known as the "All of Us" Research Program—with the goal of collecting health data from over one million participants from diverse backgrounds across the U.S. This initiative catalysed a global ripple effect, inspiring similar projects in other nations that recognized the potential of precision medicine to improve population health outcomes and reduce long-term healthcare costs. In the United Kingdom, Genomics England launched the 100,000 Genomes Project, which integrated whole-genome sequencing into the National Health Service (NHS) to study rare diseases, cancer, and infectious diseases. This program not only generated a massive genomic dataset but also established frameworks for clinical application of genomics in routine care. In Asia, efforts such as Genome Asia 100K were launched to correct the imbalance in global genomic data representation by sequencing individuals from diverse Asian ethnicities, contributing to a more inclusive foundation for precision medicine.

Across Europe, the European '1+ Million Genomes' initiative sought to link genomic databases across member countries to promote cross-border personalized care and collaborative research. Countries like China, Canada, Japan, and Australia also launched their national genome strategies, aiming to integrate genomics into cancer care, rare disease diagnosis, pharmacogenomics, and chronic disease management. These efforts were often supported by dedicated public-private partnerships, regulatory frameworks, and the integration of precision health into broader national health innovation agendas. Importantly, these global initiatives highlighted the value of public engagement and diversity in precision medicine. Recruitment strategies emphasized the inclusion of underrepresented populations to ensure that future genomic discoveries and clinical applications are equitably applicable across different demographic groups. This push for inclusivity responded to early criticisms of genomic research being too Eurocentric, thus failing to account for the genetic diversity of global populations.

The global support for precision medicine has also led to increased investment in bioinformatics infrastructure, including cloud platforms, AI algorithms, and biobanks. Governments recognized that managing, analysing, and safeguarding vast amounts of genomic and clinical data requires robust technological ecosystems and well-defined data governance policies. Additionally, ethical frameworks and data sharing guidelines were developed at national and international levels to ensure responsible use of sensitive genetic information. In medical education and clinical practice, precision medicine is increasingly being incorporated into curricula and guidelines, ensuring that future healthcare professionals are equipped to interpret genetic data, counsel patients, and make informed decisions based on molecular diagnostics. Reimbursement models and regulatory pathways are being updated to accommodate advanced molecular tests and personalized therapies, further integrating this approach into mainstream care. In summary, the Precision Medicine Initiative and its global counterparts have transformed personalized medicine from an academic concept into a policy-backed, population-scale movement. These programs underscore the global commitment to harness genomics, data science, and individual variability for a more effective, inclusive, and future-oriented healthcare system. As these initiatives continue to evolve, they are laying the groundwork for a truly personalized public health framework on a global scale.

1.2.10 Current Landscape and Future Outlook

Personalized medicine today stands at the forefront of a transformative healthcare revolution, reshaping how diseases are diagnosed, treated, and even prevented. With the convergence of genomics, biotechnology, artificial intelligence, and digital health, this approach has moved beyond theory into mainstream clinical practice. Its most notable successes have been in oncology, where therapies are routinely guided by molecular diagnostics—such as EGFR, ALK, and BRCA mutations—to match patients with treatments most likely to be effective. Similarly, rare genetic disorders, once shrouded in diagnostic uncertainty, are increasingly being identified through whole genome sequencing and treated with precision interventions, sometimes even gene therapy. In neurology, biomarkers and genetic profiling are beginning to influence the diagnosis and treatment of complex conditions like Alzheimer's, Parkinson's, and multiple sclerosis, although more work is needed. Cardiology has embraced pharmacogenomics in prescribing anticoagulants and managing cholesterol with PCSK9 inhibitors, guided by lipid-related genotypes. Even infectious diseases, such as HIV and COVID-19, have seen personalized approaches—in vaccine development, risk prediction, and tailoring antiviral therapies. Cutting-edge tools like CRISPR-Cas9 gene editing offer possibilities for correcting genetic mutations at the source, presenting potential cures for inherited diseases like sickle-cell anemia and thalassemia. Meanwhile, regenerative medicine, including stem cell therapy and tissue engineering, is evolving to restore function based on individual cellular profiles. Artificial intelligence and machine learning are enhancing diagnostics by interpreting complex datasets, including medical imaging, genomic sequences, and electronic health records, to generate personalized risk scores and treatment algorithms.

The availability of multi-omics platforms—integrating genomics, transcriptomics, proteomics, and metabolomics—provides a deep molecular view of each patient's health landscape, enabling clinicians to detect diseases early and intervene more accurately. Wearable health tech and mobile health applications now allow real-time monitoring of physiological parameters, feeding data into personalized treatment plans that adapt dynamically to patient responses.

Despite these breakthroughs, personalized medicine still faces significant challenges. Cost remains a major barrier; genetic testing, targeted therapies, and advanced diagnostics are expensive and not universally accessible. Data privacy and ethical governance are critical concerns, especially with the massive amounts of personal and genomic data being collected and stored. There are also hurdles in clinical integration, as healthcare providers need training, infrastructure, and evidence-based guidelines to interpret and act on personalized data effectively. Furthermore, health equity is a pressing issue—many underserved populations remain underrepresented in genomic studies, risking further disparities in access and treatment outcomes. Policymakers and global health organizations must ensure that personalized medicine does not become the privilege of a few but serves the many. To truly revolutionize care, innovations must be scaled, standardized, and democratized across all healthcare settings. Looking ahead, the future of medicine is unequivocally predictive, preventive, and personalized. Advances in AI-driven drug discovery, nanomedicine, and digital twins (virtual models of individual patients) are on the horizon. The ultimate vision is a healthcare system where disease is detected before symptoms arise, treatment is individualized down to the molecular level, and every person receives care tailored to their biology, behaviour, and environment. Personalized medicine is not just an evolution—it is a paradigm shift that is redefining what it means to be healthy, to be a patient, and to be treated with precision (Table-2).

Table: 2 Evolution at a Glance

Period	Key Feature	Milestone Example
Pre-modern	Constitution-based treatment	Ayurveda, Greek humoral theory
19th–20th Century	Standardized, symptom-based care	Antibiotics, RCTs
1950s–1970s	Molecular foundations	DNA structure discovery
1990–2003	Genomic revolution begins	Human Genome Project
2000s	Technological explosion in genetics	NGS, Microarrays
2000s–2010s	Targeted and pharmacogenomic therapies	HER2, Gleevec, CYP450 testing
2010s–Present	Systems biology and real-time personalization	Multi-omics, wearables, AI in diagnostics
Post-2015	Institutionalization of precision medicine	U.S. Precision Medicine Initiative

1.3 PRECISION VS. PERSONALIZED MEDICINE

Precision and personalized medicine are closely related concepts but differ in emphasis and approach. Precision medicine is a scientific strategy that focuses on classifying patients into subgroups based on genetics, molecular profiles, and disease characteristics. It aims to identify the most effective treatments for these biologically similar groups, especially useful in fields like oncology and rare diseases. In contrast, personalized medicine goes a step further by considering the whole individual—including genetic makeup, lifestyle, environment, and personal preferences—when planning treatment. While precision medicine builds the foundation with population-level data and advanced technologies like genomics and big data analytics, personalized medicine uses this foundation to create patient-specific care strategies. It emphasizes shared decision-making, patient engagement, and psychosocial context. The two approaches are not mutually exclusive but highly complementary. Precision medicine offers molecular insight and predictive power, whereas personalized medicine ensures the application is relevant and meaningful to the individual. Together, they represent the future of healthcare that is both biologically precise and humanely responsive (Table-3).

Table 3: Comparison of Precision Medicine vs. Personalized Medicine

Aspect	Precision Medicine	Personalized Medicine
Definition	Medical approach using population-level data to classify patients into subgroups.	Medical approach that considers the unique biology, lifestyle, and preferences of a person.
Focus	Stratification of groups based on genetic, molecular, and clinical characteristics.	Individual-centric customization of prevention, diagnosis, and treatment.
Data Source	Genomics, proteomics, biomarkers, big data analytics.	Combines genomic data with patient history, environment, behavior, and values.
Goal	Identify effective interventions for biologically similar patient groups.	Deliver the right care to the right individual at the right time, with holistic context.
Application	Population-based models (e.g., HER2-positive breast cancer treatment protocols).	Context-based clinical decisions (e.g., adjusting treatment based on lifestyle or beliefs).
Tools Used	High-throughput sequencing, AI algorithms, clinical databases.	Patient narratives, real-time monitoring, shared decision-making tools.
Role of Patient	Subject of data analysis; less direct input in decision-making.	Active participant in care decisions and goal setting.
Treatment Customization	Based on subgroup biology; not necessarily individual-level preferences.	Tailored to personal goals, psychosocial context, and medical needs.
Nature of Approach	More population-oriented; emphasizes biological similarity.	Deeply individual; emphasizes biological, environmental, and psychosocial uniqueness.
Integration with Care	Often applied in academic or specialized settings.	Promotes whole-person care in routine clinical practice.
Regulatory/Scientific Emphasis	Focus on standardization, evidence from clinical trials.	Emphasis on flexibility, patient engagement, and continuous feedback.
Scope of Use	More common in oncology, rare diseases, and pharmacogenomics.	Applicable across all areas of medicine including prevention, wellness, and chronic care.
Ethical Concerns	Data privacy, algorithmic bias, access to advanced diagnostics.	Informed consent, equity, cultural sensitivity in decision-making.
Outcomes Focused	Efficiency, efficacy, and safety of treatments for defined cohorts.	Patient satisfaction, adherence, and personalized health goals.
Complementarity	Provides foundational data and classification tools.	Applies those tools in a real-world, person-sensitive manner.

1.3.1 Conceptual Definitions

In modern healthcare, the shift from generalized treatment protocols to more individualized approaches has led to the emergence of two interconnected paradigms: Personalized Medicine and Precision Medicine. While the terms are often used interchangeably, they reflect distinct, though complementary, frameworks for redefining patient care in the 21st century. Personalized Medicine centers on tailoring medical treatment to the unique characteristics of each individual. It integrates a wide array of personal factors—ranging from one's genetic makeup, epigenetic profiles, environmental exposures, and lifestyle choices, to cultural background and personal preferences. This approach recognizes that no two patients are exactly alike, even if they share a diagnosis. It encourages clinicians to treat not just the disease, but the person who has the disease. In personalized medicine, care is adapted to align with a patient's values, beliefs, and behavioral patterns. For example, two patients with the same type of cancer may receive different treatment plans—not solely due to their genetic differences, but also due to their age, comorbidities, nutritional status, treatment goals, and even psychological readiness. Thus, personalized medicine reflects a holistic and patient-centric model of care. On the other hand, Precision Medicine is a more scientifically grounded and technology-driven approach. It focuses on categorizing individuals into specific subgroups based on genomic variants, molecular markers, disease phenotypes, and even socio-behavioural data. The aim is to predict disease risk more accurately, diagnose conditions more precisely, and prescribe therapies that are effective for people within a particular biological or genetic profile.

Precision medicine emerged from advances in genomic sequencing, biomarker discovery, bioinformatics, and big data analytics. It empowers physicians to select treatments that target the molecular pathways driving a patient's disease, rather than relying on one-size-fits-all protocols. For instance, in oncology, precision medicine enables the use of targeted therapies based on tumor gene expression, such as prescribing trastuzumab for breast cancer patients with HER2-positive tumors. While personalized medicine may involve the personal and contextual customization of care, precision medicine focuses more on biological accuracy and the predictive modeling of disease and treatment response. In essence, personalized medicine is a philosophy of care, while precision medicine is a scientific methodology. Together, they represent the dual pillars of future healthcare: medicine that is not only biologically precise but also personally meaningful.

1.3.2 Origin and Evolution of Terms

The conceptual and terminological evolution of personalized and precision medicine reflects broader shifts in medical thought, scientific capability, and healthcare policy over the last several decades. Although the terms are often used interchangeably, they have distinct origins and historical trajectories that continue to shape how medicine is practiced and communicated. The term Personalized Medicine began appearing in medical literature in the late 20th century, particularly as genetic and molecular sciences began to influence clinical decisions. Its core idea was to tailor treatment to the individual, considering the patient's unique characteristics—genetics, environment, behavior, and preferences. However, this terminology led to some confusion and misinterpretation. Many interpreted "personalized" to mean developing unique drugs or therapies for each individual, a notion that is logistically and economically impractical. In reality, personalized medicine aimed to customize existing treatments based on individual differences, not create one-of-a-kind pharmaceuticals. Despite its noble intent, the semantic ambiguity of the term created barriers to public understanding and policy adoption. To address this, the term Precision Medicine emerged and gained prominence, especially after the 2015 launch of the U.S. Precision Medicine Initiative under President Barack Obama. The initiative marked a pivotal moment in framing the new era of biomedicine. It clarified that the focus was on developing treatments for subgroups of patients who share genetic, bio-marker, environmental, or lifestyle characteristics—rather than treating each person entirely uniquely.

Precision medicine thus emphasizes biological accuracy, predictability, and targeted interventions, without overpromising hyper-personalization. It provides a more scientifically neutral and operationally scalable label for approaches that use large datasets, genomic information, and machine learning to guide therapeutic decisions. The shift in terminology also aligns with evolving healthcare infrastructure, regulatory standards, and data-driven innovation. Precision medicine avoids the individual-centric connotations of "personalized," making it a more acceptable term for policymakers, researchers, and pharmaceutical companies. Today, while both terms coexist, they often serve different functions. "Personalized medicine" is more commonly used in patient-centric and clinical narratives, emphasizing the human aspect of tailored care. "Precision medicine," in contrast, dominates scientific discourse, policy documents, and research funding proposals, reflecting its technological and subgroup-oriented focus. The evolution from personalized to precision medicine is less a matter of changing practice than of refining language. It represents a movement from idealist terminology to pragmatic application, helping to align expectations with capabilities in the age of genomic and data-driven healthcare.

1.3.3 Scientific Basis

The scientific foundation of personalized and precision medicine lies in understanding human variability at the molecular, clinical, and behavioural levels. Both approaches aim to move beyond generalized treatments by leveraging advances in genetics, genomics, and data science. Personalized medicine emphasizes individual-level factors like lifestyle, environment, and preferences, while precision medicine focuses on subgroup classification based on biomarkers and genetic mutations. Together, they rely on technologies such as next-generation sequencing, bioinformatics, and systems biology. These tools help decode complex disease mechanisms and identify optimal interventions. As science evolves, this dual framework continues to redefine diagnostics, therapeutics, and patient care.

- **Personalized Medicine uses tools like:** Personalized medicine integrates diverse patient-specific factors to guide healthcare decisions.It considers the individual's medical history, family background, and treatment preferences.Key tools include genomic analysis, evaluation of lifestyle habits, and behavioral health factors.This approach focuses on tailoring therapy to the whole person, not just molecular markers.It emphasizes holistic care, incorporating psychosocial and environmental influences into treatment plans.
    - Patient history
    - Preferences
    - Genomics
    - Lifestyle
    - Behaviour
- **Precision Medicine focuses on:** Precision medicine is grounded in molecular biology, genetics, and advanced analytics. It uses data on genetic mutations, such as BRCA or EGFR, to target disease-specific pathways. Molecular subtyping of diseases helps classify patients into biologically distinct subgroups. Through biomarker profiling and big data analytics, it predicts drug response and disease progression. It enables population stratification, ensuring that therapies are directed at those most likely to benefit.
    - Genetic mutations
    - Molecular subtypes
    - Biomarker profiles
    - Big data analytics
    - Population stratification

Both rely on genomic technologies, but precision medicine is more data-driven and population-based.

1.3.4 Application in Clinical Practice

The integration of personalized and precision medicine into clinical practice has significantly transformed how diseases are diagnosed, treated, and managed. Rather than relying solely on population-based protocols, modern clinicians increasingly use individual-specific data—such as genetic mutations, biomarker expression, and lifestyle factors—to inform therapeutic choices. This shift is evident across various fields, including oncology, cardiology, neurology, and infectious diseases. For instance, in cancer care, genomic testing of tumors allows doctors to select targeted therapies that are more effective and less toxic than conventional treatments. In pharmacology, pharmacogenomic testing guides medication dosing to reduce side effects and optimize response. Personalized screening programs assess individual risk for conditions like breast cancer or diabetes, enabling earlier detection and prevention. Real-time data from wearables and mobile health apps are also shaping personalized interventions for chronic diseases. Moreover, AI-driven clinical decision-support systems are aiding physicians in interpreting complex datasets for better diagnostic accuracy. Despite challenges in cost, infrastructure, and data integration, the clinical application of personalized and precision medicine is growing steadily. As these approaches become more accessible, they promise to make care more proactive, predictive, and patient-centered, ultimately improving health outcomes and quality of life.

- **Personalized Medicine:**
  - Shared decision-making
  - Customized drug regimens
  - Tailored lifestyle modifications
  - Personalized follow-up and monitoring
- **Precision Medicine:**
  - Targeted cancer therapies (e.g., EGFR inhibitors)
  - Pharmacogenomics-based prescriptions
  - Risk stratification in chronic diseases
  - Genome-guided screening programs

Example: A breast cancer patient with HER2 overexpression may receive trastuzumab—this is precision medicine. Adjusting her treatment plan based on her lifestyle, family values, or preferences is personalized medicine.

1.3.5 Technology and Tools

Technological advancements are the backbone of personalized and precision medicine, enabling the collection, analysis, and interpretation of vast health data. Next-generation sequencing (NGS) allows rapid and cost-effective decoding of entire genomes, revealing mutations and variants linked to diseases. Microarrays, CRISPR, and single-cell sequencing further refine molecular diagnostics. Bioinformatics tools process large-scale datasets, while artificial intelligence (AI) and machine learning algorithms uncover patterns and predict treatment responses. Electronic health records (EHRs) integrate clinical and genomic data, enhancing decision-making. Wearable devices and mobile apps collect real-time physiological data, supporting dynamic care models. Imaging technologies combined with molecular data offer precise disease monitoring. Cloud computing enables global data sharing and collaboration. These tools collectively drive a more informed, individualized approach to healthcare (Table-4).

Table: 4 Application of Tools in of Personalized and Precision Medicine

Tool/Aspect	Personalized Medicine	Precision Medicine
Genomic Sequencing	Used	Core diagnostic method
Wearable Devices	Frequent use for behavior monitoring	Less emphasized
Big Data Analytics	Less central	Core requirement for subgroup analysis
Electronic Health Records	Used for patient history	Integrated with algorithms

1.3.6 Scope of Use

- Personalized medicine embodies a patient-centred approach that acknowledges the entire spectrum of an individual's identity.
- It recognizes that health is influenced by emotional well-being, psychological status, and unique lifestyle choices.
- Clinicians practicing personalized medicine invest time in understanding personal goals, family history, and social contexts.
- This approach emphasizes communication, shared decision-making, and tailored care that extends beyond pure biology.
- It integrates considerations of mental health, stress management, and behavioral factors into treatment planning.
- Treatments are often modified to align with patients' values, experiences, and day-to-day realities.
- Personalized medicine thus adopts a holistic view that encompasses body, mind, and lifestyle interactions.
- It empowers patients by validating the importance of their subjective experiences and quality of life.
- In contrast, precision medicine is fundamentally disease-centered, with a focus on underlying biological mechanisms.
- It concentrates on dissecting molecular pathways, genetic mutations, and biomarker profiles associated with diseases.
- Precision medicine employs technologies like genomic sequencing and bioinformatics to categorize patient subgroups.

- This method seeks to target therapeutic interventions based on specific molecular characteristics of a disease.
- It emphasizes objective, quantifiable data, often derived from laboratory and imaging techniques.
- The molecular precision of this approach helps in designing targeted treatments that block or modify disease pathways.
- While precision medicine provides deep insights into disease mechanisms, it largely abstracts the human element.
- Its strategies are primarily driven by patterns observed in big data and molecular research rather than individual narratives.
- The humanistic scope of personalized medicine offers a broader, more empathetic perspective on patient care.
- Precision medicine, with its molecular focus, enables the development of highly specific treatment protocols.
- Together, both approaches aim to improve clinical outcomes by merging personalized patient context with scientific precision.
- Ultimately, the integration of these models promises a balanced paradigm where care is both deeply human and molecularly accurate.

1.3.7 Philosophical Orientation

Philosophically, personalized medicine is rooted in a holistic tradition that sees each patient as a unique, multifaceted individual. It draws from medical humanism and systems thinking, recognizing that biological, emotional, social, cultural, and environmental dimensions are all interconnected in shaping a person's health. This approach does not reduce the individual to a set of symptoms or molecular targets; instead, it emphasizes individuality, context, and meaning in healthcare. Personalized medicine values subjectivity, lived experience, and the therapeutic relationship between patient and provider. It seeks to understand the person behind the disease, adapting treatments to fit the patient—not the other way around. In contrast, precision medicine is philosophically aligned with systems biology and scientific reductionism. It focuses on understanding diseases by deconstructing them into their most basic molecular, cellular, and genetic components. Precision medicine relies on data, biomarkers, and measurable biological signals to inform diagnosis and treatment. This approach reflects a belief that by analysing systems at a granular level—genes, proteins, pathways—medical science can design more effective and targeted interventions. The body is treated like a machine, and illness as a disruption in its parts, repairable by targeting the specific faulty element. While personalized medicine prioritizes the individual's wholeness, preferences, and context, precision medicine emphasizes accuracy, objectivity, and molecular detail. The former is relational and patient-focused; the latter is data-driven and disease-focused. However, these orientations are not oppositional—they are complementary. By combining personalized medicine's ethical and humanistic outlook with precision medicine's analytical rigor, modern healthcare can strive toward truly comprehensive, effective, and compassionate care.

1.3.8 Limitations and Challenges

Personalized Medicine:

- While personalized medicine holds great promise in delivering patient-centered care, it also faces several significant limitations and challenges. One major concern is the risk of over-customization. Tailoring treatment plans based heavily on personal preferences, lifestyle factors, or subjective reports may sometimes lack a strong scientific foundation. This could lead to interventions that are not universally validated or reproducible across different clinical settings. In such cases, personalization might compromise the reliability and predictability of medical outcomes.
- Another challenge lies in standardization and scalability. Personalized medicine, by nature, resists "one-size-fits-all" solutions. This creates difficulties in developing standardized guidelines, protocols, or best practices, making implementation across health systems inconsistent. Moreover, the cost of personalization—including specialized diagnostics, longer consultations, and tailored interventions—can be prohibitive, especially in resource-constrained settings. Health insurance coverage may also be limited for non-standard treatments, creating inequities in access. Thus, while personalized care enhances the patient experience, its success depends on balancing individualization with evidence-based practice and healthcare efficiency.

Precision Medicine:

Precision medicine, despite its scientific rigor and technological sophistication, comes with its own set of challenges. A primary concern is the overreliance on molecular data and technology. By focusing intensely on genetic mutations, biomarkers, and algorithm-driven insights, precision medicine may sometimes neglect the broader clinical picture. Diseases are not solely rooted in biology; they are influenced by environmental, psychological, and social factors as well. When these human aspects are underrepresented, the treatment strategy might miss crucial determinants of health or patient well-being (Fig. 3).

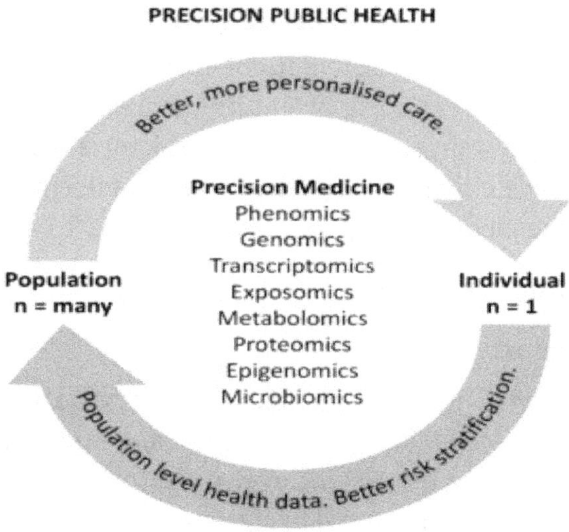

Fig. 3 Precision Medicine

Additionally, precision medicine can inadvertently overlook the social, emotional, and cultural dimensions of care. Patients are not merely biological systems—they have fears, beliefs, values, and lived experiences that influence how they perceive illness and respond to treatment. A genomics-driven approach that lacks empathetic communication or psychosocial consideration risks alienating patients or reducing their engagement with care. Furthermore, precision medicine may exacerbate health disparities if access to advanced diagnostics and targeted therapies is limited to affluent populations. Thus, the challenge lies in integrating cutting-edge science with person-centered compassion to ensure precision does not replace, but rather enhances, the art of healing.

1.3.9 Complementary Nature

Although precision medicine and personalized medicine are often used interchangeably, they each emphasize distinct but interconnected aspects of modern healthcare. Precision medicine excels in offering a molecularly informed, evidence-driven approach, using biomarkers, genomic profiling, and computational models to segment populations and predict disease behavior. It provides the scientific infrastructure, tools, and frameworks necessary to understand the underlying biological mechanisms of diseases. With this precision, healthcare professionals can better select interventions that are more likely to work for particular genetic subtypes or molecular profiles—especially in areas such as oncology, cardiology, and rare diseases. On the other hand, personalized medicine takes the outputs of precision medicine and translates them into meaningful, individual-level care. It focuses on tailoring diagnosis, treatment, and prevention strategies not just based on biology, but also incorporating a patient's values, lifestyle, culture, preferences, and psychological context. While precision medicine might identify that a certain therapy works best for a specific genetic mutation, personalized medicine ensures that the therapy is appropriate for the individual in the context of their life—considering factors such as adherence capability, emotional resilience, social support, or economic feasibility. Together, the two approaches form a synergistic alliance. Precision medicine strengthens the scientific accuracy of interventions, while personalized medicine enhances their relevance and acceptability. For instance, a precision-based cancer treatment might be biologically optimal, but only becomes truly effective when a personalized approach ensures the patient is emotionally prepared, supported, and able to follow through with the therapy plan. As medicine evolves, integrating these approaches is key to delivering care that is both clinically effective and deeply humane. Their collaboration ensures that we not only treat the disease with molecular precision, but also heal the person with empathy, context, and care (Table-5).

Table 5: Concise summary of Personalized and Precision medicine

Aspect	Personalized Medicine	Precision Medicine
Focus	Individual patient	Subgroup of patients
Orientation	Patient-centred	Data-driven, disease-focused
Origin of Term	Earlier (clinical tradition)	Modern (scientific standard)
Tools Used	EHR, wearables, patient feedback	Genomics, biomarkers, bioinformatics
Example	Tailoring treatment based on lifestyle	Choosing drug based on mutation profile
Scope	Broad, includes preferences	Specific to biological mechanisms
Common Use Cases	Chronic disease management	Oncology, pharmacogenomics

1.4DRIVERSOFPERSONALIZEDMEDICINE:TECHNOLOGY,BIOLOGY, AND DATA

1.4.1 Technological Drivers

The explosive growth of technology has been a cornerstone in the rise of personalized medicine. Tools such as next-generation sequencing (NGS) have enabled rapid and cost-effective analysis of entire genomes, uncovering individual genetic variations that can influence disease susceptibility and drug response. Technologies like CRISPR-Cas9 now allow for precise gene editing, holding promise for correcting genetic mutations at their source. In parallel, digital diagnostics and wearable devices (e.g., fitness trackers, ECG-enabled smartwatches, continuous glucose monitors) are reshaping how health data is collected—passively, in real-time, and outside clinical settings. These innovations, when coupled with AI and machine learning, allow for the prediction of health outcomes and personalized intervention strategies, bringing personalized care closer to everyday life.

1.4.2 Biological Drivers

Biological understanding of human diversity has significantly deepened, thanks to advancements in genomics, transcriptomics, proteomics, metabolomics, and epigenomics. These fields reveal that individuals differ not just genetically, but also in protein expression, metabolic processing, and gene-environment interactions. The identification of disease-associated genes, such as BRCA1/2 in breast cancer or EGFR in lung cancer, enables targeted treatments tailored to an individual's molecular makeup. Microbiome research has also highlighted the unique ecosystem of each person's gut, skin, and oral microbiota, showing how these communities influence disease and therapy response. Systems biology integrates this knowledge, offering a holistic view of disease processes and therapeutic targets, thus enabling biologically grounded personalized interventions.

1.4.3 Data Science and Informatics

Personalized medicine thrives on data—big, diverse, and complex. The explosion of electronic health records (EHRs), biobanks, genomic databases, and real-world patient data demands sophisticated computational tools. Bioinformatics, cloud computing, and AI allow for the integration and analysis of these vast datasets. Researchers now use machine learning models to identify patterns in genotype-phenotype relationships, predict disease risk, and personalize treatment options. These capabilities are transforming healthcare from a reactive model—treating illness after it appears—to a proactive one that anticipates and prevents disease. Importantly, such data-driven models support clinical decision-making at the point of care, bringing statistical rigor to individualized treatment planning.

1.4.4 Interdisciplinary Integration

Personalized medicine is inherently collaborative. It relies on the convergence of biology, computer science, engineering, statistics, ethics, and clinical medicine. For instance, geneticists and data scientists may decode mutations, but clinicians and ethicists are crucial in determining how and when to apply that knowledge responsibly in practice. This cross-disciplinary integration ensures that discoveries in the lab translate into clinically actionable and ethically sound treatments. Medical innovation now depends not just on one specialty, but on ecosystems of professionals co-creating healthcare solutions that are scientifically grounded and socially relevant.

1.4.5 Patient Engagement and Health Consumerism

Today's patients are not passive recipients of care—they are informed participants. The rise of health consumerism is a powerful social driver of personalized medicine. Direct-to-consumer genetic testing platforms like 23andMe, AncestryDNA, and

Color Genomics have given individuals access to their genetic data, fostering curiosity and engagement. Moreover, patients increasingly use mobile apps to track symptoms, monitor chronic conditions, and access telehealth services. This heightened self-awareness and digital empowerment has led to growing demand for personalized care plans, transparency, and shared decision-making. As patients expect treatments that align with their values, preferences, and data, healthcare providers are being pushed to move from one-size-fits-all models to truly individualized care.

1.5 SOCIETAL AND CLINICAL IMPORTANCE

Personalized medicine holds transformative potential not only for individual patients but also for society and healthcare systems at large. Clinically, it moves medicine away from reactive, generalized treatment toward a proactive, precise, and preventive model. By understanding a patient's genetic makeup, lifestyle, and environmental exposures, clinicians can select treatments with higher efficacy and fewer side effects. This improves patient outcomes, reduces trial-and-error prescribing, and minimizes adverse drug reactions—which are among the leading causes of hospitalizations globally. For example, pharmacogenomic testing can identify whether a patient will respond positively or negatively to a specific drug, allowing for safer and more effective prescribing. In cancer care, therapies like trastuzumab or pembrolizumab are now routinely chosen based on tumour biomarkers, dramatically improving survival in select groups (Fig.4).

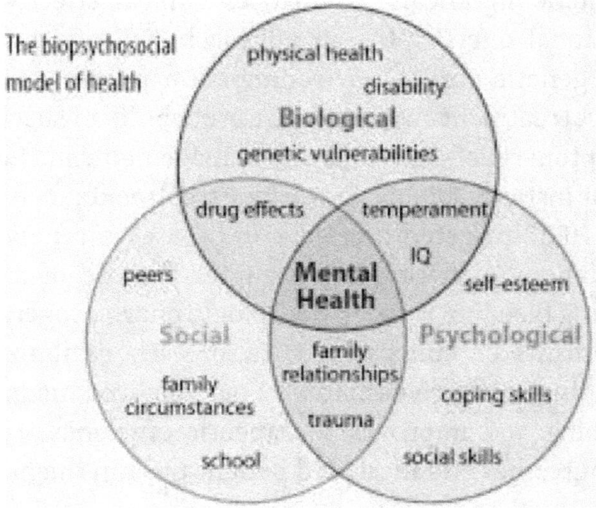

Fig. 4 The Biopsychosocial model of health

From a societal perspective, personalized medicine promises greater efficiency in healthcare resource allocation. It reduces wasteful spending on ineffective treatments and unnecessary procedures by tailoring care to those most likely to benefit. It also supports earlier diagnosis through predictive genetic testing, which can delay or prevent the onset of chronic diseases such as diabetes, cardiovascular conditions, and inherited cancers. As a result, long-term healthcare costs can be lowered while improving quality of life and productivity. Moreover, the widespread adoption of personalized approaches fosters innovation across sectors—biotechnology, diagnostics, informatics, and pharmaceuticals—spurring economic growth and job creation. Personalized medicine also plays a vital role in promoting health equity when implemented responsibly. It offers the opportunity to address disparities by including diverse populations in research and tailoring care to underserved communities who may have distinct genetic or environmental risk factors. Furthermore, by empowering patients with personalized data, it strengthens trust, adherence, and engagement in their own care. However, societal benefits also come with ethical responsibilities. Ensuring equitable access, maintaining data privacy, and addressing social determinants of health are essential to avoid widening health disparities. The clinical and societal importance of personalized medicine lies in its ability to deliver smarter, safer, and more inclusive healthcare. It redefines the patient-doctor relationship, reframes healthcare economics, and reshapes the future of public health. With continued investment, education, and regulation, it holds the promise of a healthier, more efficient, and more equitable healthcare system for all.

1.5.1 Clinical Effectiveness

Personalized medicine significantly enhances clinical effectiveness by moving beyond the traditional one-size-fits-all approach. By tailoring therapies based on an individual's genetic profile, environmental exposures, and lifestyle habits, clinicians can select treatments with a higher probability of success. This precision leads to faster symptom relief, better disease management, and improved quality of life. In oncology, for instance, biomarker-driven treatments such as EGFR inhibitors in lung cancer or HER2-targeted therapies in breast cancer have revolutionized outcomes. In cardiology, genetic testing guides the use of anticoagulants like warfarin, minimizing bleeding risks. In neurology, pharmacogenomics helps select optimal antidepressants or epilepsy medications. By minimizing adverse drug reactions and avoiding ineffective therapies, personalized medicine reduces trial-and-error prescribing and improves therapeutic efficiency, resulting in better long-term health outcomes and increased patient trust in the healthcare system.

1.5.2 Prevention and Early Diagnosis

Personalized medicine shifts the paradigm from reactive treatment to proactive prevention. Tools like polygenic risk scores, carrier screening, and predictive genetic testing enable early identification of individuals at high risk for conditions such as breast cancer (BRCA mutations), Alzheimer's disease (APOE), or diabetes.

These individuals can undergo regular monitoring, lifestyle modifications, or prophylactic interventions to delay or prevent disease onset. Real-time physiological monitoring through wearables and mobile health apps further strengthens early detection by flagging abnormal trends before clinical symptoms manifest. This early diagnosis allows for timely intervention and reduces disease burden. Furthermore, newborn screening, prenatal genetic diagnostics, and family history analysis expand prevention opportunities across the lifespan. The result is a shift from expensive, invasive treatments to personalized health maintenance strategies that improve both individual wellbeing and public health outcomes.

1.5.3 Healthcare Efficiency and Cost Reduction

One of the most tangible societal benefits of personalized medicine is its ability to optimize healthcare efficiency and reduce overall system costs. By precisely matching therapies to patient profiles, unnecessary diagnostic tests, ineffective treatments, and hospital readmissions are minimized. For example, selecting the correct chemotherapy based on tumour genomics spares patients from toxic regimens with low efficacy. Similarly, pharmacogenomic insights prevent adverse drug reactions that often lead to emergency visits or prolonged hospital stays. Chronic diseases such as diabetes, hypertension, and asthma benefit from tailored care plans that reduce disease complications and reliance on emergency services. Over time, these targeted interventions reduce the economic burden on both healthcare providers and patients. While the initial investment in genetic testing and data infrastructure may be high, the long-term cost savings from streamlined care and improved outcomes are substantial, positioning personalized medicine as a sustainable model for future healthcare systems.

1.5.4. Empowerment and Patient Engagement

Personalized medicine fosters a shift from passive patient compliance to active participation. With greater access to health data—including genomic reports, fitness tracking, and real-time biosensor feedback—patients become empowered to understand and manage their health. This transparency encourages informed decision-making, shared goal-setting, and improved adherence to treatment plans. Digital health platforms and mobile applications allow patients to track symptoms, report outcomes, and communicate with providers, reinforcing engagement. Genetic counsellors and health coaches also play a critical role in helping individuals interpret complex data and act on it meaningfully. As patients gain insight into their unique risks and responses, they feel more in control, which improves mental well-being and health literacy. This cultural shift not only enhances clinical outcomes but also builds stronger therapeutic alliances between patients and providers, fostering a more collaborative, respectful, and responsive healthcare environment.

1.5.5 Innovation and Economic Growth

The rise of personalized medicine is a powerful engine for innovation and economic development. Advances in genomics, diagnostics, bioinformatics, artificial intelligence, and biotechnology are being driven by the need to support individualized care. This momentum fuels job creation in emerging sectors such as data science, precision pharmacology, molecular diagnostics, and telehealth. Start-ups and large pharmaceutical firms alike are investing in targeted therapies, companion diagnostics, and AI-powered decision-support tools. Personalized approaches reduce R&D failure rates by focusing on well-defined subpopulations, increasing trial success and speeding up regulatory approvals. Moreover, the global market for personalized medicine is expanding rapidly, attracting venture capital and public funding. The economic impact extends beyond the lab, benefiting healthcare providers, insurance models, and even policy innovation. Thus, personalized medicine is not only transforming care but also reshaping the global biomedical landscape and driving knowledge-based economies.

1.5.6 Equity and Inclusion

When developed and implemented equitably, personalized medicine can address long-standing health disparities. Historically, biomedical research has overrepresented populations of European descent, leading to biases in diagnostics and therapeutics. Personalized medicine recognizes the need for inclusive research that reflects genetic diversity across ethnic, regional, and socio-economic groups. Initiatives like Genome Asia 100K, All of Us Research Program, and H3Africa are helping to diversify genomic datasets and inform more culturally competent care. Furthermore, individualized care considers not just molecular profiles but also social determinants of health such as access to care, education, and environmental exposures. When deployed responsibly, personalized medicine can empower underserved populations with tailored interventions and culturally relevant health strategies. However, equity requires deliberate action—ensuring affordability, avoiding algorithmic bias, and promoting digital access. The goal is a healthcare system where precision does not come at the cost of inclusion, but rather ensures it.

1.5.7 Ethical and Regulatory Implications

The societal integration of personalized medicine raises profound ethical and legal challenges. Central among these is genetic privacy—who owns the data, how it is shared, and how consent is managed. Patients may worry about misuse of their genomic information by insurers or employers, necessitating robust safeguards. Informed consent must be dynamic, especially in cases where data may be re-analyzed or shared in future research. Additionally, incidental findings—genetic risks unrelated to the original testing purpose—require sensitive communication strategies. The rise of direct-to-consumer testing also blurs regulatory boundaries, often lacking clinical oversight. Policymakers and regulators must adapt frameworks to keep pace with technological advances, ensuring safety without stifling innovation. Guidelines from bodies like the FDA, EMA, and national ethics boards must balance individual rights with scientific progress. Ultimately, the success of personalized medicine depends on trust, transparency, and a shared commitment to ethical stewardship.

1.5.8 Public Health Transformation

Personalized medicine is redefining the scope and strategies of public health. Rather than relying on population-level averages, public health programs can now stratify risk and target interventions to high-risk subgroups. For example, vaccination campaigns or screening programs can be customized based on genetic susceptibilities or geographic data. Precision public health tools enable community-level interventions tailored to local environmental and genomic factors. This shift enhances effectiveness, reduces waste, and strengthens disease prevention efforts. Additionally, digital health platforms and data analytics support real-time surveillance and early outbreak detection, enabling rapid responses. Personalized medicine also enhances chronic disease prevention through population risk modelling and lifestyle modification strategies. When integrated with social policy, it can improve food systems, urban planning, and occupational health. In essence, personalized medicine is evolving from individual treatment to population-wide transformation—blending biology with public good to achieve more equitable, efficient, and effective health systems.

2 Chapter GENOMICS AND MOLECULAR FOUNDATIONS

2.0 INTRODUCTION: AN OVERVIEW

Personalized medicine represents a paradigm shift in modern healthcare, moving away from the traditional "one-size-fits-all" model to an approach that considers individual variability in genes, environment, and lifestyle. At the heart of this transformation lies the field of genomics—the study of the entire genome—and its close companion, molecular biology, which examines the structure and function of biomolecules essential to life. Together, these disciplines provide the scientific backbone for understanding the biological uniqueness of each individual and translating that knowledge into precise, patient-centred care. The sequencing of the human genome in the early 2000s marked a historical milestone, unveiling approximately 20,000–25,000 protein-coding genes and revealing the vast complexity of human genetic variation. This achievement laid the groundwork for uncovering how subtle differences in DNA sequences—such as single nucleotide polymorphisms (SNPs), insertions, deletions, and structural variants—can influence disease susceptibility, drug metabolism, and treatment response. The ability to decode a person's genetic blueprint has revolutionized disease risk assessment, diagnosis, and therapy development. Beyond genomics, molecular foundations also include transcriptomics, proteomics, metabolomics, and epigenomics. These "-omics" technologies offer a layered understanding of how genes are expressed, how proteins are synthesized and modified, how metabolites fluctuate with physiological changes, and how external factors can epigenetically alter gene function without changing the DNA sequence. Collectively, these tools are integral to personalized medicine, allowing clinicians to view health and disease through a multidimensional lens.

One of the central applications of genomics in personalized medicine is pharmacogenomics, which investigates how genetic variants affect individual responses to medications. This enables tailored prescriptions that maximize efficacy and minimize adverse effects. For example, patients with certain CYP450 gene variants may metabolize drugs like warfarin, clopidogrel, or antidepressants differently, requiring dosage adjustments or alternative therapies. This genetic insight reduces trial-and-error prescribing and enhances patient safety (Fig. 1).

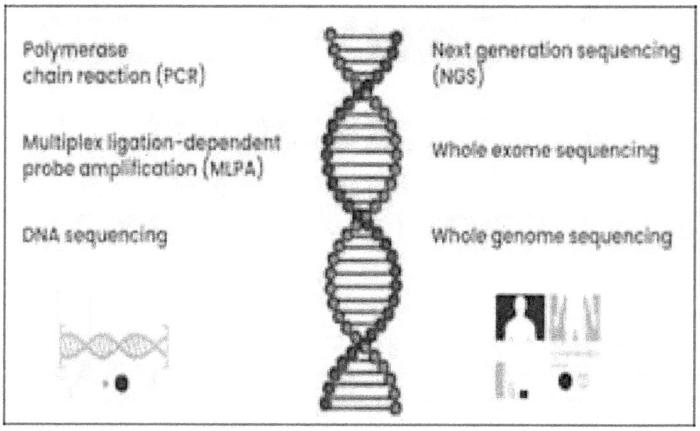

Fig. 1 Personalized medicine represents a paradigm shift in modern healthcare

Cancer care has been at the forefront of genomics-driven personalization. Oncogenomics—focused on the genetic alterations in tumours—has enabled the classification of cancers based on molecular profiles rather than tissue of origin. Targeted therapies, such as HER2 inhibitors for breast cancer or EGFR inhibitors for lung cancer, have shown remarkable success in improving survival and reducing toxicity by directly interfering with the mutated pathways driving tumour growth. This molecular approach is now expanding to other complex diseases, including cardiovascular, neurological, and autoimmune conditions. The integration of genomics into clinical practice is also transforming preventive medicine. Through genetic screening and predictive testing, individuals at high risk for hereditary diseases such as BRCA-related breast and ovarian cancer, Lynch syndrome, or familial hypercholesterolemia can be identified early. This allows for proactive interventions, lifestyle modifications, and enhanced surveillance, shifting the focus from reactive treatment to proactive prevention. Moreover, advances in next-generation sequencing (NGS), bioinformatics, and computational biology have made genomic data generation faster, cheaper, and more accurate. The cost of sequencing a human genome has dropped from billions of dollars to just a few hundred, making it accessible to routine clinical use. High-throughput data analysis tools can now process vast datasets, identify disease-associated variants, and guide clinical decision-making in near real-time. However, the power of genomics and molecular science in personalized medicine is not without challenges. Interpretation of genetic data remains complex due to the vast number of variants of unknown significance (VUS), limited population diversity in genetic databases, and the need for clinical validation. Ethical, legal, and social issues surrounding genetic privacy, informed consent, and potential discrimination also require careful consideration. Furthermore, the equitable implementation of genomic medicine across diverse populations and healthcare systems remains a critical priority.

Despite these challenges, the integration of genomics and molecular foundations continues to accelerate, propelled by global research collaborations, patient advocacy, and interdisciplinary innovation. Large-scale initiatives such as the 100,000 Genomes Project, All of Us Research Program, and international biobanks are expanding the diversity and depth of genomic data available for analysis. These efforts are paving the way for more accurate risk stratification, individualized treatment pathways, and the development of novel therapeutics based on genetic and molecular insights.

In summary, genomics and molecular biology are the bedrock of personalized medicine, offering unprecedented opportunities to decode the biological individuality of each patient. By harnessing the power of DNA, RNA, proteins, and metabolites, personalized medicine aims to deliver safer, more effective, and more proactive healthcare. As technology continues to evolve and our molecular understanding deepens, the dream of truly personalized care is becoming an achievable reality. The following sections will explore the structure and function of the human genome, key molecular mechanisms, and how this knowledge is translated into clinical applications that redefine the future of medicine.

2.1 HUMAN GENOME PROJECT AND ITS LEGACY

The Human Genome Project (HGP) stands as one of the most ambitious and transformative scientific undertakings in modern history. Initiated in 1990, the project was a collaborative international effort involving research institutions and scientists from across the globe, with the primary objective of mapping and sequencing the entire human genome, which comprises more than 3 billion DNA base pairs. After 13 years of intensive work, the project was successfully completed in April 2003—two years ahead of schedule. The result was the first comprehensive, high-resolution draft of the human genetic code, providing unprecedented insights into the blueprint of human life. At its core, the HGP aimed to identify and map all the genes present in human DNA—estimated to be between 20,000 and 25,000. By sequencing the entire genome, researchers hoped to uncover the molecular underpinnings of human biology and to gain a deeper understanding of how genetic variations contribute to health and disease. One of the most surprising findings from the project was that humans have far fewer protein-coding genes than previously assumed, suggesting that gene regulation, non-coding regions, and epigenetic factors play a far more complex role than expected. The HGP revealed that while only about 1.5% of the genome codes for proteins, the remaining non-coding portion—once dismissed as "junk DNA"—is rich in regulatory sequences and other functional elements.

The completion of the HGP marked the beginning of a new era in biomedical science. The genomic data generated through the project have become foundational for countless research initiatives, including disease gene discovery, cancer genomics, and population genetics. One of the most immediate and powerful impacts has been in the field of personalized medicine. By enabling a better understanding of genetic variation, the HGP has allowed scientists and clinicians to begin tailoring treatments to the genetic makeup of individual patients. This has led to the emergence of pharmacogenomics, a discipline that examines how genetic differences influence drug metabolism, efficacy, and toxicity. For example, variants in genes like CYP2C19 or TPMT can affect how patients respond to medications such as clopidogrel or thiopurines, guiding personalized dosing strategies. Another major legacy of the HGP is the rapid advancement of sequencing technologies. During the early stages of the project, sequencing a single human genome cost nearly $3 billion and took over a decade. Today, thanks to innovations such as next-generation sequencing (NGS) and improvements in bioinformatics, entire genomes can be sequenced in a matter of hours for less than a thousand dollars. This dramatic reduction in cost and time has made genomic analysis increasingly accessible for clinical, research, and even consumer applications. It has also facilitated large-scale population sequencing efforts and the establishment of vast genomic databases.

The Human Genome Project also played a key role in highlighting the importance of addressing ethical, legal, and social issues (ELSI) associated with genomic information. Questions around genetic privacy, potential misuse of genetic data, informed consent, and discrimination were brought to the forefront. As a result, frameworks were developed to protect individuals from genetic discrimination, such as the Genetic Information Non-discrimination Act (GINA) in the United States. Additionally, public engagement and policy discussions around responsible genomic data use became an integral part of the project's vision. Despite its tremendous success, the HGP also revealed the complexity of translating genomic data into clinical applications. The interpretation of genetic variants remains challenging, especially when considering variants of uncertain significance (VUS) that lack clear functional or phenotypic correlation. Moreover, early genomic datasets were disproportionately representative of individuals of European ancestry, limiting the global applicability of findings. These limitations have driven a new wave of research focused on improving diversity and representation in genomic studies.

The HGP's influence continues to grow through numerous successor projects. Initiatives like the ENCODE (Encyclopedia of DNA Elements) project have worked to identify and catalog functional elements in the human genome, while the 1000 Genomes Project and the Human Cell Atlas aim to catalog genetic variation and cellular diversity across populations and tissues. The UK Biobank, All of Us Research Program (USA), and other efforts are building rich repositories of genetic, clinical, and lifestyle data to enable precision health research on an unprecedented scale.In cancer research, the genomic blueprint provided by the HGP has fueled a revolution in molecular oncology. Tumor genome sequencing has enabled the identification of driver mutations and the development of targeted therapies that specifically address the molecular aberrations present in an individual's cancer. This has shifted oncology from a tissue-based to a molecular-based classification system, improving outcomes and reducing unnecessary side effects. Similarly, genetic testing for inherited conditions—such as BRCA1 and BRCA2 mutations in breast and ovarian cancer—allows for early detection and risk-reducing interventions. Ultimately, the Human Genome Project laid the scientific and technological foundation for personalized medicine. It transformed biology into a data-driven discipline and established genomics as a central pillar of healthcare innovation. Its legacy is not just in the genome sequence itself, but in the culture of collaboration, openness, and ethical responsibility it fostered. By decoding the language of life, the HGP empowered humanity to begin understanding the intricate interplay between genes and health, setting in motion a future where medicine can be as unique as each individual (Table-1).

Table-1 Concise Summary of Human Genome Project and Its Legacy

Heading	Description
Name of Project	Human Genome Project (HGP)
Launch Year	1990
Completion Year	2003 (completed two years ahead of schedule)
Main Objective	To map and sequence the entire human genome (3 billion DNA base pairs); identify all human genes (~20,000–25,000)
Participating Bodies	International collaboration involving USA, UK, Japan, France, Germany, China, and others
Key Milestones	2000: Working draft published 2003: Final sequence completed
Major Outcomes	- Complete human genome sequence - Fewer protein-coding genes than expected - Recognition of functional non-coding DNA
Technological Advancements	- Development of high-throughput and next-generation sequencing (NGS) - Improved bioinformatics and data storage systems
Scientific Contributions	- Foundation for disease gene discovery - Enhanced understanding of human genetic variation - Comparative genomics
Impact on Personalized Medicine	- Enabled pharmacogenomics - Guided targeted therapies - Supported predictive genetic testing - Enabled genome-based diagnostics
Ethical, Legal, Social Impact	- Raised issues of genetic privacy and discrimination - Informed laws like GINA - Promoted ethical genomic research

Heading	Description
Limitations Identified	- Difficulty interpreting variants of uncertain significance (VUS) - Limited diversity in early datasets - Complex gene-environment interactions
Follow-Up Projects	- ENCODE (functional elements) - 1000 Genomes Project - UK Biobank - All of Us (USA) - Human Cell Atlas
Influence on Cancer Genomics	- Identification of driver mutations - Molecular classification of cancers - Targeted and personalized oncology treatments
Economic Impact	- Lowered genome sequencing cost (from ~$3B to <$1K) - Stimulated biotech and health industries
Data Accessibility	- Open-source data sharing enabled global scientific progress
Legacy	- Shifted biology to a data-driven science - Established foundation for modern genomics - Empowered personalized, predictive, and preventive healthcare

2.1.1 Objectives of the HGP

The Human Genome Project (HGP), launched in 1990, was a landmark international scientific effort aimed at unlocking the complete genetic blueprint of human life. Its overarching goal was to map, sequence, and understand the entire human genome, comprising over 3 billion DNA base pairs. Central to this mission was the identification of all human genes, estimated to be around 20,000–25,000, to gain insights into their functions and roles in health and disease. Beyond sequencing, the project also aimed to store genomic information in publicly accessible databases, fostering global collaboration and data sharing. Another key objective was to improve computational tools for analyzing genetic data, enabling meaningful interpretation of vast sequences. Recognizing the societal impact of such powerful knowledge, the HGP included a dedicated focus on ethical, legal, and social implications (ELSI), addressing concerns like privacy, consent, and potential discrimination. The project's goals were not only scientific but also transformative—paving the way for innovations in medicine, biotechnology, and our understanding of human biology. Through its multi-faceted objectives, the HGP laid the foundation for the genomic revolution that continues to shape modern science and personalized healthcare.

- **Gene Identification:** Mapping the Blueprint of Life: One of the primary goals of the Human Genome Project was to identify all the approximately 20,000 to 25,000 genes that make up the human genome. This involved not only locating the genes within the vast expanse of DNA but also characterizing their structure, function, and regulatory mechanisms. Understanding the position and role of each gene was critical for deciphering how genetic instructions govern cellular processes, influence development, and contribute to disease. By revealing the precise genetic architecture, the HGP provided researchers with the ability to explore gene expression patterns and link specific genes to hereditary conditions, offering a foundation for diagnosis, treatment, and prevention.

- **Sequencing the Human Genome:** Unravelling 3 Billion Base Pairs: Another cornerstone of the HGP was to determine the complete nucleotide sequence of all 3 billion base pairs in human DNA. This task required innovative sequencing technologies and massive computational power to read, align, and assemble vast stretches of genetic information. By decoding the full genome, scientists gained an unprecedented view of both coding and non-coding regions, regulatory elements, repetitive sequences, and structural motifs. This monumental effort revealed not only the genetic script of human life but also provided insight into evolutionary biology, gene-environment interactions, and the molecular roots of health and disease.
- **Data Storage and Accessibility:** Building a Genomic Knowledge Infrastructure: The enormous amount of genetic data generated by the HGP necessitated robust systems for data management and accessibility. One of the project's crucial objectives was to store all genomic information in publicly available and well-organized databases. Repositories such as GenBank, Ensembl, and the UCSC Genome Browser were developed to ensure that researchers worldwide could freely access, retrieve, and utilize this data. These open-access platforms became essential tools for academic and clinical research, enabling collaboration, cross-validation, and continuous discovery in genomics, bioinformatics, and systems biology.
- **Advancing Analytical Tools:** Empowering Genomic Interpretation: Interpreting the vast and complex data generated by genome sequencing required powerful analytical tools. The HGP invested significantly in the development of bioinformatics methods and software to analyse genetic sequences, detect mutations, annotate genes, and predict functional elements. These tools facilitated large-scale comparisons across species, the identification of disease-associated variants, and the modelling of genetic networks. They also laid the groundwork for technologies such as genome-wide association studies (GWAS), personalized risk profiling, and precision drug development, helping transform raw sequence data into actionable medical insights.
- **Ethical, Legal, and Social Implications (ELSI):** Safeguarding Humanity in the Genomic Era: Recognizing the transformative potential of genetic

information, the HGP incorporated a pioneering focus on ethical, legal, and social implications (ELSI). This component aimed to address the challenges posed by genetic testing, privacy, discrimination, and informed consent. It also considered broader societal questions regarding the equitable access to genomic technologies, the potential misuse of genetic data, and the cultural impact of predictive genetic knowledge. The ELSI program was the first of its kind in large-scale science and became a model for integrating ethics into cutting-edge research. It influenced policies such as the Genetic Information Non-discrimination Act (GINA) and set a precedent for responsible genomics worldwide.

- **Foundation for Future Medicine and Science:** Together, these five objectives formed the backbone of the Human Genome Project. Their successful execution not only led to the complete mapping and understanding of the human genome but also catalysed revolutions in biotechnology, healthcare, and life sciences. The legacy of the HGP lives on in personalized medicine, where genetic information is now routinely used to guide treatment decisions, assess disease risk, and tailor prevention strategies. By combining scientific ambition with ethical foresight, the Human Genome Project has become a landmark in the history of science—one that continues to shape the future of health, medicine, and humanity itself.

2.1.2 Major Milestones

The Human Genome Project (HGP) was a landmark scientific initiative that unfolded over more than a decade, achieving a series of groundbreaking milestones that forever changed the landscape of biology and medicine. From its launch in 1990 to its successful completion in 2003, the project progressed through carefully planned phases, each contributing significantly to our understanding of human genetics. These milestones were not isolated events, but cumulative achievements built upon technological innovation, international collaboration, and visionary leadership. The launch of the HGP in 1990 marked the beginning of a new era in genomic science. It laid out an ambitious roadmap to decode the entire human genome and identify all human genes. By the year 2000, the release of the working draft of the human genome signalled a major breakthrough—offering scientists an initial, although incomplete, map of our genetic material. Just three years later, in April 2003, the completion of the final genome sequence was announced, two years ahead of schedule, marking the official end of the project and fulfilling its central objective. In parallel with sequencing the human genome, researchers also undertook the sequencing of model organisms such as the mouse, fruit fly, and yeast. This provided essential comparative data and insights into gene function and evolution. Each milestone reflected a step forward not just in knowledge, but in the development of new tools, global data sharing, and public trust in genomics. Together, these achievements represent a foundation on which modern personalized medicine and genomic science are built.

- **1990: Project Launch:** The Human Genome Project officially commenced in 1990, marking the beginning of one of the most ambitious and collaborative scientific endeavours in human history. Spearheaded by the U.S. Department of Energy (DOE) and the National Institutes of Health (NIH), the project also received strong international support from research institutions in the United Kingdom, France, Germany, Japan, China, and others. The central goal was to map and sequence the entire human genome, which consists of over 3 billion DNA base pairs. Scientists anticipated that decoding the genome would revolutionize biomedical research and lead to new insights into human biology, evolution, and disease. The project was initially estimated to take 15 years, with an allocated budget of approximately $3 billion. From the start, the HGP embraced values of open data sharing, ethical foresight, and global cooperation. It also catalysed investments in sequencing technologies, computational biology, and bioinformatics. The launch of the HGP marked a turning point for molecular biology, transforming it into a big-data science and laying the foundation for personalized medicine and genomics-driven healthcare.
- **2000: Completion of the Working Draft of the Human Genome:** By June 2000, the Human Genome Project achieved a major milestone: the successful completion of a working draft of the human genome. This version represented around 90% of the genome sequence and was a significant step forward in understanding the structure and organization of human DNA. The announcement, made jointly by U.S. President Bill Clinton and U.K. Prime Minister Tony Blair, highlighted the international and collaborative nature of the project. The draft revealed an initial map of genes, regulatory elements, and repetitive sequences, allowing researchers to begin exploring gene function and genetic variation. Although gaps and ambiguities remained in the sequence, the draft provided a critical platform for immediate use by scientists and clinicians worldwide. The availability of this data accelerated gene discovery, facilitated the identification of disease-associated loci, and enabled comparative studies with other species. It also marked a shift toward functional genomics and systems biology. Importantly, the release of the draft version signalled a commitment to data transparency and accessibility, as the information was made publicly available in real-time for global research and innovation.

- **2003: Completion of the Final Sequence and Official End of the Project:** In April 2003, the Human Genome Project was declared complete, coinciding with the 50th anniversary of the discovery of the DNA double helix by Watson and Crick. The final version of the human genome sequence covered 99% of the euchromatic (gene-rich) regions with an accuracy exceeding 99.99%. The project concluded two years ahead of schedule and within budget—an extraordinary achievement given the complexity of sequencing 3 billion DNA base pairs. This final sequence enabled a much more detailed and accurate understanding of gene locations, structures, and functions. It allowed researchers to better study non-coding regions, which were increasingly recognized as essential for gene regulation and genome stability. The completed genome sequence paved the way for advances in medical genetics, including risk prediction, early diagnosis, and the development of gene-targeted therapies. It also helped unravel the genetic basis of complex traits and diseases such as diabetes, cancer, and heart disease. The successful conclusion of the HGP marked a monumental step forward for science, signifying the dawn of the genomic era and redefining how we approach human health and biology.
- **Initiation of Parallel Model Organism Sequencing:** While sequencing the human genome was the centrepiece of the HGP, a complementary milestone was the simultaneous sequencing of the genomes of several model organisms. These included the mouse (Mus musculus), yeast (Saccharomyces cerevisiae), the fruit fly (Drosophila melanogaster), and the roundworm (Caenorhabditis elegans). The rationale behind this parallel effort was to enable comparative genomics—examining the similarities and differences in gene structure and function across species. Because many genes and biological pathways are conserved through evolution, studying simpler organisms helped identify genes of interest in humans and predict their function. For example, the mouse genome, sharing approximately 85% of its genes with humans, became an invaluable tool for creating disease models and testing therapeutic interventions. Yeast and worms provided insights into cell division, aging, and genetic regulation. Sequencing model organisms also enhanced our understanding of evolution, developmental biology, and genome organization. This strategy of multi-species analysis enriched the utility of the human genome data, making it more interpretable and functionally meaningful. Ultimately, model organism research became a vital pillar supporting genomics-driven discovery and translational science.

2.1.3 Technological Advancements

Technological advancements have been the driving force behind the rapid evolution of genomics and the realization of personalized medicine. The Human Genome Project (HGP) not only aimed to decode the human genome but also served as a catalyst for innovation in sequencing technologies, data analysis tools, and molecular techniques. As the demand for faster, more accurate, and cost-effective genome sequencing grew, it led to the development of high-throughput and automated methods that transformed biological research into a data-rich, scalable science. These innovations made it possible to sequence entire genomes in days instead of years and at a fraction of the original cost. Alongside this, the emergence of bioinformatics empowered scientists to store, manage, and interpret massive genomic datasets with precision and speed. The post-HGP era witnessed the rise of next-generation sequencing (NGS), which opened new possibilities for studying gene expression, epigenetics, and disease mechanisms at unprecedented resolution. Automation, miniaturization, and portable sequencing platforms have further revolutionized genomic workflows, bringing genomic capabilities from centralized labs to point-of-care settings. Collectively, these technological breakthroughs have made personalized medicine not only possible but increasingly practical, enabling genetic insights to guide prevention, diagnosis, and treatment tailored to the individual.

- **Development of High-Throughput Sequencing Techniques:** One of the most significant technological advancements driven by the Human Genome Project was the development of high-throughput sequencing techniques. Prior to the HGP, sequencing DNA was slow, labour-intensive, and costly. To sequence over 3 billion base pairs in the human genome, scientists needed faster and more efficient methods. This demand led to the refinement of automated Sanger sequencing, allowing researchers to process large volumes of DNA simultaneously across multiple samples. High-throughput platforms drastically increased the speed of sequencing while lowering error rates and cost. These systems used capillary electrophoresis and fluorescently labelled nucleotides to read DNA at unprecedented scales. This innovation not only enabled the HGP to meet its timeline but also laid the groundwork for post-genomic applications. High-throughput sequencing remains a cornerstone of molecular biology, now used for diagnostics, microbial studies, cancer genomics, and more.
- **Emergence of Bioinformatics Tools and Genome Databases:** The vast amount of data generated by the HGP necessitated a parallel leap in computational biology, resulting in the emergence of bioinformatics tools and genome databases. Without advanced software and data infrastructure, it would have been impossible to manage, analyze, and interpret billions

of DNA bases. Bioinformatics evolved as a critical discipline, enabling sequence alignment, gene annotation, variant analysis, and genome visualization. Key platforms such as GenBank, UCSC Genome Browser, and Ensembl were developed to store and distribute genomic data globally. These databases provided open access to scientists, accelerating discoveries across disciplines. Additionally, new algorithms and pipelines were created for comparing sequences, predicting gene functions, and identifying evolutionary patterns. The integration of biology with computational science not only supported the HGP but also launched a new era of data-driven research in genomics, systems biology, and personalized medicine.

- **Initiation of Next-Generation Sequencing (NGS) Technologies Post-HGP:** While high-throughput sequencing powered the HGP, its conclusion catalysed the initiation of next-generation sequencing (NGS) technologies that would go on to revolutionize genomics. NGS refers to a set of advanced platforms that can sequence millions to billions of DNA fragments in parallel, dramatically lowering costs and turnaround time. Unlike Sanger sequencing, NGS is based on massively parallel short-read sequencing, enabling the whole genome, transcriptome, or targeted regions to be analysed rapidly and at scale. Platforms like Illumina, Roche 454, and later, Oxford Nanopore and PacBio, transformed research and clinical diagnostics. These technologies allowed for whole-genome sequencing, RNA sequencing (RNA-seq), epigenetic profiling, and metagenomics. Importantly, NGS made personal genome sequencing feasible, opening doors to individualized risk assessment, pharmacogenomics, and cancer profiling. The post-HGP sequencing revolution thus empowered both large-scale population studies and bedside applications.

- **Miniaturization and Automation of Genomic Technologies:** To support the scale and complexity of the Human Genome Project, researchers pursued the miniaturization and automation of genomic technologies, turning labour-intensive lab protocols into streamlined, high-efficiency systems. Automated DNA extraction, library preparation, PCR amplification, and sequencing reactions became standard, reducing human error and increasing reproducibility. Robotic platforms and microfluidics allowed for the handling of thousands of samples with minimal volumes, conserving reagents and lowering costs. The miniaturization of devices also enabled the creation of portable sequencing machines, like the Oxford Nanopore MinION, that could be used in clinical settings or field research. Automation accelerated experimental workflows and made large-scale genomic projects feasible, from national biobanks to pandemic surveillance. This integration of engineering with biology reflected a new era of biotechnological convergence, making genomic science faster, smarter, and more accessible across research and healthcare sectors.

2.1.4 Scientific Discoveries

The completion of the Human Genome Project (HGP) marked a monumental turning point in the history of science, laying bare the complete blueprint of human life encoded in our DNA. While its initial goal was to sequence the entire human genome, the project went far beyond generating raw data—it uncovered profound biological insights that continue to transform our understanding of genetics, evolution, and disease. Perhaps most surprising was the discovery that the human genome contains only around 20,000–25,000 protein-coding genes, a number far lower than anticipated and surprisingly close to those found in simpler organisms. This challenged the assumption that gene quantity determines biological complexity, redirecting scientific focus toward gene regulation, epigenetics, and post-transcriptional mechanisms. Another key revelation was the discovery that most of the genome—over 98%—does not code for proteins, yet plays crucial functional roles. Once dismissed as "junk DNA," these non-coding regions are now understood to house essential regulatory elements and non-coding RNAs that orchestrate when, where, and how genes are expressed. These elements are vital in development, differentiation, and disease progression, shifting attention from the gene-centric model to a more integrated, systems-level view of the genome.

In addition, the HGP highlighted the immense genetic variation among individuals. Scientists identified millions of single nucleotide polymorphisms (SNPs), along with structural variations such as insertions, deletions, and copy number variants (CNVs). These variations help explain differences in traits, disease susceptibility, and drug response, forming the basis of genome-wide association studies (GWAS) and the emerging field of personalized medicine.

Finally, through comparative genomics, the HGP uncovered evolutionary relationships by identifying conserved sequences shared across species. These highly preserved regions reveal common biological pathways and underscore the shared ancestry of life on Earth. Model organisms such as mice, fruit flies, and yeast were validated as crucial systems for studying human genes and diseases. Together, these discoveries have not only revolutionized genomics but also reshaped medicine, biotechnology, and evolutionary biology. They laid the foundation for personalized approaches to healthcare, deepened our understanding of life's complexity, and opened new frontiers for future scientific exploration.

- **Fewer Protein-Coding Genes Than Expected (~20,000):** One of the most unexpected and profound discoveries from the Human Genome Project was that the human genome contains far fewer protein-coding genes than scientists had anticipated. Prior to sequencing, estimates suggested that humans would have over 100,000 genes to account for our biological complexity. However, the HGP revealed that the number of protein-coding genes is only around 20,000 to 25,000—surprisingly close to that of simpler organisms like mice and fruit flies. This finding challenged the long-held assumption that gene quantity equated to biological sophistication. It suggested that complexity in humans arises not from gene number alone, but from how genes are regulated, expressed, and interact with one another. Mechanisms such as alternative splicing, post-translational modifications, and gene regulatory networks were recognized as critical contributors to proteomic diversity and functional complexity. This insight has reshaped the way researchers view human biology and has underscored the importance of looking beyond protein-coding regions to understand disease and individual variation.

- **Functional Significance of the Non-Coding Genome:** Another major revelation from the Human Genome Project was the recognition that the vast majority of the human genome—over 98%—does not code for proteins, yet is functionally significant. Previously labelled as "junk DNA," these non-coding regions were once thought to be evolutionary remnants with no biological role. However, subsequent research demonstrated that many non-coding elements serve essential regulatory functions. These include promoters, enhancers, silencers, insulators, and various non-coding RNAs such as microRNAs, long non-coding RNAs (lncRNAs), and circular RNAs. These elements play crucial roles in controlling gene expression, timing, tissue specificity, and response to environmental signals. Epigenetic modifications, like DNA methylation and histone modification, also operate within these non-coding regions to regulate gene accessibility. Understanding the non-coding genome has opened new avenues in disease research, especially in cancer and neurological disorders, where regulatory dysfunction often occurs without mutations in protein-coding genes. This discovery has fundamentally expanded the scope of functional genomics and deepened our appreciation of genome complexity.
- **Discovery of Genetic Variation: SNPs, CNVs, Structural Variants:** The Human Genome Project and its follow-up initiatives unveiled the immense diversity within the human genome, revealing that no two individuals (except identical twins) share exactly the same DNA sequence. Among the most common forms of variation are single nucleotide polymorphisms (SNPs)—single-base changes in the DNA sequence that occur roughly once every 1,000 base pairs. SNPs can influence traits, disease susceptibility, and drug response. In addition to SNPs, scientists discovered copy number variants (CNVs)—larger segments of DNA that are duplicated or deleted—

and other structural variants, such as inversions and translocations. These variations can affect gene dosage, disrupt coding sequences, or alter gene regulation, contributing to a wide range of health conditions. Understanding genetic variation has been foundational to the development of genome-wide association studies (GWAS), which link specific variants to complex traits and diseases. These discoveries also form the basis of personalized medicine, allowing risk prediction, targeted therapies, and pharmacogenomic profiling based on an individual's unique genetic makeup.

- **Identification of Conserved Sequences and Evolutionary Links:** The Human Genome Project also enabled researchers to compare the human genome with those of other species, leading to the discovery of conserved sequences—regions of DNA that remain relatively unchanged throughout evolution. These sequences are often associated with essential biological functions, such as development, cellular regulation, and survival. Comparative genomics showed that humans share a significant portion of their genome with other organisms: for instance, over 98% similarity with chimpanzees, 85% with mice, and notable conservation with even more distant species like yeast. These findings highlighted the shared evolutionary ancestry of life on Earth and allowed scientists to identify functionally important genes and pathways. Studying conserved genes and regulatory elements has helped identify genes involved in congenital disorders, immune responses, and brain development. Additionally, it validated the use of model organisms in research, as they offer insight into human physiology and disease mechanisms. This evolutionary perspective reinforced the unity of life and demonstrated how small genetic differences can lead to major phenotypic variation across species.

2.1.5 Impact on Personalized Medicine

The Human Genome Project (HGP) has had a transformative impact on the evolution and realization of personalized medicine. By successfully mapping and sequencing the complete human genome, the HGP provided the foundational blueprint that allows healthcare to shift from a generalized, population-based model to a tailored, individual-centric approach. Personalized medicine is rooted in the understanding that each person's genetic makeup profoundly influences their susceptibility to diseases, progression patterns, and response to treatment. This paradigm shift has been made possible by the wealth of genomic information unlocked by the HGP, which enables clinicians and researchers to identify genetic variants associated with complex diseases, uncover molecular subtypes of conditions, and match treatments to individual genetic profiles. One of the most significant impacts has been the integration of genomic data into clinical practice, particularly in areas such as oncology, pharmacology, and rare disease diagnosis. With insights from the HGP, doctors can now utilize genetic screening and predictive testing to assess disease risk, implement preventive measures, and detect conditions earlier. Moreover, pharmacogenomics—a field born from the HGP—has revolutionized drug prescription by ensuring that therapies are safer and more effective, based on how an individual metabolizes or responds to specific drugs. The project also enabled the development of targeted therapies and companion diagnostics that have redefined how diseases, especially cancers, are treated.

- **Laid the Foundation for Genomics-Driven Healthcare:** The Human Genome Project (HGP) established the fundamental knowledge base upon which genomics-driven healthcare has been built. By providing the complete sequence of the human genome and identifying the vast array of human genes, the project allowed researchers and clinicians to better understand how genetic variations contribute to health and disease. This genomic insight shifted medicine from a reactive, symptom-based model to a predictive and preventive framework. It opened new pathways to identify disease risk, refine diagnoses, and anticipate patient responses to treatments. Genomics-driven healthcare now integrates data from an individual's genome to guide clinical decision-making, helping physicians select the most appropriate interventions with improved accuracy and fewer side effects. From rare monogenic disorders to complex diseases like diabetes, asthma, and cardiovascular disease, the HGP enabled personalized approaches that account for individual biological variation. Ultimately, this genomic foundation has led to more precise, efficient, and patient-centered care—marking a transformative era in modern medicine.
- **Enabled the Development of Pharmacogenomics:** Pharmacogenomics—the study of how genes influence an individual's response to drugs—emerged directly from insights gained through the Human Genome Project. Before this advancement, drug therapy largely followed a one-size-fits-all approach, often resulting in adverse drug reactions or suboptimal treatment efficacy. By identifying gene variants that affect drug metabolism, transport, and targets, pharmacogenomics allows clinicians to personalize drug prescriptions based on a patient's genetic profile. For example, variations in the CYP450 enzyme family influence how patients metabolize drugs like warfarin, clopidogrel, and antidepressants. By testing for such variants, clinicians can tailor dosages to minimize side effects and improve outcomes. The integration of pharmacogenomics into clinical practice enhances drug safety, improves therapeutic effectiveness,

and reduces trial-and-error prescribing. Today, pharmacogenomic testing is increasingly used in oncology, cardiology, psychiatry, and infectious diseases, representing a key pillar of personalized medicine and a direct application of genomic research in patient care.

- **Facilitated Molecular Classification of Diseases, Especially Cancers:** Traditionally, diseases—especially cancers—were classified based on anatomical location and histological appearance. However, the Human Genome Project transformed this model by enabling molecular classification based on genetic and genomic alterations. Cancer, in particular, has benefited enormously from this shift. Through genome sequencing, researchers identified key mutations, gene fusions, and expression profiles unique to different cancer subtypes. This allowed oncologists to distinguish, for example, between HER2-positive and HER2-negative breast cancers, or between different genetic forms of leukaemia, even if they appeared similar under a microscope. Molecular profiling now guides diagnosis, risk assessment, and treatment strategy, ensuring that patients receive therapies most likely to work for their specific tumour type. It also enables early detection and monitoring of minimal residual disease. This genetic stratification marks a paradigm shift from organ-based to mutation-based oncology, and it continues to drive the development of next-generation precision therapies.
- **Advanced Genetic Screening and Predictive Testing for Inherited Disorders:** The HGP made it possible to develop powerful genetic screening and predictive testing tools for a wide range of inherited disorders. Before the genome was mapped, diagnosing genetic diseases was often difficult, time-consuming, and imprecise. Now, clinicians can identify mutations responsible for conditions such as cystic fibrosis, Huntington's disease, Tay-Sachs disease, and BRCA1/2-linked breast and ovarian cancers with high accuracy. These tests allow individuals to understand their genetic risks before symptoms arise, enabling preventive strategies or early interventions. In reproductive health, carrier screening helps identify couples at risk of passing on inherited conditions. Prenatal and newborn screening programs have expanded dramatically, improving early diagnosis and care. Importantly, predictive testing also empowers patients to make informed lifestyle, reproductive, and medical decisions. While such testing raises ethical considerations, it remains one of the most impactful clinical applications of genomics, highlighting the preventive power of personalized medicine.

- **Encouraged Development of Targeted Therapies and Companion Diagnostics:** One of the most powerful legacies of the Human Genome Project is the acceleration of targeted therapy—the design of drugs that act on specific molecular targets involved in disease. By understanding the genetic mutations and pathways driving diseases, especially cancers, pharmaceutical researchers can develop therapies that interfere with those specific mechanisms. Drugs like imatinib for chronic myeloid leukaemia (targeting BCR-ABL), trastuzumab for HER2-positive breast cancer, and vemurafenib for BRAF-mutated melanoma are landmark examples of this precision approach. These therapies are often more effective and less toxic than conventional treatments. Alongside targeted drugs, companion diagnostics—tests that identify whether a patient carries the relevant mutation or biomarker—ensure that the right patients receive the right therapy. This co-development model has become standard in precision oncology and is expanding into other fields like immunology and infectious diseases. Together, targeted therapy and companion diagnostics embody the essence of personalized medicine, transforming clinical outcomes and driving future innovation.

2.1.6 Ethical, Legal, and Social Implications (ELSI)

The Human Genome Project (HGP) was not only a scientific and technological milestone—it was also a profound social experiment that raised unprecedented ethical, legal, and social questions. As researchers prepared to decode the entire human genome, it became evident that such knowledge would have far-reaching implications beyond the laboratory. The ability to access, interpret, and manipulate genetic information introduced complex dilemmas related to privacy, consent, discrimination, and societal equity. Recognizing these challenges early, the HGP uniquely allocated a portion of its funding—approximately 3–5%—to the study of Ethical, Legal, and Social Implications (ELSI), marking the first time such a major scientific initiative embedded ethics into its core design. Among the foremost concerns was the privacy of genetic data. With the power to predict future health risks, family histories, and even behavioural tendencies, genetic information became highly sensitive, raising questions about who could access it and for what purposes. Alongside privacy, the potential for genetic discrimination by insurers or employers became a major public concern, fuelling calls for protective legislation. Furthermore, issues around informed consent, particularly in research involving vulnerable populations or complex data-sharing practices, added layers of ethical complexity. The HGP also initiated global dialogues on responsible genetic testing, the limits of human enhancement, and the societal consequences of unequal access to genomic technologies. The ELSI program's work laid the groundwork for laws like the Genetic Information non-discrimination Act (GINA) in the U.S.

and informed ethical standards worldwide. Ultimately, the ELSI framework set a precedent for embedding ethical inquiry within scientific progress—ensuring that as we uncover the secrets of the genome, we do so with a commitment to fairness, accountability, and human dignity.

Raised Questions About Genetic Privacy, Discrimination, and Consent: The Human Genome Project brought to light the immense power—and potential risk—of genetic information, raising pressing ethical concerns about how this sensitive data should be accessed, shared, and protected. As genetic testing and sequencing became more widespread, fears emerged that individuals could be subjected to genetic discrimination by employers, insurers, or even social institutions based on predispositions to certain diseases. Concerns also centred on privacy, especially regarding who has the right to access a person's genomic information and under what conditions. Moreover, informed consent became a complex issue, especially in large-scale genomic research and biobanking, where individuals may not fully understand how their data will be used, stored, or linked to other datasets. These concerns highlighted the need for new ethical standards and frameworks to ensure that individuals retain autonomy and control over their genetic information while still benefiting from scientific progress. Without clear guidelines, the misuse of genomic data could reinforce social inequalities and erode public trust in genomic medicine.

Led to the Establishment of Protective Legislation (e.g., GINA in the U.S.): In response to the ethical and legal concerns brought forward by the Human Genome Project, several countries began enacting legislation to protect individuals from the misuse of genetic data. One landmark example is the Genetic Information non-discrimination Act (GINA), passed in the United States in 2008. GINA prohibits health insurers and employers from using genetic information to make decisions about coverage, rates, hiring, or job assignments. It was a pivotal step in ensuring that people could undergo genetic testing without fear of being penalized based on their inherited traits or disease risks. GINA and similar laws serve as legal safeguards to support both patient autonomy and public confidence in genomic research and personalized medicine. However, these laws are not without limitations—GINA, for example, does not apply to life insurance or long-term care insurance, and enforcement varies by jurisdiction. Nevertheless, such legislation is a critical component of ethical genomics, ensuring that medical innovation is accompanied by robust human rights protections.

Initiated Public Dialogue on the Responsible Use of Genetic Information: One of the most enduring impacts of the Human Genome Project was its proactive approach to ethical, legal, and social issues—most notably by allocating a portion of its budget specifically to explore these dimensions. This led to the creation of dedicated ELSI programs, which not only supported academic research but also fostered public education and engagement. These initiatives helped spark widespread dialogue around the responsible use of genetic data, encouraging society to confront challenging questions: Who owns genetic information? How should we balance scientific advancement with individual rights? What safeguards are necessary for vulnerable populations? Public debates also emerged around prenatal genetic screening, direct-to-consumer genetic tests, and the ethical implications of gene editing technologies like CRISPR. These conversations were vital in democratizing the ethics of genomics and ensuring that policy decisions were informed by public values. The HGP thus played a central role in making bioethics a public concern, encouraging transparency, accountability, and ethical foresight in the genomic era.

2.1.7 Legacy and Continuing Impact

The Human Genome Project (HGP) stands as a landmark achievement that has forever altered the course of biomedical science, healthcare, and biotechnology. Its successful completion in 2003 provided the first complete map of the human genome, catalysing a series of global initiatives that continue to expand our understanding of genetics and human health. Projects such as the 1000 Genomes Project, ENCODE, and the All of Us Research Program were born from the vision and success of the HGP, each building on its foundation to explore genetic diversity, functional genomics, and population-wide health data. These initiatives are crucial in advancing precision medicine and ensuring that genomic science benefits diverse communities. The project also revolutionized genome sequencing by dramatically reducing its cost and time. What once took billions of dollars and years can now be done in days for a fraction of the cost, opening the door for routine clinical applications and large-scale population studies. This affordability has brought genome sequencing into hospitals, enabling early diagnosis, risk assessment, and personalized treatments. Furthermore, the HGP fostered unprecedented interdisciplinary collaboration, merging biology with computer science, mathematics, and medicine, and leading to the emergence of new fields such as bioinformatics, systems biology, and genomic medicine. Beyond research and medicine, the HGP sparked innovation across the biotechnology industry, fuelling the development of targeted therapies, gene editing tools, and molecular diagnostics. Its legacy is not just scientific but also cultural—it normalized data sharing, emphasized ethical inquiry through the ELSI program, and engaged the public in discussions about the future of health. In essence, the HGP laid the genomic foundation for the 21st century, and its influence continues to shape the trajectory of science, healthcare, and society in profound ways.

- **Catalysed the Launch of Global Genomics Initiatives:** The Human Genome Project laid the foundation for a new era of collaborative, global genomics research. By proving that large-scale DNA sequencing was feasible and scientifically valuable, the HGP inspired the launch of subsequent initiatives aimed at expanding our understanding of human genetic diversity and genome function. Notable among these is the 1000 Genomes Project, which sought to catalogue genetic variation across populations; ENCODE (Encyclopaedia of DNA Elements), which focused on identifying all functional elements in the human genome; and the All of Us Research Program, a U.S.-based initiative aiming to collect health data from one million diverse individuals to advance precision medicine. These projects build directly on the HGP's achievements and continue to evolve our understanding of the genome in ways that improve global health equity, disease prevention, and personalized care. Each initiative underscores the HGP's enduring influence in encouraging open science, data sharing, and population-inclusive genomic research.

- **Reduced the Cost and Time of Genome Sequencing Dramatically:** At the start of the HGP, sequencing a single human genome cost nearly $3 billion and took over a decade. By the time it concluded in 2003, costs had already begun to decline due to technological innovation. In the years that followed, building on HGP-driven breakthroughs, genome sequencing experienced a dramatic drop in cost and a corresponding increase in speed. Today, whole genome sequencing can be performed in under 24 hours for less than $1,000—a reduction that has made genomic analysis accessible to both researchers and clinicians around the world. This cost revolution was made possible through the development of next-generation sequencing (NGS) platforms, automation, miniaturization, and improved bioinformatics. These changes democratized access to genomics, empowering projects in low-resource settings and enabling clinical use of genome sequencing for diagnosis, cancer profiling, pharmacogenomics, and more. Thus, the HGP served as a springboard for the rapid technological scaling that underpins modern precision medicine.
- **Encouraged Interdisciplinary Collaboration Across Biology, Computer Science, and Medicine:** One of the most profound impacts of the Human Genome Project was its role in dissolving boundaries between scientific disciplines. Sequencing and analysing the human genome required the integration of molecular biology, genetics, informatics, mathematics, engineering, and clinical medicine, leading to the emergence of genomics as an interdisciplinary field. The massive data sets generated by the HGP could not be understood or utilized without advanced computational tools, sparking a surge in bioinformatics and computational biology. Clinicians, too, became vital collaborators as the implications of genomics for disease

understanding and treatment became clear. This convergence fostered a new research culture built on collaboration, data sharing, and systems thinking. Universities and research institutions began training scientists who were "bilingual" in biology and computer science, giving rise to hybrid disciplines like systems genomics and computational medicine. The HGP thus reshaped the scientific workforce and laid the groundwork for today's highly collaborative biomedical research ecosystem.

- **Revolutionized Medical Research, Diagnostics, and Biotechnology Industries:** The legacy of the HGP can be most clearly seen in the transformation of medicine and biotechnology. With the human genome mapped, researchers gained unprecedented insight into the genetic underpinnings of thousands of diseases, particularly complex, multifactorial conditions like cancer, diabetes, and neurodegenerative disorders. Genetic markers discovered through HGP data enabled early disease detection, risk prediction, and patient stratification for clinical trials. The HGP also paved the way for the rise of personalized and precision medicine, where therapies can be tailored to an individual's genetic profile. In diagnostics, molecular testing has become a standard practice in areas such as oncology and prenatal screening. Biotech companies have leveraged this genomic knowledge to develop targeted drugs, gene therapies, and biologics, leading to an explosion of innovation in therapeutic development. The project essentially redefined the commercial landscape of medicine and biotechnology, anchoring future progress in genomic knowledge and personalized care.

2.1.8 Challenges and Limitations

While the Human Genome Project (HGP) marked a monumental scientific achievement, unlocking the entire sequence of the human genome, it also revealed a landscape filled with unresolved complexities and emerging limitations. The initial optimism that decoding our genetic blueprint would rapidly translate into cures, precise diagnostics, and universally personalized medicine has been tempered by the intricate reality of human biology. Many of the approximately 20,000–25,000 protein-coding genes identified remain only partially understood, with vast regions of non-coding DNA still functionally enigmatic. This limited understanding constrains our ability to link genetic information with disease mechanisms or clinical outcomes. A major conceptual challenge lies in the misconception of genetic determinism—the belief that genes alone govern health and disease. In truth, gene expression is deeply influenced by environmental, lifestyle, and epigenetic factors, making disease prediction and treatment far more complex than originally anticipated. Compounding this issue is the lack of genetic diversity in early genomic databases, which were predominantly built on European populations. This imbalance has resulted in reduced accuracy of genomic tools for underrepresented groups, raising concerns about equity and applicability in global health contexts. Another critical barrier is the difficulty in interpreting variants of uncertain significance (VUS)—genetic changes whose impact remains unclear. These ambiguous findings often provide little clinical guidance, leaving patients and healthcare providers in a diagnostic grey zone. Additionally, ethical, legal, and social concerns—such as data privacy, informed consent, and potential misuse of genetic information—remain ongoing issues that need constant vigilance. Despite its transformative legacy, the HGP serves as both a triumph and a starting point—a reminder that while the map of the genome is complete, the journey toward fully understanding and applying it is far from over.

- **Many Gene Functions Still Remain Unknown or Poorly Understood:** Despite the enormous achievement of sequencing the entire human genome, a substantial portion of our genetic code remains poorly understood. While the HGP identified approximately 20,000–25,000 protein-coding genes, the function of many of these genes—and their interactions with each other and the environment—remains largely uncharacterized. Furthermore, vast regions of non-coding DNA, once dismissed as "junk," are now known to play vital regulatory and structural roles, yet their precise biological significance is still being unravelled. These knowledge gaps limit the translation of genomic data into actionable clinical insights. Without a clear understanding of gene function, it becomes difficult to predict how specific mutations lead to disease or how they may be targeted therapeutically. Progress in functional genomics, systems biology, and experimental validation is essential to fully unlock the genome's potential. Thus, while the HGP mapped the sequence, interpreting the biological meaning of that sequence remains an ongoing and complex scientific challenge.
- **Genetic Determinism Concerns:** Genes Are Not the Sole Determinants of Health: The Human Genome Project, while groundbreaking, inadvertently fuelled a widespread misconception known as genetic determinism—the belief that genes alone dictate an individual's health, traits, and behaviours. This simplistic view overlooks the complexity of human biology, which is shaped by a dynamic interplay of genetic, environmental, lifestyle, and epigenetic factors. For many common diseases such as diabetes, heart disease, and depression, genes contribute only a portion of the risk, and their expression is heavily influenced by external factors like diet, stress, pollutants, and socioeconomic conditions. The danger of genetic determinism lies in overselling the power of genetics while underappreciating broader determinants of health, potentially leading to

fatalism or reduced emphasis on preventive care. The HGP revealed the genome's complexity but also emphasized the need for integrative models of health that consider the full biological and social context. Genomics must be framed as one piece of the puzzle—not the sole answer.

- **Need for Diversity:** Early Data Skewed Toward Populations of European Descent: One of the major limitations of the original Human Genome Project was its lack of representation of global genetic diversity. The majority of early genomic data came from individuals of European ancestry, which skewed the reference genome and initial genetic studies. This imbalance has had lasting implications: genetic variants important in non-European populations may be underrepresented or misinterpreted, and polygenic risk scores developed from Eurocentric data often perform poorly in other groups. Such disparities threaten to exacerbate health inequities, as people from underrepresented backgrounds may not benefit equally from genomic medicine. Recognizing this, more recent efforts—such as the Human Heredity and Health in Africa (H3Africa) initiative and the All of Us program in the U.S.—aim to expand genomic research across diverse populations. Addressing this challenge is essential for ensuring the equity, validity, and utility of genomic science across all communities, not just a privileged few.
- **Difficulty in Interpreting Variants of Uncertain Significance (VUS):** As genome sequencing becomes more widespread, clinicians and researchers frequently encounter Variants of Uncertain Significance (VUS)—genetic changes whose impact on health is unknown. These ambiguous results present significant challenges for diagnosis, counseling, and treatment decisions. A VUS may occur in a gene associated with a disease, but without sufficient evidence, it is unclear whether the variant is benign or pathogenic. This uncertainty can cause anxiety for patients and leave clinicians with limited guidance. The interpretation of VUS depends heavily on context—family history, functional studies, population databases, and predictive models—all of which are still evolving. Moreover, the interpretation may change over time as new data emerge, requiring continuous updates to medical records and patient communication. The prevalence of VUS highlights the limitations of our current knowledge and the need for improved databases, international data sharing, and functional assays to move uncertain variants into clearer categories. Until then, VUS will remain a barrier to fully leveraging genomics in clinical care.

2.2 GENOMIC VARIABILITY AND POPULATION DIVERSITY

Genomic variability refers to the natural differences in DNA sequences that exist among individuals and across populations. This variation is fundamental to the diversity of human traits, health conditions, and biological responses. From single nucleotide polymorphisms (SNPs) to larger structural changes such as insertions, deletions, and copy number variants (CNVs), these genetic differences play a critical role in influencing how people respond to diseases, medications, and environmental exposures. Understanding this variability is essential to advancing personalized medicine, where prevention, diagnosis, and treatment are tailored to an individual's unique genetic makeup. Population diversity adds an important dimension to genomic variability. Each human population has a distinct genetic signature shaped by its unique history of migration, adaptation, and evolution. For instance, African populations exhibit the highest level of genetic diversity, reflecting their ancestral origins, while other groups possess unique mutations that reflect their specific environments and historical selection pressures. Unfortunately, early genomic research focused heavily on individuals of European descent, resulting in significant knowledge gaps and unequal benefits of genomic medicine. Recognizing the need for inclusivity, recent efforts in global genomics have emphasized diversifying genetic research to better represent the global population. Projects like the 1000 Genomes Project, H3Africa, and All of Us are building rich, multi-ethnic genomic databases to ensure that medical discoveries are equitable and relevant to all. Addressing this diversity is not just a scientific necessity but a moral imperative in ensuring fairness, accuracy, and access in healthcare. As personalized medicine advances, integrating genomic variability and population diversity will be vital in delivering truly individualized and globally applicable care.

2.2.1 Understanding Genomic Variability

Genomic variability encompasses the natural and heritable differences found in the DNA sequences among individuals and across populations. This variation forms the biological foundation of human uniqueness, influencing everything from eye color and metabolism to disease susceptibility and immune responses. These genetic differences arise due to mutations, recombination, and evolutionary forces, accumulating over generations. The spectrum of variability ranges from the smallest changes—such as single nucleotide polymorphisms (SNPs)—to large-scale structural alterations like insertions, deletions, and chromosomal rearrangements. Such variations are not always pathological; many are benign or even beneficial, depending on the context and environment. In modern biomedicine, identifying and cataloguing these variations is critical for understanding the relationship between genotype and phenotype. Importantly, this understanding is essential for the advancement of personalized medicine, where diagnosis, treatment, and disease prevention are tailored to an individual's unique genetic profile. Moreover, the study of variability contributes to population genetics, evolutionary biology, and forensic science. It also plays a pivotal role in reconstructing ancestry and human migration patterns. Ultimately, genomic variability is the gateway to deciphering human diversity at the molecular level and unlocking precision-based healthcare.

2.2.2 Types of Genetic Variations

Genetic variations are broadly categorized based on the size and nature of the change in the DNA sequence. The most common type is the single nucleotide polymorphism (SNP), which involves a single base pair alteration and accounts for the majority of human genetic differences. These may have functional consequences or serve as neutral markers. Insertions and deletions (indels) represent small additions or losses of nucleotides, potentially causing frameshifts or affecting gene expression. Copy Number Variants (CNVs) are larger segments of DNA that are duplicated or deleted, influencing gene dosage and potentially leading to disorders such as autism or developmental delays. Structural variants encompass major chromosomal changes like inversions, duplications, and translocations, which can disrupt regulatory networks or fusion genes, sometimes contributing to cancers or genetic syndromes. Each type of variation has the potential to be benign, beneficial, or detrimental, depending on its location and context. These variations shape our biology and are used as biomarkers for disease prediction, ancestry tracing, and therapeutic decision-making. Advances in sequencing and bioinformatics have made it possible to detect, catalogue, and interpret these variations at population scale, strengthening the genomic basis of precision medicine.

2.2.3 Importance in Health and Disease

Genomic variability has profound implications for understanding human health and the ethology of disease. While some genetic variations are harmless, others contribute to a spectrum of disorders, ranging from monogenic conditions like cystic fibrosis to complex diseases such as cardiovascular disorders, diabetes, and cancer. Variants in specific genes can increase susceptibility or confer resistance to infections, influence the progression of disease, and determine an individual's response to treatment. For instance, BRCA1/2 mutations elevate the risk for breast and ovarian cancers, while variants in HLA genes influence immune response. In the realm of complex diseases, polygenic risk scores aggregate the impact of many variants to estimate a person's overall risk. Understanding these genetic contributions allows for earlier interventions, better stratification of patients, and improved therapeutic targeting. Personalized medicine utilizes this knowledge to move from population-wide treatment strategies to more precise, individualized care plans. As genetic testing becomes more accessible and affordable, its integration into routine clinical practice is expanding, enabling a more nuanced approach to diagnosis, prognosis, and therapy selection based on each patient's unique genomic makeup.

2.2.4 Population Diversity and Global Genomics

The genetic diversity observed in global populations reflects centuries of human evolution, migration, adaptation, and interbreeding. This diversity is not just an anthropological curiosity—it has real biological and clinical implications. African populations, as the oldest and most genetically diverse, contain a vast array of unique alleles, while populations that underwent bottlenecks or founder effects, such as those in isolated island communities, display reduced variability but high frequencies of specific variants. Environmental pressures, such as high altitude or exposure to pathogens, have driven adaptive evolution resulting in traits like sickle cell resistance to malaria or EPAS1 variants in Tibetan populations. Understanding these differences enhances our grasp of disease mechanisms, pharmacogenetics, and gene-environment interactions. Comparative population genomics enables the identification of conserved versus population-specific disease alleles, thereby improving diagnostics and interventions. A comprehensive understanding of population diversity is necessary for inclusive medical research and equitable health outcomes. Neglecting such diversity may lead to the development of biased diagnostic tools and interventions that are ineffective or even harmful in non-European populations. Thus, integrating diverse genomic data is foundational to the success of global personalized medicine.

2.2.5 Underrepresentation in Genomic Research

A significant limitation in the early phases of genomic research was its overwhelming focus on populations of European descent. More than 80% of genomic data used in biomedical research comes from individuals of European ancestry, despite the fact that they comprise less than 20% of the global population. This imbalance has led to biased findings, misclassification of genetic variants, and limited applicability of genomic tests for underrepresented groups. Tools like polygenic risk scores, which are trained on Eurocentric data, often perform poorly when applied to individuals from African, Asian, or Indigenous populations. Such disparities compromise the goals of personalized medicine and risk reinforcing health inequities. There is now increasing recognition of the need for inclusivity and representativeness in genomic studies. Funding agencies, research institutions, and public health organizations are calling for diversity in genomic cohorts. Diversification is not only an ethical imperative but a scientific necessity, ensuring the accuracy, generalizability, and fairness of genetic-based diagnostics and therapies. Addressing this imbalance will require collaborative international efforts, community engagement, capacity-building in low-resource settings, and ethical frameworks that respect cultural sensitivities.

2.2.6 Role in Drug Response and Pharmacogenomics

Genomic variability plays a pivotal role in how individuals respond to medications—a concept at the core of pharmacogenomics. Genetic differences in drug-metabolizing enzymes, transporters, and receptors influence the efficacy and toxicity of various treatments. For instance, polymorphisms in the CYP2C19 gene affect how individuals metabolize clopidogrel, a blood thinner, potentially rendering it ineffective in some patients. Similarly, variations in TPMT or NUDT15 genes can lead to severe toxicity when patients are treated with thiopurines unless dose adjustments are made. These gene-drug interactions are increasingly being integrated into clinical guidelines and decision-support tools. Moreover, different populations exhibit distinct frequencies of pharmacogenomic variants, necessitating population-specific considerations in drug development and prescription. Personalized medicine aims to use this information to avoid adverse drug reactions, enhance therapeutic efficacy, and reduce trial-and-error prescribing. Advances in genome sequencing and pharmacogenomic profiling have made it feasible to implement such personalized approaches, especially in oncology, cardiology, and psychiatry. As precision prescribing becomes standard practice, understanding the link between genetic diversity and drug response will be critical for improving patient outcomes globally.

2.2.7 Ethical and Social Implications

Conducting genomic research in diverse populations raises several ethical, legal, and social issues that must be carefully managed. Chief among these are concerns around informed consent, privacy, data ownership, and potential misuse of genetic information. Historically marginalized communities may harbour mistrust due to past exploitation or unethical research practices. Therefore, researchers must engage in culturally sensitive dialogue, ensuring transparency, respect, and community benefit. Genetic data must be protected to prevent discrimination in employment, insurance, or social standing—issues addressed in part by laws such as the Genetic Information Non-discrimination Act (GINA) in the U.S. There is also the risk of stigmatization when certain variants are incorrectly associated with racial or ethnic groups, perpetuating stereotypes or fuelling eugenic ideologies. Ethical frameworks must therefore prioritize participant autonomy, data sovereignty, and equitable access to the benefits of research. Additionally, capacity-building efforts should empower local scientists and healthcare systems to participate fully in the genomic revolution. Only by embedding ethics into every phase of population genomics can we ensure that science serves all of humanity fairly and respectfully.

2.2.8 Initiatives to Increase Diversity

In response to the imbalance in genomic research, numerous global initiatives have been launched to capture a broader representation of human diversity. The

1000 Genomes Project was among the first to catalogue human genetic variation across multiple continents. H3Africa (Human Heredity and Health in Africa) supports genomic research led by African scientists, fostering infrastructure, training, and culturally sensitive practices. The All of Us Research Program in the United States aims to enrol over a million diverse participants to drive equity in precision health. Genome Asia 100K focuses on sequencing Asian populations to build regional genomic resources. These initiatives contribute to comprehensive reference databases that enhance variant interpretation, facilitate equitable drug development, and improve diagnostic precision for all populations. Furthermore, they promote international collaboration and empower underrepresented communities through capacity-building and ethical governance. By prioritizing diversity, these programs ensure that personalized medicine becomes a globally relevant and inclusive endeavour. They also serve as models for integrating social justice with scientific innovation in the era of genomics.

2.3 SINGLE NUCLEOTIDE POLYMORPHISMS (SNPS) AND DISEASE RISK

Single Nucleotide Polymorphisms (SNPs) are the most prevalent and well-studied form of genetic variation in the human genome. These variations arise when a single nucleotide—adenine (A), thymine (T), cytosine (C), or guanine (G)—is altered at a specific position in the DNA sequence. For example, one individual may have a cytosine (C) at a particular locus, while another may have a thymine (T). Such changes occur approximately once every 300 base pairs, resulting in an estimated 10 million SNPs dispersed throughout the human genome. Although most SNPs are found in non-coding regions and were initially assumed to be biologically inert, growing evidence shows they can influence gene regulation, chromatin structure, and RNA splicing. When located in coding regions, SNPs may lead to amino acid substitutions (missense mutations) or premature stop codons (nonsense mutations), potentially altering protein structure and function. SNPs in promoters, enhancers, or untranslated regions can affect gene expression by modifying transcription factor binding or mRNA stability. This makes them important in modulating phenotypic traits and susceptibility to complex diseases such as cancer, diabetes, cardiovascular disorders, and neurological conditions. Furthermore, SNPs can influence how individuals respond to environmental stimuli, infections, and drugs. They form the basis of personalized medicine by enabling the prediction of disease risk, identification of therapeutic targets, and optimization of treatment strategies tailored to individual genetic profiles. High-throughput genotyping technologies, such as SNP arrays and next-generation sequencing, have made it feasible to analyse millions of SNPs rapidly, supporting large-scale studies on human health and genetic diversity. The continued exploration of SNPs holds promise for advancing predictive genomics, risk stratification, and precision healthcare worldwide.

2.3.1 SNPs as Genetic Markers

Single Nucleotide Polymorphisms (SNPs) are exceptionally valuable as genetic markers due to their abundance, stability, and uniform distribution across the genome. Their presence at predictable locations allows researchers to track the inheritance of genomic regions across generations. One of their most powerful applications is in genome-wide association studies (GWAS), where hundreds of thousands to millions of SNPs are scanned across genomes of large populations to identify correlations with specific traits or diseases. These associations help pinpoint genomic regions that may harbour causal genes or regulatory elements contributing to conditions such as diabetes, cancer, asthma, or schizophrenia. Unlike rare mutations, SNPs occur frequently and are often shared among individuals, making them ideal for statistical analysis in diverse populations. They also aid in the construction of haplotypes—clusters of SNPs that tend to be inherited together—which can reveal ancestral linkages and evolutionary relationships. SNPs are instrumental in studying linkage disequilibrium, a phenomenon where certain alleles are inherited together more frequently than expected by chance, which provides clues about gene locations and disease mechanisms. The advent of SNP arrays or "SNP chips" has revolutionized genotyping, allowing researchers to analyse hundreds of thousands of SNPs in a single experiment quickly and affordably. These arrays enable population-scale analyses and the identification of genetic variants associated with complex diseases or traits. Moreover, SNPs play a role in forensic science, anthropology, and agriculture, where they are used to identify individuals, trace ancestry, and assist in crop and livestock breeding. In the context of personalized medicine, SNPs guide diagnostic tools, risk stratification, and therapeutic decision-making. Their robust reproducibility, informativeness, and ease of analysis continue to make SNPs indispensable in the field of human genetics and biomedical research.

2.3.2 Functional Impact of SNPs

While the majority of single nucleotide polymorphisms (SNPs) are considered neutral and do not impact health or development, a significant subset can have profound biological and clinical consequences. Functional SNPs are those that alter the behaviour or expression of genes, often affecting cellular pathways and disease processes. In coding regions of genes, SNPs can cause missense mutations, where a single nucleotide change results in a different amino acid being incorporated into the protein. This can alter the protein's structure, stability, or function—potentially leading to gain- or loss-of-function effects. Nonsense mutations, another outcome of SNPs, introduce premature stop codons, leading to truncated, non-functional proteins that may disrupt key cellular processes. Beyond the coding sequences, SNPs in regulatory regions such as promoters, enhancers, and silencers can impact gene expression by modifying how transcription factors bind to DNA, or by affecting chromatin accessibility. These changes may upregulate or downregulate gene activity, contributing to disease risk or progression. Intronic SNPs, located within non-coding segments of genes, may seem inconsequential at first glance, but they can disrupt splicing mechanisms, leading to aberrant mRNA transcripts and faulty protein products. Moreover, some SNPs affect mRNA stability, polyadenylation, or translation efficiency, influencing how much protein is produced from a gene. Functional SNPs are also key components in expression quantitative trait loci (eQTL) studies, which correlate SNPs with changes in gene expression levels across tissues. Such SNPs provide mechanistic insights into complex traits and are increasingly used to uncover causal variants behind genome-wide associations. Importantly, understanding the function of these SNPs helps researchers identify therapeutic targets and develop precision interventions tailored to a patient's genetic profile. Thus, functional SNPs represent a crucial link between genetic variation and phenotypic expression, with direct relevance to diagnostics, therapeutics, and the advancement of personalized medicine.

2.3.3 SNPs and Disease Susceptibility

Single Nucleotide Polymorphisms (SNPs) play a pivotal role in modulating individual and population-level susceptibility to a wide array of diseases. These tiny genomic alterations can influence how genes function or are expressed, thereby impacting biological pathways involved in disease processes. Genome-Wide Association Studies (GWAS) have uncovered thousands of SNPs that correlate with increased or decreased risk for common and complex diseases. For example, SNPs near the FTO gene have been repeatedly linked to obesity, likely affecting energy metabolism and appetite regulation. The APOE ε4 allele, a well-known SNP variant, is strongly associated with late-onset Alzheimer's disease, influencing amyloid-beta accumulation in the brain. Variants in the 5p15 region, including TERT, have been tied to lung cancer susceptibility, as they affect telomerase activity and cellular aging. Beyond these, SNPs have been linked to conditions such as type 2 diabetes, coronary artery disease, schizophrenia, Crohn's disease, and rheumatoid arthritis. These associations are often polygenic, meaning no single SNP causes the disease, but rather a constellation of variants exerts cumulative effects. Many SNPs exert modest effects individually, altering disease risk by a small percentage, but their combined influence—captured in polygenic models—can be substantial. Disease-associated SNPs can reside in coding regions, affecting protein structure, or in non-coding regions, influencing gene regulation and expression. Moreover, SNP-disease associations often vary across populations, due to differences in allele frequencies, environmental exposures, and gene-gene interactions. Understanding these variants allows researchers to identify at-risk individuals, uncover biological pathways underlying disease, and inform preventive or therapeutic strategies.

Importantly, SNP studies have advanced the movement toward personalized medicine, enabling risk stratification and early interventions. However, translating SNP findings into clinical practice requires deeper insight into the mechanistic roles of these variants and validation across diverse ancestries to ensure equitable healthcare outcomes.

2.3.4 Polygenic Risk Scores (PRS)

Polygenic Risk Scores (PRS) have emerged as a powerful tool in the field of genomic medicine, offering a comprehensive approach to assess an individual's genetic predisposition to complex diseases. Unlike single SNPs, which typically have minimal predictive power, PRS combine the weighted effect of thousands—or even millions—of SNPs across the genome to estimate an individual's overall disease risk. These scores are calculated using data from large-scale genome-wide association studies (GWAS), where each SNP's contribution to disease risk is quantified and summed. PRS are particularly useful for polygenic diseases such as breast cancer, type 2 diabetes, coronary artery disease, and schizophrenia, where no single variant determines outcome but a constellation of small-effect variants collectively influences susceptibility. By stratifying individuals into different genetic risk percentiles, PRS enable predictive risk modelling, allowing for early identification of high-risk individuals even before symptoms manifest. In preventive medicine, PRS can inform personalized screening protocols, lifestyle modifications, and targeted interventions, potentially delaying or avoiding disease onset. For example, individuals with a high PRS for cardiovascular disease may benefit from earlier cholesterol testing or proactive statin therapy. However, one of the key challenges in the implementation of PRS is their limited generalizability across populations. Most GWAS datasets are disproportionately composed of individuals of European ancestry, meaning that PRS derived from such data often perform poorly in non-European populations, potentially leading to inequitable risk assessments. This underlines the urgent need for diversity in genomic research to build equitable PRS models that reflect global populations. Additionally, while PRS are a promising tool, they are not deterministic—environmental factors, lifestyle, and gene–gene interactions also play critical roles. As methods evolve, integrating PRS with clinical, environmental, and family history data could enhance risk prediction models, making them more robust and clinically actionable.

2.3.5 SNPs and Pharmacogenomics

Single Nucleotide Polymorphisms (SNPs) play a pivotal role in determining how individuals metabolize and respond to various drugs, making them a key focus in pharmacogenomics. These genetic variations can influence drug absorption, distribution, metabolism, and excretion, thereby affecting both therapeutic efficacy and the risk of adverse reactions. For instance, polymorphisms in the CYP2C19 gene significantly alter the metabolic activation of clopidogrel, a common antiplatelet drug, which can lead to reduced effectiveness in poor metabolizers. Similarly, variations in TPMT and NUDT15 are crucial in determining patient tolerance to thiopurines, drugs used in cancer and autoimmune diseases—deficiency in enzyme activity can result in life-threatening toxicity. Another critical example is the VKORC1 gene, where SNPs modulate sensitivity to warfarin, necessitating precise dose adjustments to prevent bleeding or clotting complications. By analysing such SNP profiles through pharmacogenomic testing, clinicians can personalize drug prescriptions to match an individual's genetic makeup. This SNP-guided approach reduces trial-and-error in prescribing, minimizes adverse drug reactions, and optimizes therapeutic outcomes. It exemplifies the shift from generalized medicine to highly individualized care, anchoring pharmacogenomics as a foundational pillar of personalized medicine.

2.3.6 Population-Specific SNP Patterns

The frequency and distribution of Single Nucleotide Polymorphisms (SNPs) differ significantly across global populations due to evolutionary forces such as genetic drift, natural selection, migration, and founder effects. These processes shape the genetic landscape uniquely within each population, resulting in some SNPs being highly prevalent in certain groups while rare or entirely absent in others. Such variability has profound implications for biomedical research and clinical practice. In disease risk prediction, SNPs associated with specific conditions may show varying predictive power across populations, potentially leading to underestimation or overestimation of risk in certain ethnic groups. In pharmacogenomics, these differences influence how populations respond to drugs; for example, a SNP affecting drug metabolism in one population may be irrelevant in another, necessitating population-tailored prescribing guidelines. Consequently, the development of accurate, inclusive, and effective precision medicine approaches must account for these inter-population differences. The historical underrepresentation of diverse ancestries in genomic research limits the generalizability of findings and perpetuates health disparities. Addressing this gap requires deliberate efforts to include diverse populations in genomic studies, ensuring that the benefits of personalized medicine are equitably distributed and scientifically robust across all global communities.

2.3.7 Limitations and Challenges

Despite the immense utility of SNPs in advancing our understanding of complex diseases, interpreting SNP-disease associations remains a challenging endeavour. A major complication arises from the fact that many SNPs identified through genome-wide association studies (GWAS) are located in non-coding regions of the genome, such as introns or intergenic regions. These areas do not code for proteins, and their biological roles are often poorly understood, making it difficult to determine how they influence disease mechanisms. Additionally, SNPs often exist in linkage disequilibrium—clusters of inherited variants that are genetically correlated—complicating efforts to pinpoint which specific variant is truly causal. This creates ambiguity in identifying the functional variant responsible for disease risk.The complexity is further compounded by environmental influences and lifestyle factors, which can modulate genetic predispositions in ways that are difficult to disentangle statistically. Gene–gene interactions, or epistasis, also obscure the independent effects of individual SNPs, as multiple variants may act synergistically or antagonistically to influence disease phenotypes. Another critical limitation is the lack of ancestral diversity in GWAS datasets. The vast majority of SNP associations have been derived from individuals of European descent, raising concerns about the applicability of these findings to non-European populations. This Eurocentric bias not only reduces the predictive power of SNP-based risk scores in diverse groups but also perpetuates health disparities in genomic medicine. Addressing these interpretive challenges requires more functional genomics research, improved statistical methods, and a concerted global effort to include underrepresented populations in genomic studies. Only then can SNP-based insights translate into universally effective and equitable healthcare solutions.

2.3.8 Future Directions

Emerging techniques such as fine-mapping, expression quantitative trait loci (eQTL) analysis, and functional genomics are helping to uncover how SNPs influence gene regulation and disease pathways. Integration of SNP data with multi-omic layers (e.g., transcriptomics, epigenomics) and machine learning approaches will enhance risk prediction and therapeutic targeting. There's also a push to develop population-specific PRS and increase representation in SNP databases through inclusive global research initiatives.

- **Fine-Mapping of Causal Variants:** Fine-mapping techniques are being developed to distinguish true causal variants from correlated SNPs in linkage disequilibrium. By narrowing down associated genomic regions, researchers can more accurately identify SNPs that have a direct biological effect on disease risk or drug response.
- **eQTL and Regulatory SNP Analysis:** Expression Quantitative Trait Loci (eQTL) analysis links SNPs to gene expression levels, helping clarify how non-coding variants regulate genes. These studies are key to understanding the functional consequences of SNPs and their role in disease biology, especially for variants in enhancer or promoter regions.
- **Functional Genomics and CRISPR Screening:** Functional genomics tools—including CRISPR/Cas9 and massively parallel reporter assays—are

used to validate the biological impact of candidate SNPs. These approaches can experimentally test how specific SNPs alter gene function, cellular pathways, or phenotype expression.

- **Multi-Omics Integration:** Future research increasingly focuses on integrating SNP data with other 'omics' layers such as transcriptomics, proteomics, metabolomics, and epigenomics. This multi-dimensional approach provides a more holistic view of disease mechanisms and enables more accurate biomarker discovery.
- **Machine Learning and Predictive Modelling:** Advanced computational tools, including machine learning and artificial intelligence, are being applied to large-scale genomic datasets. These methods can identify complex patterns and interactions among SNPs, enhancing disease risk prediction, drug response modelling, and therapeutic stratification.
- **Development of Population-Specific Polygenic Risk Scores (PRS):** There is a growing effort to create and validate polygenic risk scores that are specific to diverse populations. Tailored PRS can improve risk prediction accuracy for non-European groups, addressing current biases in genomic risk assessment tools.
- **Global Representation in Genomic Research:** To ensure equitable healthcare outcomes, global research initiatives are prioritizing the inclusion of underrepresented populations in SNP databases and GWAS. Expanding genetic diversity in research cohorts improves the generalizability and clinical utility of SNP-based tools across populations.
- **Clinical Translation and SNP-Based Therapies:** The ultimate goal is to integrate SNP insights into clinical decision-making. This includes not only refining diagnostics and prognostics but also guiding personalized interventions and drug development based on validated SNP targets.

2.4 WHOLE GENOME, EXOME, AND TRANSCRIPTOME SEQUENCING

2.4.1. Whole Genome Sequencing (WGS)

Whole Genome Sequencing provides a comprehensive view of an individual's entire DNA sequence, covering both coding (exons) and non-coding regions (introns, intergenic regions, regulatory elements). It enables detection of all types of genetic variations including SNPs, insertions/deletions, structural variants, and copy number variations. WGS is particularly valuable for uncovering rare or novel variants, mapping complex traits, and investigating regulatory elements that influence gene expression. While its cost has decreased significantly, it still requires substantial computational resources and generates massive datasets demanding advanced bioinformatics analysis.

2.4.2 Whole Exome Sequencing (WES)

Whole Exome Sequencing focuses specifically on the protein-coding regions of the genome, which constitute approximately 1–2% of the total DNA but harbour nearly 85% of known disease-causing mutations. WES is more cost-effective than WGS and allows for efficient identification of clinically relevant variants, especially in Mendelian disorders. However, it misses important information from non-coding regions and may fail to detect deep intronic or regulatory mutations. WES is widely used in both clinical diagnostics and research due to its high diagnostic yield and affordability.

2.4.3 Transcriptome Sequencing (RNA-Seq)

Transcriptome sequencing, or RNA-Seq, profiles all RNA molecules expressed in a specific tissue or cell type at a given time. It offers insight into gene expression patterns, splicing variants, fusion transcripts, and non-coding RNAs. RNA-Seq is crucial for understanding gene regulation, disease mechanisms, and cellular responses to environmental or therapeutic stimuli. Unlike DNA sequencing, it reflects the functional output of the genome and is sensitive to temporal and spatial biological conditions. It also complements WGS and WES by validating whether detected genetic variants affect gene expression.

2.4.4 Comparative Advantages and Limitations

WGS provides complete genomic information but is costly and complex. WES is more affordable with a focus on exons, but overlooks regulatory variants.

RNA-Seq captures functional activity, but does not detect genomic DNA changes and is tissue-dependent.

2.4.5 Integration in Personalized Medicine

Combining WGS, WES, and RNA-Seq offers a powerful framework for personalized medicine. WGS/WES identifies genetic predispositions and mutations, while RNA-Seq reveals their functional impact. This multi-layered approach enhances diagnosis, risk assessment, treatment planning, and biomarker discovery—especially in cancer genomics, rare diseases, and pharmacogenomics.

2.5 EPIGENOMICS, PROTEOMICS, AND METABOLOMICS IN PERSONALIZATION

2.5.1. Epigenomics- Beyond the DNA Sequence

Epigenomics explores chemical modifications to DNA and histones that regulate gene expression without altering the DNA sequence. These modifications include DNA methylation, histone acetylation, and chromatin remodelling, which can switch genes on or off in response to developmental cues or environmental exposures. In personalized medicine, epigenomic profiling helps understand individual differences in disease susceptibility, treatment response, and aging. For example, aberrant methylation patterns are linked to cancers, neurodegeneration, and autoimmune diseases. Epigenetic markers can serve as diagnostic tools and therapeutic targets, offering personalized strategies based on reversible modifications of gene regulation.

2.5.2 Proteomics- The Dynamic Protein Landscape

Proteomics involves the large-scale study of proteins—the functional molecules that execute genetic instructions. Unlike genomics, which is static, the proteome is highly dynamic and influenced by time, tissue type, disease state, and external factors. Proteomics provides insights into protein expression levels, post-translational modifications, and protein–protein interactions. In personalized medicine, proteomic profiling enables the identification of disease-specific biomarkers and therapeutic targets. It is particularly valuable in oncology, where protein signatures guide diagnose is, prognosis, and drug selection. Proteomics also supports real-time monitoring of treatment efficacy and toxicity.

2.5.3 Metabolomics- Capturing the Chemical Fingerprint

Metabolomics is the comprehensive analysis of metabolites—small molecules involved in cellular processes such as energy production, signalling, and detoxification. The metabolome reflects both genetic and environmental influences, providing a real-time snapshot of an individual's physiological and pathological state. In personalized medicine, metabolomic data can detect early disease markers, predict treatment response, and guide dietary or lifestyle interventions. For instance, specific metabolic profiles are used in diagnosing inborn errors of metabolism or assessing response to cancer therapies. Metabolomics bridges the gap between genotype and phenotype, offering a powerful tool for individualized care.

2.5.4 Integrated Omics for Precision Health

While each omics field offers unique insights, their integration—commonly referred to as multi-omics—provides a holistic understanding of human biology. Combining genomic, epigenomic, proteomic, and metabolomic data enhances disease modelling, improves biomarker discovery, and supports truly personalized interventions. Systems biology approaches and AI-driven analytics are being used to synthesize this complex data, allowing clinicians to tailor prevention, diagnosis, and treatment to the unique molecular makeup of each patient (Table-2).

Table: 2 Concise Summary of Epigenomics, Proteomics, and Metabolomics in Personalized Medicine

S. No.	Field	Description	Role in Personalized Medicine	Examples/ Applications
1	Epigenomics Beyond the DNA Sequence	Studies chemical modifications (e.g., DNA methylation, histone acetylation) that regulate gene expression without changing DNA sequence	Helps understand individual variation in disease susceptibility, aging, and therapy response	Methylation markers for cancer, neurodegeneration; reversible gene regulation as therapeutic targets
2	Proteomics The Dynamic Protein Landscape	Analyses large-scale protein expression, modifications, and interactions	Identifies disease-specific biomarkers, drug targets; enables dynamic monitoring of therapy	Protein signatures in cancer for diagnosis and drug selection; real-time treatment efficacy
3	Metabolomics Capturing the Chemical Fingerprint	Profiles small molecule metabolites reflecting cellular activity and environment	Detects early disease markers; guides nutritional and lifestyle interventions; predicts drug response	Metabolic profiling for cancer therapy, inborn errors of metabolism diagnosis
4	Integrated Omics for Precision Health	Combines genomic, epigenomic, proteomic, and metabolomic data	Provides a systems-level understanding; supports highly tailored diagnosis, prevention, and treatment	AI-driven multi-omics analysis for individualized care in complex diseases

3 Chapter
BIOMARKERS AND DIAGNOSTICS

3.0 INTRODUCTION: AN OVERVIEW

Biomarkers are measurable biological indicators that reflect physiological or pathological processes, or responses to therapeutic interventions. In the context of personalized medicine, biomarkers serve as critical tools for early detection, diagnosis, prognosis, treatment selection, and disease monitoring. They can take many forms, including genetic variants, proteins, metabolites, RNA transcripts, epigenetic marks, or imaging signals. The integration of biomarkers into clinical diagnostics enables a shift from a one-size-fits-all approach to a more individualized model of care, where decisions are guided by a patient's unique molecular profile. For example, the presence of HER2 overexpression in breast cancer guides the use of trastuzumab, while EGFR mutations in lung cancer predict response to tyrosine kinase inhibitors. Advances in high-throughput technologies such as next-generation sequencing, proteomics, and metabolomics have exponentially increased the number and types of biomarkers available. Moreover, multi-modal biomarker panels, incorporating data from different biological layers, offer enhanced accuracy in complex disease assessment. Companion diagnostics—tests developed alongside targeted therapies—are now essential components of personalized treatment pathways. The use of biomarkers not only improves diagnostic precision but also reduces trial-and-error prescribing, minimizes adverse effects, and enhances therapeutic outcomes. As research continues to uncover novel biomarkers, their role in transforming healthcare into a more predictive, preventive, and precise system becomes increasingly central (Fig. 1).

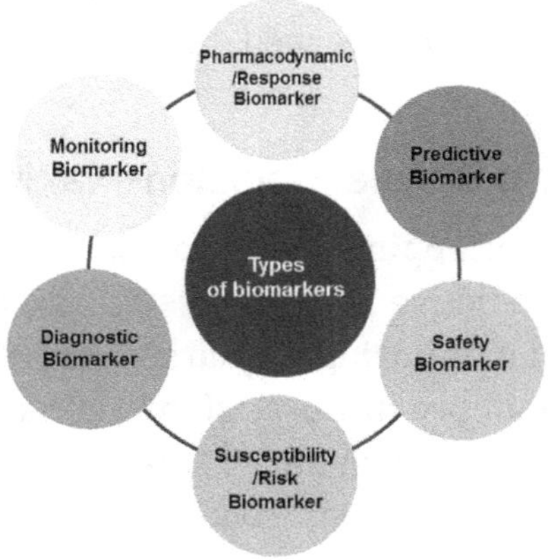

Fig. 1 Types and Relevance of Biomarkers

3.1 ROLE OF BIOMARKERS IN DIAGNOSIS, PROGNOSIS, AND MONITORING

3.1.1 Biomarkers in Diagnosis

Diagnostic biomarkers help identify the presence or absence of a disease, often before symptoms appear. They enable early and accurate detection, facilitating timely intervention and improving outcomes. For example, prostate-specific antigen (PSA) is used for prostate cancer screening, while elevated troponin levels indicate myocardial infarction. In infectious diseases, molecular biomarkers such as viral RNA (e.g., SARS-CoV-2) are critical for confirming infection. Diagnostic biomarkers are increasingly integrated with imaging and clinical data to enhance specificity and sensitivity.

3.1.2 Biomarkers in Prognosis

Prognostic biomarkers provide information about the likely course, severity, or outcome of a disease, independent of treatment. They help stratify patients based on risk, guiding decisions on surveillance intensity or aggressive therapy. For instance, BRCA1/BRCA2 mutations not only indicate cancer risk but also suggest a more aggressive tumor phenotype. Similarly, high levels of B-type natriuretic peptide (BNP) in heart failure patients are associated with poorer prognosis. Prognostic biomarkers are essential in identifying high-risk individuals who may benefit from preventive strategies.

3.1.3 Biomarkers in Monitoring Disease Progression and Treatment Response

Monitoring biomarkers are used to track disease progression, detect relapse, and assess therapeutic response over time. They provide real-time feedback on the effectiveness of a given treatment and help guide dosage adjustments or therapy changes. For example, HbA1c is routinely used to monitor long-term glucose control in diabetes, and C-reactive protein (CRP) levels are used to evaluate inflammation in autoimmune diseases. In oncology, circulating tumour DNA (ctDNA) and tumour markers like CA-125 or CEA are tracked to monitor treatment response and recurrence.

3.1.4 Combined Utility in Clinical Decision-Making

Many biomarkers serve overlapping roles—for example, HER2 in breast cancer is both diagnostic and predictive of response to targeted therapy. Combining diagnostic, prognostic, and monitoring biomarkers enables a more holistic view of the patient's disease status, improving precision in clinical decision-making. These integrated approaches support personalized treatment plans, reduce unnecessary interventions, and optimize patient outcomes. Role of biomarkers in diagnosis, prognosis, and monitoring are summarised in Table-1.

Table:1 Biomarkers in Diagnosis, Prognosis, and Monitoring

S. No.	Biomarker Role	Function	Examples	Clinical Impact
1	Biomarkers in Diagnosis	Identify presence or absence of disease, often before symptoms arise	PSA (prostate cancer), Troponin (heart attack), SARS-CoV-2 RNA (COVID-19)	Enables early detection, timely intervention, and improved outcomes
2	Biomarkers in Prognosis	Predict disease course, severity, or outcome, independent of treatment	BRCA1/BRCA2 (cancer risk), BNP (heart failure)	Guides risk stratification, surveillance, and preventive strategies
3	Biomarkers in Monitoring	Track disease progression, detect relapse, and assess treatment response	HbA1c (diabetes), CRP (inflammation), ctDNA, CA-125, CEA (cancer)	Supports real-time therapy adjustment and disease management
4	Combined Utility	Biomarkers may serve multiple roles—diagnostic, prognostic, and monitoring	HER2 in breast cancer (diagnostic + predictive)	Enables holistic assessment, personalized treatment, and optimized care

3.2 COMPANION DIAGNOSTICS IN DRUG DEVELOPMENT

3.2.1 Companion Diagnostics: An Overview

Companion diagnostics (CDx) represent a cornerstone of personalized medicine, offering a bridge between molecular diagnostics and targeted therapy. These specialized laboratory tests are developed in parallel with specific therapeutic drugs to guide treatment decisions by identifying individuals who are most likely to benefit from, or potentially experience harm due to, a particular medical intervention. By stratifying patients based on their genetic, proteomic, or molecular profile, companion diagnostics help deliver the right drug to the right patient at the right time—transforming traditional trial-and-error medicine into a more precise, efficient, and patient-centred model of care.

The fundamental principle behind companion diagnostics lies in the concept of biological variability. Not all patients respond to a given therapy in the same way. Differences in genetic makeup, tumour biology, or protein expression can profoundly influence a drug's efficacy and toxicity profile. For example, a patient with a mutation in the EGFR gene may respond well to tyrosine kinase inhibitors in non-small cell lung cancer, whereas those lacking this mutation may derive little or no benefit. Similarly, patients with HER2-positive breast cancer are more likely to respond to trastuzumab, an anti-HER2 monoclonal antibody, while HER2-negative patients would not benefit and may be unnecessarily exposed to risks. Companion diagnostics make it possible to detect these key biomarkers before treatment is initiated, ensuring that medical decisions are evidence-based and individualized.

In the pharmaceutical and biotechnology industries, the development of CDx is closely integrated with the drug development pipeline. Drug developers and diagnostic companies often collaborate from the preclinical or early clinical trial phases to co-develop a therapeutic agent alongside its corresponding diagnostic tool. This coordinated approach allows for the enrichment of clinical trial populations by selecting individuals with the relevant biomarker profile, thereby increasing the likelihood of demonstrating drug efficacy and reducing trial costs and timelines. Regulatory agencies such as the U.S. Food and Drug Administration (FDA) and the European Medicines Agency (EMA) now often require companion diagnostics to be approved or cleared concurrently with their associated drugs, especially in oncology and targeted therapy fields. Regulatory oversight of companion diagnostics is stringent, given their influence on critical treatment decisions. These tests are generally classified as high-risk in vitro diagnostic devices and must demonstrate not only analytical validity (accurate and reliable test performance) but also clinical validity (accurate association with therapeutic response) and clinical utility (demonstrated improvement in patient outcomes). The FDA has issued specific guidelines on co-development and approval processes for CDx, emphasizing the need for robust clinical evidence, transparent labelling, and well-defined intended use. The clinical applications of companion diagnostics are most prominent in oncology, where tumour heterogeneity and mutation-driven therapies dominate treatment paradigms. Beyond the examples of HER2, EGFR, and BRAF, CDx are also used to guide immunotherapy decisions—such as assessing PD-L1 expression to determine eligibility for immune checkpoint inhibitors like pembrolizumab or nivolumab. These diagnostics are also gaining traction in other areas, including cardiology (e.g., CYP2C19 genotyping for antiplatelet therapy), infectious diseases (e.g., HIV tropism assays), and rare genetic disorders, where precision medicine can be life-saving. The benefits of companion diagnostics are multifaceted. They enable a more rational use of medicines by reducing exposure to ineffective or harmful treatments. They improve therapeutic efficacy by identifying responsive subpopulations. They enhance patient safety and satisfaction through reduced side effects and better clinical outcomes. From an economic perspective, CDx can reduce healthcare costs by minimizing unnecessary treatments and hospitalizations. For drug developers, CDx increases the probability of regulatory approval by optimizing trial design and demonstrating efficacy in a targeted cohort. However, despite their advantages, companion diagnostics face significant challenges. The co-development process can be complex and resource-intensive, requiring close coordination between drug and diagnostic developers. The regulatory landscape is still evolving, with differing standards across countries. Many companion diagnostics are single-analyte tests tied to a single therapy, limiting their flexibility in multi-drug decision contexts. Furthermore, disparities in access to molecular testing, especially in low- and middle-income countries, can widen global health inequities if CDx-guided therapies are not made universally accessible.

Looking ahead, the future of companion diagnostics is rapidly evolving with the integration of next-generation sequencing (NGS), liquid biopsy technologies, and artificial intelligence-driven analytics. Multi-gene panels and pan-cancer assays are replacing single-biomarker tests, allowing for more comprehensive and cost-effective profiling. Liquid biopsies, which detect circulating tumor DNA or exosomes from blood samples, offer a minimally invasive alternative for real-time monitoring and companion testing. AI and machine learning are enhancing data interpretation and predictive accuracy, bringing CDx into the realm of real-time clinical decision support. Companion diagnostics are essential enablers of personalized medicine. They redefine the way we diagnose, treat, and monitor disease by embedding molecular precision into every clinical decision. As technology advances and global access improves, companion diagnostics will continue to drive the evolution of safer, smarter, and more personalized healthcare.

3.2.2 Role in Personalized Medicine

Companion diagnostics (CDx) are indispensable tools in personalized medicine, offering a targeted approach that tailors treatment decisions to the unique molecular characteristics of each individual. By identifying specific biomarkers, such as gene mutations, protein overexpression, or enzymatic activity, CDx help clinicians determine which patients are most likely to benefit from a particular therapeutic intervention. This biomarker-guided selection ensures that the right drug is administered to the right patient at the right dose and time, fundamentally transforming the traditional "one-size-fits-all" model of healthcare. The primary strength of companion diagnostics lies in their ability to enhance therapeutic efficacy. By matching patients with treatments known to work for their particular molecular profiles, CDx eliminate much of the uncertainty and trial-and-error associated with conventional prescribing. For example, drugs like trastuzumab are only effective in breast cancer patients with HER2 overexpression; without HER2 testing, these treatments might be administered ineffectively, delaying appropriate care and exposing patients to unnecessary toxicity. Similarly, CDx for EGFR mutations in non-small cell lung cancer guide the use of tyrosine kinase inhibitors, improving survival outcomes and quality of life. Beyond improving treatment outcomes, companion diagnostics significantly reduce the risk of adverse drug reactions. Many drugs interact differently in patients based on genetic factors such as polymorphisms in metabolizing enzymes. CDx can identify individuals at risk for severe side effects, allowing clinicians to modify treatment plans, reduce dosages, or choose alternative therapies. This pre-emptive personalization minimizes harm and improves safety profiles.

From an economic standpoint, CDx contribute to cost-effective healthcare delivery. By directing expensive therapies only to those most likely to benefit, they reduce spending on ineffective treatments and decrease the costs associated with managing complications from inappropriate drug use. Payers, providers, and health systems all benefit from the resource optimization and value-based care that CDx enables. Companion diagnostics also promote patient empowerment and engagement. Patients armed with knowledge about their biomarker status can make informed choices about their treatment options, aligning medical decisions with their preferences, values, and lifestyle considerations. This shared decision-making leads to better adherence, satisfaction, and overall clinical outcomes. As the field of personalized medicine expands, the role of CDx continues to grow—extending beyond oncology into cardiology, psychiatry, infectious diseases, and autoimmune conditions. With advances in technologies such as next-generation sequencing, liquid biopsy, and multiplex assays, companion diagnostics are becoming more accessible, comprehensive, and integral to clinical decision-making. In this evolving landscape, CDx are not merely supporting tools but cornerstones of precision medicine—ushering in a new era of safe, effective, and individualized healthcare.

3.2.3 Integration into Drug Development Pipeline

The integration of companion diagnostics (CDx) into the drug development pipeline has become a strategic and scientific imperative in the era of precision medicine. Increasingly, pharmaceutical companies recognize the value of incorporating CDx early in the drug discovery process to identify patient subgroups most likely to respond to investigational therapies. This approach not only increases the probability of clinical success but also aligns with the growing regulatory emphasis on biomarker-driven treatment strategies. Co-development of drugs and diagnostics has evolved into a parallel, collaborative model where therapeutic development and biomarker identification occur simultaneously. Rather than treating diagnostics as afterthoughts, drug developers now partner with diagnostic companies from the outset, selecting or discovering biomarkers during preclinical studies, then validating their predictive power in clinical trials. This integration allows early stratification of trial participants, focusing enrolment on biomarker-positive individuals, which enhances signal detection, reduces trial size, shortens timelines, and lowers costs. In regulatory terms, agencies like the U.S. Food and Drug Administration (FDA) and the European Medicines Agency (EMA) now often require co-approval of both the therapeutic product and its associated CDx, especially when the diagnostic is critical to ensuring the drug's safety or efficacy. The FDA's framework for In Vitro Companion Diagnostic Devices mandates that such diagnostics be approved or cleared concurrently with the therapeutic product if the test is essential for the drug's intended use. This regulatory co-dependence ensures that clinical implementation of the drug is contingent on the availability of a validated and approved diagnostic test. The integration of CDx into the pipeline also improves trial design efficiency. Biomarker-enriched trials—those enrolling only biomarker-positive patients—yield more definitive efficacy signals and reduce the risk of negative results due to heterogeneity in patient response. Adaptive trial designs, enabled by real-time biomarker data, further refine dosing and eligibility criteria mid-trial, improving agility and precision. Beyond the trial phase, CDx influence post-market surveillance and lifecycle management. Real-world data collected through CDx usage can provide insights into long-term drug performance, resistance mechanisms, or new indications, informing post-marketing commitments and label expansions. Moreover, this integration fosters a more collaborative ecosystem between drug manufacturers, diagnostic firms, regulators, and clinicians. It demands shared data systems, coordinated timelines, and mutual alignment of scientific and commercial goals. Challenges such as assay standardization, analytical validation, and intellectual property management must be addressed collaboratively to ensure success. In sum, the co-development and regulatory integration of companion diagnostics within the drug development pipeline represent a paradigm shift in how medicines are discovered, evaluated, and delivered. This integrated model not only supports regulatory compliance but also accelerates innovation, enhances therapeutic precision, and ensures that new drugs reach the right patients—faster, safer, and more effectively.

3.2.4 Regulatory Consideration

Regulatory considerations play a pivotal role in the development, approval, and clinical implementation of companion diagnostics (CDx), which are classified as high-risk medical devices due to their direct impact on patient care and treatment decisions. Given their function in determining eligibility for targeted therapies, CDx must meet stringent regulatory requirements to ensure their safety, reliability, and effectiveness. Regulatory agencies worldwide—such as the U.S. Food and Drug Administration (FDA), the European Medicines Agency (EMA), and Japan's Pharmaceuticals and Medical Devices Agency (PMDA)—treat CDx as essential tools for risk stratification, thereby necessitating thorough scrutiny during approval.

In the United States, the FDA requires companion diagnostics to be reviewed through the Premarket Approval (PMA) pathway, the most rigorous evaluation route for medical devices. This pathway demands comprehensive evidence for analytical validity (i.e., the test accurately and reliably measures the intended biomarker), clinical validity (i.e., the biomarker is meaningfully associated with a clinical outcome or drug response), and clinical utility (i.e., the test result improves clinical decision-making or patient outcomes). A CDx must be approved or cleared before the corresponding therapeutic can be prescribed to patients with the targeted biomarker. This co-approval ensures that the drug is only used in populations where it is proven to be safe and effective. In the European Union, CDx are regulated under the In Vitro Diagnostic Regulation (IVDR), which came into full effect in 2022. The IVDR imposes stricter standards compared to its predecessor (IVDD), reclassifying CDx as Class C devices—reflecting their medium-to-high risk level. Under this regulation, CDx manufacturers must undergo notified body assessment and provide evidence for clinical benefit, in consultation with relevant medicinal product authorities. This requirement ensures a harmonized approach between the drug and diagnostic approval processes, similar to the FDA's coordinated model.

Japan's PMDA has also established a co-review system, requiring simultaneous evaluation of both the drug and the associated diagnostic. Like other regulators, the PMDA emphasizes the need for population-specific validation, particularly important in ethnically diverse or genetically distinct populations. Global regulatory convergence is improving through initiatives such as the International Medical Device Regulators Forum (IMDRF) and International Council for Harmonisation (ICH), which seek to align standards for CDx development and approval. However, regional differences in evidentiary thresholds, clinical trial design, and biomarker prevalence continue to pose challenges for multinational CDx deployment. Additionally, regulators are increasingly accommodating emerging technologies, such as next-generation sequencing (NGS)-based CDx and liquid biopsies. These platforms pose unique challenges, including the need for standardization of complex data outputs and continuous validation across evolving drug targets. Regulators also consider labelling and post-market surveillance critical. CDx must include clear instructions for use, defined patient populations, and interpretative criteria. Post-market obligations may include performance monitoring, adverse event reporting, and periodic re-evaluation in the light of new evidence. Regulatory frameworks for companion diagnostics are designed to ensure that only well-validated, clinically actionable tests reach patients. By setting high standards for clinical and analytical performance, these regulations safeguard patient safety, uphold therapeutic efficacy, and support the foundational goals of personalized medicine. Regulatory foresight and harmonization will be crucial as CDx technologies evolve and become central to future healthcare models.

3.2.5 Examples of Approved Companion Diagnostics

- **HER2 Testing – For Trastuzumab (Herceptin) in HER2-Positive Breast Cancer:** HER2 (human epidermal growth factor receptor 2) is a transmembrane receptor tyrosine kinase overexpressed in approximately 15–20% of breast cancers. HER2 amplification is associated with aggressive tumour behaviour and poor prognosis. HER2 testing (via IHC or FISH) identifies patients who may benefit from trastuzumab, a monoclonal antibody that targets the HER2 receptor. The drug inhibits downstream signalling, suppresses tumour growth, and enhances immune-mediated cytotoxicity. Only HER2-positive patients respond effectively, making this test essential for therapeutic selection. HER2 testing has become a model for biomarker-driven oncology and remains integral to breast cancer management. Without this test, patients may undergo ineffective treatment or miss a life-saving therapy.
- **EGFR Mutation Testing – For Use of EGFR Inhibitors in Non-Small Cell Lung Cancer:** EGFR (epidermal growth factor receptor) mutations, particularly in exons 19 and 21, are common in non-small cell lung cancer (NSCLC), especially among non-smokers and Asian populations. EGFR mutation testing (typically via PCR or NGS) is used to determine eligibility for EGFR tyrosine kinase inhibitors (TKIs) such as erlotinib, gefitinib, or osimertinib. These drugs block aberrant EGFR signalling, which drives uncontrolled cell proliferation in mutated tumours. Patients with wild-type EGFR do not benefit and may experience unnecessary toxicity if treated. This test has revolutionized lung cancer treatment by enabling targeted, genotype-specific therapies that improve progression-free survival and quality of life.
- **BRAF V600E Mutation Testing – To Guide Vemurafenib Therapy in Melanoma:** The BRAF V600E mutation results in a constitutively active serine/threonine kinase, found in about 50% of cutaneous melanomas. BRAF testing identifies patients eligible for treatment with BRAF inhibitors like vemurafenib, which selectively block the mutant protein's signalling, halting cell proliferation. Testing is performed using PCR, Sanger sequencing, or NGS platforms. Only patients with the V600E mutation benefit significantly from vemurafenib; others are likely to suffer side effects without therapeutic benefit. This biomarker-guided approach exemplifies how CDx can transform melanoma, a once notoriously treatment-resistant cancer, into a condition amenable to effective targeted therapy.
- **PD-L1 Expression Assays – To Determine Eligibility for Immunotherapies Like Pembrolizumab:** Programmed death-ligand 1 (PD-L1) expression on tumour or immune cells can suppress T-cell-mediated anti-tumour

responses. PD-L1 expression assays—performed via immunohistochemistry (IHC)—are used to assess suitability for immune checkpoint inhibitors such as pembrolizumab. High PD-L1 levels often correlate with better response rates to PD-1/PD-L1 inhibitors in cancers like NSCLC, melanoma, and bladder cancer. However, PD-L1 is an imperfect biomarker with dynamic expression and variable predictive power. Despite this, PD-L1 testing helps prioritize patients likely to benefit from expensive and potentially toxic immunotherapies, ensuring resource-efficient, targeted intervention.

These examples illustrate how companion diagnostics guide drug use in oncology, which remains the leading field for CDx implementation.

3.2.6 Benefits and Impact on Drug Development

Companion diagnostics (CDx) have transformed the traditional model of drug development by introducing a precision-based approach that aligns drug efficacy with individual patient biology. One of their most profound benefits lies in the enrichment of clinical trial populations. By selecting only those individuals who express the relevant biomarker or genetic profile, CDx increases the likelihood of demonstrating significant therapeutic efficacy, thereby reducing trial size, duration, and cost. This biomarker-driven patient stratification leads to cleaner data sets, more robust statistical outcomes, and greater confidence in the treatment's clinical value. As a result, pharmaceutical companies experience a higher success rate in clinical trials, mitigating the historically high risk and expense associated with late-stage drug development failures. Moreover, the integration of CDx into drug trials facilitates faster regulatory approval. Regulatory agencies such as the FDA and EMA increasingly endorse co-development models where the diagnostic and therapeutic are reviewed in tandem. This parallel approval pathway ensures that the therapy reaches the appropriate patient population as soon as it becomes available, streamlining market entry. Beyond approval, CDx significantly enhances post-market performance by reducing the rate of adverse drug reactions, which are a major cause of patient morbidity, litigation, and drug withdrawals. Targeted treatment also improves real-world efficacy, supporting better health outcomes and increased cost-effectiveness across healthcare systems. For clinicians and patients, the availability of a validated CDx boosts confidence in treatment decisions. When a diagnostic test confirms that a patient is a likely responder, both the prescriber and patient are more assured of the therapy's benefit, encouraging adherence and shared decision-making. From a business perspective, CDx helps pharmaceutical companies optimize their return on investment by reducing the need for broad-spectrum marketing and enabling premium pricing for niche, high-value therapeutics. In essence, companion diagnostics bridge the gap between drug discovery and personalized care, making drug development more strategic, economical, and patient-centred than ever before.

3.2.7 Challenges and Limitations

While companion diagnostics (CDx) have emerged as powerful tools in the era of personalized medicine, their development and implementation are accompanied by significant challenges. One of the foremost hurdles is the high cost and extended timeline required for co-development. Designing, validating, and clinically integrating a diagnostic test alongside a therapeutic agent demands substantial investment in infrastructure, cross-disciplinary collaboration, and regulatory compliance. This dual-path development process is not only resource-intensive but also complex, often leading to delays in bringing both the drug and diagnostic to market. Furthermore, regulatory pathways for CDx are stringent; agencies such as the FDA classify them as high-risk medical devices, requiring rigorous demonstration of analytical validity, clinical validity, and clinical utility—standards that can be difficult to meet, especially when biomarker prevalence is low or heterogeneous. Another limitation stems from the narrow focus of many existing CDx, which are typically developed for a single drug or a limited class of therapies. This "one-drug-one-test" model restricts clinical flexibility and may require patients to undergo multiple tests to determine treatment options, increasing both burden and cost. Additionally, many CDx have been developed and validated predominantly in populations of European descent, raising serious concerns about their generalizability and efficacy in other ethnic or genetically diverse groups. The lack of inclusivity in clinical validation can lead to disparities in access to personalized therapies and inaccurate test results in underrepresented populations. Technical challenges also exist in terms of platform compatibility and reproducibility. CDx must function reliably across different laboratory settings, instrumentation, and biospecimen conditions, which is not always guaranteed. Lack of standardization in assay procedures and result interpretation further complicates their clinical integration. Moreover, as the number of available targeted therapies grows, there is increasing demand for multiplexed or comprehensive testing solutions rather than fragmented, single-marker diagnostics. Without broader, adaptable diagnostic platforms, healthcare providers face workflow inefficiencies and decision-making bottlenecks. Finally, market and reimbursement barriers can inhibit the widespread adoption of CDx. Payers may hesitate to cover expensive tests, especially when clinical utility has not been clearly demonstrated or quantified. In many regions, regulatory and reimbursement frameworks have not yet evolved to accommodate the fast pace of innovation in personalized medicine, creating uncertainty for developers and clinicians alike. Addressing these multifaceted limitations will be critical for the sustainable and equitable integration of CDx into modern healthcare.

3.2.8 Future Directions

The future of companion diagnostics (CDx) is poised to evolve beyond the traditional one-drug-one-test paradigm, moving toward more comprehensive, efficient, and inclusive approaches. One of the most promising advancements lies in the development of multi-analyte assays that assess several biomarkers simultaneously. These panels enable clinicians to determine eligibility for multiple targeted therapies from a single test, streamlining diagnosis and expanding treatment options. Powered by next-generation sequencing (NGS), these multiplex assays can analyse genetic mutations, expression levels, copy number variations, and even epigenetic markers in one integrated platform. This not only enhances the efficiency of clinical decision-making but also reduces turnaround time and cost, making personalized medicine more practical and scalable.

Liquid biopsies represent another transformative innovation. By analysing circulating tumour DNA (ctDNA), exosomes, or other biomolecules in blood or other bodily fluids, liquid biopsies offer a non-invasive alternative to traditional tissue sampling. This approach is especially valuable in cases where tumours are inaccessible or tissue biopsies pose a risk. Liquid biopsies can be used for real-time monitoring of treatment response, early detection of resistance mutations, and longitudinal disease tracking—enabling dynamic treatment adjustments and truly adaptive care strategies. As technologies improve, their sensitivity and specificity are expected to rival those of tissue-based diagnostics, further solidifying their role in the CDx ecosystem. From a regulatory and clinical integration perspective, harmonization of global regulatory frameworks is a pressing need. Differences in approval requirements across regions (e.g., FDA in the U.S., EMA in Europe, PMDA in Japan) currently create fragmentation and delays in CDx access. Establishing unified, transparent, and collaborative regulatory pathways would accelerate global adoption, reduce duplication of effort, and foster innovation. Additionally, alignment between drug and diagnostic approval processes is critical for ensuring simultaneous availability of both components, especially in international markets. Equally important is the urgent need for inclusivity in CDx development. Historically, most biomarker studies have been conducted in populations of European ancestry, limiting the applicability of these diagnostics in genetically diverse groups. Future CDx must be validated across broad demographic and ethnic populations to ensure equitable access to precision medicine. This includes adapting trial recruitment strategies, enhancing representation in genetic databases, and building culturally competent clinical infrastructures. Addressing these disparities is not only a scientific necessity but also a moral imperative. As companion diagnostics become more central to drug development and healthcare delivery, integration with digital technologies and AI will also gain traction. Machine learning algorithms can analyse vast multi-omic datasets to identify novel biomarker combinations, predict treatment response, and personalize therapy selection with increasing accuracy. In clinical settings, AI-enhanced diagnostic platforms may assist in interpreting complex test results and guiding physicians in evidence-based treatment decisions. In sum, the next generation of companion diagnostics will be defined by technological convergence, regulatory innovation, and global inclusivity. By enabling broader biomarker profiling, minimizing invasiveness, and tailoring therapies with unprecedented precision, these advancements promise to make personalized medicine a truly accessible and global reality.

3.3 LIQUID BIOPSIES AND NON-INVASIVE TESTING

3.3.1 Liquid Biopsies: An Overview

Liquid biopsies represent a groundbreaking advancement in modern diagnostics, offering a minimally invasive means of assessing molecular changes within the body by analysing circulating biomarkers present in various biofluids—most commonly blood, but also urine, saliva, and cerebrospinal fluid. These biomarkers include circulating tumour DNA (ctDNA), circulating tumour cells (CTCs), cell-free RNA, and extracellular vesicles like exosomes, each providing a snapshot of ongoing physiological and pathological processes, particularly in the context of cancer. Unlike traditional tissue biopsies, which are often invasive, painful, and limited to a single anatomical site and time point, liquid biopsies can be performed repeatedly with minimal risk, allowing for real-time monitoring of disease progression, therapeutic response, and emergence of resistance mutations. The non-invasive nature of liquid biopsies makes them exceptionally valuable in clinical practice. They can be used in patients who are not candidates for surgery, those with inaccessible tumours, or those requiring serial monitoring. By capturing the heterogeneity of tumours—often missed by localized tissue sampling—liquid biopsies offer a more comprehensive view of cancer evolution. For instance, ctDNA analysis can identify genetic mutations and chromosomal alterations associated with specific cancers, guiding the selection of targeted therapies. CTCs provide phenotypic data and can even be cultured for drug sensitivity testing, offering functional insights into the tumour's behaviour. Exosomes, containing DNA, RNA, and proteins, reflect the molecular signature of parent cells, further enriching diagnostic capabilities (Fig. 2).

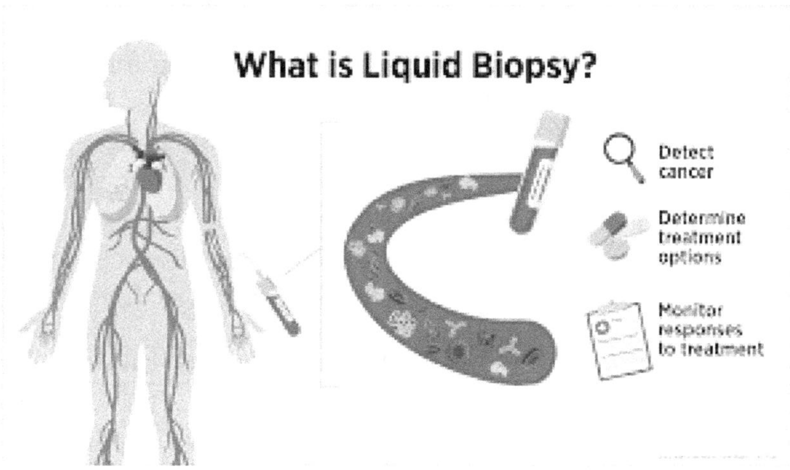

Fig. 2 Liquid biopsy

Clinically, liquid biopsies are transforming cancer care across the continuum—from early detection and prognosis to treatment selection and post-treatment surveillance. They have demonstrated particular utility in tracking minimal residual disease (MRD) and detecting early recurrence before clinical or radiographic signs emerge. In diseases like non-small cell lung cancer and colorectal cancer, liquid biopsy-guided mutation profiling informs decisions on tyrosine kinase inhibitors or anti-EGFR therapies. Moreover, the ability to monitor resistance mechanisms through serial blood draws allows for timely adjustments in therapy, potentially improving patient outcomes and prolonging survival. Technological advances such as digital PCR and next-generation sequencing (NGS) have significantly enhanced the sensitivity and specificity of liquid biopsy platforms. These innovations enable detection of even low-frequency mutations in ctDNA, making the test suitable not just for advanced-stage malignancies but also for early detection efforts. Several liquid biopsy-based companion diagnostics, like Guardant360 CDx and Foundation One Liquid CDx, are now FDA-approved, validating their clinical relevance and paving the way for broader adoption. Despite their promise, challenges remain. Liquid biopsies may not detect all mutations present in a tumour due to low shedding rates or technical limitations in early-stage disease. Standardization of assays, clinical interpretation frameworks, and integration into clinical workflows are still evolving. Nevertheless, the field is rapidly advancing, with ongoing research aimed at expanding the applications of liquid biopsy to non-oncological diseases such as organ rejection, prenatal testing, and neurodegenerative disorders. Liquid biopsies exemplify the convergence of molecular biology, genomics, and patient-centred innovation. By offering a safer, faster, and more dynamic approach to disease characterization and monitoring, they are reshaping the landscape of precision medicine. As technologies mature and evidence mounts, liquid biopsies are poised to become a cornerstone of diagnostic and therapeutic decision-making in routine clinical care.

3.3.2 Biomarkers Analysed

- **Circulating Tumour DNA (ctDNA):** Small fragments of DNA shed by cancer cells into the bloodstream, used to detect mutations, resistance markers, and tumour burden.
- **Circulating Tumour DNA (ctDNA):** Circulating tumour DNA (ctDNA) refers to small fragments of DNA released into the bloodstream by apoptotic or necrotic tumour cells. ctDNA carries tumour-specific genetic and epigenetic alterations, including point mutations, copy number variations, rearrangements, and methylation patterns. Because it mirrors the molecular profile of the tumour, ctDNA is a powerful tool for real-time monitoring of cancer dynamics. Its utility spans early detection, assessing tumour burden, predicting prognosis, identifying actionable mutations for targeted therapy, and detecting resistance mutations that emerge during treatment. For example, EGFR T790M mutation detection in lung cancer using ctDNA can inform second-line therapy decisions without requiring a repeat biopsy. ctDNA analysis is minimally invasive, allowing frequent sampling to track disease evolution or minimal residual disease (MRD). Advanced platforms like digital PCR and next-generation sequencing (NGS) have significantly improved ctDNA detection sensitivity and specificity. However, its reliability depends on tumour type and burden, as some cancers shed less DNA into the circulation. Despite this limitation, ctDNA continues to gain ground as a surrogate for tissue biopsy in both clinical trials and routine oncology practice.
- **Circulating Tumour Cells (CTCs):** Circulating tumour cells (CTCs) are intact, viable cancer cells that detach from a primary or metastatic tumour and enter the bloodstream. Though rare—often just one CTC per billion blood cells—these cells provide rich phenotypic and genotypic information about the tumour. CTCs can be isolated and analysed to assess epithelial-to-mesenchymal transition (EMT), mutations, gene expression patterns, and protein markers, offering insights into metastatic potential and resistance mechanisms. Unlike ctDNA, which only provides nucleic acid fragments, CTCs can reveal cellular behaviours, morphological features, and the tumour's functional state. This makes them valuable for both prognostic assessments and guiding treatment strategies, especially in breast, prostate, and colorectal cancers. Furthermore, CTCs may be cultured ex vivo to test drug sensitivity, enabling truly personalized therapy approaches. Technologies like the Cell Search® system—FDA-approved for some cancers—have standardized CTC detection, but challenges remain due to their low abundance and heterogeneity. Nonetheless, CTCs represent

a vital component of liquid biopsy, bridging the gap between molecular biology and whole-cell analysis in cancer management.

- **Exosomes and microRNAs (miRNAs):** Exosomes are nanoscale extracellular vesicles (30–150 nm in size) secreted by nearly all cell types, including tumour cells. They carry diverse molecular cargo such as DNA, RNA (including microRNAs), proteins, and lipids, which reflect the physiological or pathological state of their cell of origin. microRNAs (miRNAs), which are small non-coding RNAs regulating gene expression, are often enriched in exosomes and are particularly stable in circulation. Together, exosomes and miRNAs serve as key mediators of intercellular communication and play a role in promoting tumour progression, metastasis, and immune evasion. Their molecular content can be profiled to detect cancer-specific signatures, monitor treatment response, or predict recurrence. Due to their stability in body fluids and early release by tumours, exosome miRNAs are being explored for use in early cancer detection. For instance, specific miRNA panels have been associated with lung, pancreatic, and ovarian cancers. Isolation and analysis of exosomes require sophisticated methods like ultracentrifugation and immunocapture, but ongoing innovations are improving clinical applicability. As research advances, exosomes and miRNAs may unlock new frontiers in cancer diagnostics, prognostics, and even therapeutic delivery.

3.3.3 Applications in Personalized Medicine:

- **Early Detection:** Liquid biopsies offer a transformative approach to early cancer detection by identifying tumour-specific alterations in circulating biomarkers—often before clinical symptoms become apparent. This is particularly crucial for cancers that are asymptomatic in early stages, such as pancreatic, ovarian, or lung cancers, where early diagnosis can significantly improve survival outcomes. Circulating tumour DNA (ctDNA), exosome miRNAs, and methylation patterns can serve as early biomarkers, reflecting the presence of malignancy at a molecular level. Unlike conventional imaging or serum protein markers, which may miss small or non-secretory tumours, liquid biopsies provide a molecular snapshot of tumour activity. Early detection via blood or urine sampling also facilitates screening in high-risk populations, potentially allowing for preventive interventions or curative treatments at an earlier stage. Commercial tests like Galleri and Cancer SEEK are already leveraging multi-analyte liquid biopsy strategies for pan-cancer screening. As technology advances, liquid biopsy is poised to redefine cancer screening paradigms with greater accuracy, accessibility, and patient compliance.

- **Real-Time Monitoring:** Liquid biopsies enable dynamic, real-time tracking of tumour burden and treatment response throughout the course of therapy. By sampling ctDNA or CTCs at multiple time points, clinicians can observe changes in mutation frequencies, tumour load, or molecular signatures—providing insight into whether a therapy is effective or whether the tumour is evolving. This helps avoid prolonged use of ineffective treatments and allows for timely modification of therapeutic strategies. For example, a declining ctDNA level may indicate a favourable response, while stable or rising levels could signal resistance or progression. Moreover, liquid biopsies can detect minimal residual disease (MRD)—small amounts of cancer that remain after treatment and could lead to relapse. MRD detection is increasingly used to guide decisions on adjuvant therapy and patient surveillance, particularly in haematological malignancies and colorectal cancer. The ability to monitor disease in near real time makes liquid biopsy a key component of adaptive treatment planning and personalized oncology.
- **Resistance Mutation Identification:** One of the most impactful applications of liquid biopsy is its ability to detect emerging resistance mutations, which often develop under selective pressure from targeted therapies. For instance, in non-small cell lung cancer (NSCLC), the EGFR T790M mutation frequently arises during treatment with first-generation EGFR inhibitors, rendering them ineffective. Liquid biopsy allows for early and non-invasive detection of such mutations, enabling clinicians to switch to appropriate next-line therapies (e.g., osimertinib for T790M-positive tumours) without requiring a repeat tissue biopsy, which can be risky or infeasible. This real-time molecular surveillance helps stay ahead of tumour evolution, delaying or preventing clinical relapse. Moreover, in cases of polyclonal resistance or heterogeneous tumours, liquid biopsies may offer a more comprehensive mutation profile than a single-site tissue biopsy. Incorporating resistance profiling into treatment algorithms enhances precision and ensures the continuity of effective therapy.
- **Therapy Selection:** Liquid biopsy facilitates personalized therapy selection by identifying actionable genetic alterations or predictive biomarkers in a minimally invasive manner. This is particularly beneficial when traditional tissue biopsy is not feasible due to tumour location, patient comorbidities, or insufficient sample material. By analysing ctDNA or exosomal RNA, clinicians can detect driver mutations (e.g., EGFR, BRAF, ALK, KRAS), gene fusions, or alterations in tumour mutational burden (TMB) or microsatellite instability (MSI) that guide the use of targeted therapies or immunotherapies. For example, identifying ALK or ROS1 rearrangements

in lung cancer patients allows for the use of tyrosine kinase inhibitors tailored to those mutations. Importantly, therapy selection via liquid biopsy supports treatment personalization not just at baseline but continuously throughout disease progression. As the tumour evolves, repeat liquid biopsies can help reassess molecular status and inform new therapeutic paths. Thus, liquid biopsy bridges molecular diagnostics with therapeutic precision, enhancing treatment outcomes and patient safety.

3.3.4 Advantages Over Traditional Biopsies

- **Non-Invasive:** Liquid biopsies are significantly less invasive than traditional tissue biopsies, which often require surgical procedures, needle aspirations, or endoscopic interventions. By analysing circulating tumour DNA (ctDNA), circulating tumour cells (CTCs), or exosomal RNA in body fluids—most commonly blood—liquid biopsies eliminate the need for physically accessing the tumour site. This not only minimizes procedural risks such as bleeding, infection, and pain, but also improves patient compliance and comfort. For patients with inoperable tumours or fragile health conditions, this non-invasive approach offers a practical and safe alternative for molecular profiling. It is especially beneficial in paediatric, geriatric, and critically ill populations where invasive procedures may be contraindicated. Overall, the non-invasive nature of liquid biopsy enhances accessibility and broadens diagnostic reach across diverse patient groups.
- **Repeatable:** A key strength of liquid biopsy is its suitability for repeated sampling over the course of a patient's treatment. Unlike tissue biopsies, which are limited by anatomical, clinical, and ethical considerations, liquid biopsies can be performed frequently with minimal risk or discomfort. This enables longitudinal monitoring of tumour dynamics, allowing clinicians to track changes in mutational profiles, treatment response, and disease progression in real time. Serial testing is particularly useful for detecting the emergence of resistance mutations or minimal residual disease (MRD) after therapy, thereby guiding timely modifications in treatment. Repeatability also supports precision medicine by tailoring therapy based on evolving tumour biology, not just a single static snapshot. This dynamic monitoring facilitates adaptive treatment strategies that respond to the cancer's changing molecular landscape.
- **Faster Turnaround Time:** Liquid biopsy workflows typically offer faster processing and results compared to tissue biopsies, which require time-consuming steps such as surgical extraction, histological analysis, and molecular testing. In contrast, the isolation and analysis of ctDNA or exosome biomarkers from blood can be completed within a few days, and

sometimes even within 24–48 hours in urgent clinical situations. This speed is critical in oncology, where timely treatment decisions can significantly impact patient outcomes. For instance, rapid identification of actionable mutations allows prompt initiation of targeted therapy, avoiding delays that could lead to disease progression. Faster turnaround times also enhance patient throughput and reduce anxiety associated with long diagnostic waits. As analytical technologies continue to evolve, the efficiency and reliability of liquid biopsy testing are expected to improve even further.

- **Broad Representation:** Liquid biopsies may provide a more comprehensive picture of tumour heterogeneity than tissue biopsies obtained from a single site. Solid tumours often exhibit spatial and temporal heterogeneity, meaning different parts of the tumour or metastatic sites may harbour distinct genetic mutations. A tissue biopsy samples only a small, localized region and may miss relevant sub clonal mutations present elsewhere in the tumour or in metastases. In contrast, ctDNA and CTCs released into the bloodstream originate from various tumour regions, offering a pooled, systemic view of the tumour's genetic landscape. This broader molecular insight supports more informed therapeutic decisions and improves the likelihood of detecting resistance mechanisms or actionable targets. As a result, liquid biopsy enhances the accuracy of molecular diagnostics in complex, heterogeneous cancers.

3.3.5 Role in Companion Diagnostics

Liquid biopsies are playing an increasingly transformative role in the realm of companion diagnostics (CDx), offering a non-invasive yet highly informative method to match patients with the most appropriate targeted therapies. Traditionally, companion diagnostics relied on tissue biopsies to assess the presence of actionable biomarkers that predict response to specific drugs. However, the integration of liquid biopsy technologies—particularly the analysis of circulating tumour DNA (ctDNA)—has introduced a new dimension of accessibility, real-time monitoring, and comprehensive tumour profiling. These advancements allow clinicians to make timely, evidence-based therapeutic decisions, especially in cases where tissue samples are insufficient, inaccessible, or carry procedural risks. One of the most well-established examples of this integration is plasma-based EGFR mutation testing in non-small cell lung cancer (NSCLC). When tumour tissue is unavailable, liquid biopsy allows the detection of activating EGFR mutations, enabling the selection of patients eligible for tyrosine kinase inhibitors (TKIs) like erlotinib, gefitinib, or osimertinib. This is particularly valuable in monitoring the emergence of resistance mutations, such as T790M, which can guide a switch to second- or third-generation TKIs without the need for repeated tissue biopsies. Similarly, in metastatic colorectal cancer (mCRC), ctDNA analysis helps assess KRAS and NRAS mutation status, ensuring anti-EGFR therapies like cetuximab or panitumumab are given only to patients with RAS wild-type tumours. These insights are crucial because patients with RAS mutations derive no benefit from these treatments and may experience unnecessary toxicity. In breast cancer, liquid biopsies are used to monitor HER2 amplification and PIK3CA mutations to determine eligibility for HER2-targeted therapies or PI3K inhibitors like alpelisib. The non-invasive nature of liquid biopsies allows for serial testing throughout the disease course, supporting dynamic therapy adjustment based on evolving molecular profiles. This is particularly relevant in metastatic settings, where the biology of the tumour may shift over time due to treatment pressure or clonal evolution. Additionally, liquid biopsy-guided CDx are being explored in other malignancies, including prostate, pancreatic, and bladder cancers, broadening their applicability across oncology. By enabling biomarker-driven therapy selection, resistance monitoring, and response assessment, liquid biopsies enhance the flexibility, timeliness, and precision of companion diagnostics. Their integration into CDx platforms is also accelerating the pace of clinical trials, allowing for easier patient enrolment based on molecular eligibility and facilitating adaptive trial designs. As the technology matures, and regulatory frameworks evolve to accommodate liquid biopsy-based diagnostics, their role in guiding personalized cancer therapy will become even more central—bridging molecular diagnostics and targeted therapeutics with greater speed, safety, and scalability.

3.3.6 Emerging Technologies and Innovations

- **Ultra-Deep Sequencing and Digital PCR:** Ultra-deep sequencing and digital PCR (dPCR) are revolutionizing the analytical sensitivity of liquid biopsy assays by enabling the detection of extremely low-frequency variants in circulating tumour DNA (ctDNA). These technologies can identify rare mutations present at as low as 0.01% variant allele frequency, making them especially valuable in early cancer detection, minimal residual disease (MRD) assessment, and monitoring emerging resistance mutations. dPCR, with its high precision and absolute quantification capability, is ideal for tracking known mutations over time, such as EGFR T790M or KRAS G12C. On the other hand, ultra-deep next-generation sequencing (NGS) can capture a broader spectrum of alterations—including point mutations, insertions/deletions, and copy number changes—across hundreds of genes in a single assay. These approaches significantly reduce the risk of false negatives and allow for early therapeutic intervention, even when tumour burden is low. As a result, both technologies are becoming foundational tools for sensitive, reliable, and personalized companion diagnostics in oncology and beyond.

- **AI-Powered Interpretation Tools:** The complexity of liquid biopsy data, especially from multiplex NGS panels, demands robust interpretation frameworks that can accurately decode a wealth of genomic alterations in real time. Artificial intelligence (AI) and machine learning (ML) algorithms are being increasingly employed to enhance the diagnostic and predictive value of liquid biopsies. These tools are trained on large datasets comprising genomic profiles, treatment responses, and clinical outcomes, allowing them to identify actionable mutations, suggest optimal therapies, and even predict resistance patterns. AI-powered platforms can also distinguish between tumour-derived mutations and background noise, which is crucial for early detection or when analysing samples with low tumour content. Moreover, by integrating clinical variables, radiological data, and treatment histories, AI systems can generate more holistic and personalized interpretations. These innovations are streamlining decision-making for oncologists, reducing turnaround time, and improving patient outcomes through precise, data-driven companion diagnostic insights.
- **Multiplex Panels for Comprehensive Profiling:** Multiplex panels are emerging as powerful tools that allow simultaneous detection of multiple genetic alterations from a single blood sample, transforming how companion diagnostics are conducted. Instead of targeting just one or two mutations, these panels can assess dozens to hundreds of cancer-related genes—capturing point mutations, gene fusions, amplifications, and more. This comprehensive molecular profiling is particularly beneficial in heterogeneous tumours or advanced-stage cancers where resistance mechanisms are diverse and evolve rapidly. By delivering a panoramic view of the tumour's genomic landscape, multiplex panels empower clinicians to make informed, upfront decisions regarding therapy selection, including enrolment in biomarker-matched clinical trials. Additionally, these assays are increasingly being designed to monitor disease progression, predict relapse, and adjust treatment regimens dynamically over time. With advancements in sequencing chemistry, bioinformatics, and regulatory acceptance, multiplex panels are poised to become the standard in next-generation companion diagnostics—offering breadth, depth, and precision in a single, non-invasive test.

3.3.7 Current Limitations

- **Analytical Sensitivity:** One of the foremost challenges in liquid biopsy is its limited ability to detect low-frequency mutations, particularly in early-stage cancers or minimal residual disease. Since the amount of tumour-derived material such as ctDNA in circulation can be extremely low, especially when the tumour burden is small, conventional assays may fail to identify clinically relevant alterations. This can lead to false negatives and missed opportunities for early intervention. Enhancing sensitivity requires advanced platforms like ultra-deep sequencing or digital PCR, but these come with higher costs and technical demands. Furthermore, biological variability—such as uneven ctDNA shedding across tumour types—adds complexity. Thus, while liquid biopsy holds promise, improving detection thresholds remains critical for expanding its utility across disease stages.

- **Standardization:** A significant barrier to the widespread adoption of liquid biopsy is the absence of standardized protocols for sample collection, processing, assay methodology, and result interpretation. Different laboratories may use varying techniques for DNA extraction, sequencing platforms, and bioinformatics pipelines, resulting in inconsistent outcomes. Moreover, there is no universal agreement on cut-off values for mutation detection or clinical significance thresholds. This lack of harmonization undermines reproducibility, complicates cross-study comparisons, and erodes clinician confidence in test results. Establishing consensus-driven guidelines through collaboration among regulatory bodies, professional societies, and industry stakeholders is essential to ensure the reliability and comparability of liquid biopsy-based companion diagnostics.
- **Regulatory Hurdles:** Despite rapid technological advances, only a handful of liquid biopsy-based companion diagnostics have received formal approval from regulatory agencies like the FDA or EMA. These tests are classified as high-risk devices because treatment decisions based on their results can significantly impact patient outcomes. Therefore, approval requires comprehensive evidence demonstrating analytical validity, clinical validity, and clinical utility. However, generating such evidence through large-scale, multicentre studies is both time-consuming and expensive. Additionally, global regulatory frameworks differ, which complicates market access and scalability across regions. Harmonized and adaptive regulatory pathways are needed to accelerate the approval of high-quality, evidence-backed liquid biopsy diagnostics.
- **Clinical Validation:** For liquid biopsies to be adopted as routine tools in personalized medicine, robust clinical validation across diverse populations and disease contexts is essential. Most existing data on their utility comes from studies focused on specific cancers or limited patient demographics, often lacking ethnic, geographic, or socioeconomic diversity. As a result, the generalizability of these findings remains uncertain. Moreover, the prognostic and predictive value of many detected mutations remains to be

fully understood in real-world clinical settings. Expanding clinical trials, incorporating real-world evidence, and ensuring inclusive research designs will be crucial to validate and refine the role of liquid biopsy companion diagnostics across broader patient groups and therapeutic indications.

3.3.8 Regulatory and Clinical Integration

The clinical and regulatory landscapes are rapidly evolving to accommodate the growing utility of liquid biopsies as companion diagnostics (CDx). Regulatory bodies such as the U.S. Food and Drug Administration (FDA) and the European Medicines Agency (EMA) are progressively recognizing the scientific validity and clinical importance of non-invasive molecular diagnostics. A landmark development in this trajectory has been the approval of comprehensive liquid biopsy panels such as Guardant360 CDx and Foundation One Liquid CDx. These multi-gene assays are now FDA-approved to identify actionable mutations in advanced solid tumours and guide the use of specific targeted therapies, such as EGFR inhibitors in non-small cell lung cancer (NSCLC) or PARP inhibitors in prostate and breast cancer. These approvals are significant because they represent a shift from viewing liquid biopsies merely as experimental or adjunctive tools to fully validated diagnostics integrated into formal treatment pathways. Importantly, these tests were granted regulatory approval based on robust analytical validation and clinical evidence, including their ability to detect genomic alterations with high sensitivity and correlate results with treatment outcomes. Their use has been embedded in official drug labels, meaning that therapeutic decisions—such as selecting osimertinib for EGFR T790M-positive NSCLC—can now be based on liquid biopsy results rather than tissue biopsy alone.

On the clinical front, adoption is steadily increasing across major cancer centres and academic hospitals. Oncologists are beginning to utilize liquid biopsies not only for initial therapy selection but also for longitudinal disease monitoring, resistance mutation tracking, and re-stratifying patients whose disease progresses. This has led to improvements in the timeliness of clinical decision-making, especially for patients unable to undergo repeat tissue biopsies due to tumour inaccessibility or health limitations. In particular, liquid biopsies are proving invaluable in dynamic treatment environments like metastatic cancer, where tumour genomics evolve and new resistance mechanisms frequently emerge. The integration of liquid biopsy into clinical guidelines is further supporting its uptake. Organizations like the National Comprehensive Cancer Network (NCCN) have begun to include liquid biopsy recommendations in their protocols, especially when tissue is unavailable or insufficient. Additionally, expanding payer coverage and inclusion in value-based care models are making these diagnostics more accessible to patients. However, to reach their full potential, continued regulatory flexibility, harmonization of international approval frameworks, and expanded clinical validation—especially in underrepresented populations—will be essential. Liquid biopsies are transitioning from cutting-edge innovation to established clinical reality. With growing regulatory endorsements and increasing integration into everyday oncologic care, they are poised to become cornerstone tools in the personalized medicine era—enabling safer, faster, and more precise treatment strategies tailored to each patient's molecular profile.

3.4 PHARMACOGENOMICS

Pharmacogenomics (PGx) is the study of how an individual's genetic makeup affects their response to medications. By analysing genetic variations, particularly in drug-metabolizing enzymes, transporters, and targets, pharmacogenomics enables the selection of drugs and dosages that are optimized for safety and efficacy. This field is foundational to personalized medicine, offering a pathway to avoid adverse drug reactions (ADRs), improve therapeutic outcomes, and reduce trial-and-error prescribing (Fig. 3).

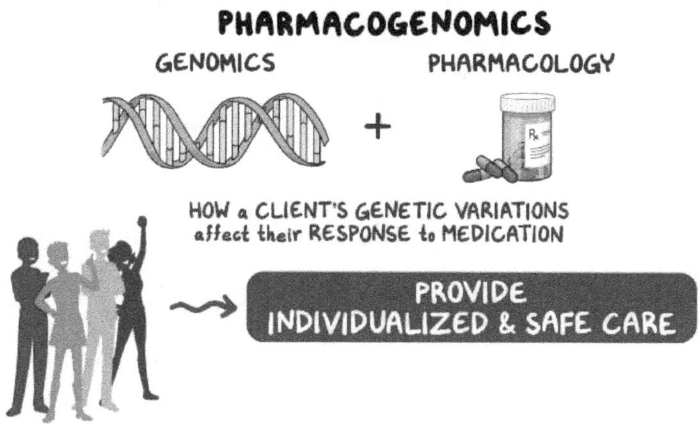

Fig.3 Pharmacogenomics

3.4.1 Genetic Variability and Drug Response

Genetic polymorphisms—particularly single nucleotide polymorphisms (SNPs)—influence how drugs are absorbed, distributed, metabolized, and excreted. For example:

- **CYP450 Family- CYP2D6, CYP2C19, and CYP3A4:** The cytochrome P450 (CYP450) enzyme family plays a central role in the metabolism of over 70% of clinically used drugs. Genetic variants in CYP2D6, CYP2C19, and CYP3A4 significantly affect drug metabolism capacity. Individuals can be classified into poor, intermediate, normal (extensive), rapid, or ultra-rapid metabolizers depending on their allele combinations. For example, poor metabolizers of CYP2D6 may experience toxicity from standard doses of tricyclic antidepressants or opioids, while ultra-rapid metabolizers may derive little benefit due to accelerated drug clearance. Similarly, CYP2C19 variation influences the activation of clopidogrel, where loss-of-function alleles reduce its efficacy, increasing the risk of cardiovascular events. CYP3A4, although less polymorphic, affects the metabolism of statins and immunosuppressants like tacrolimus. Understanding a patient's CYP450 genotype can guide drug selection and dosage to improve treatment outcomes and avoid adverse effects. PGx testing for these genes is increasingly incorporated into clinical guidelines.

- **TPMT and NUDT15- Thiopurine Metabolism:** Thiopurine drugs such as azathioprine, 6-mercaptopurine (6-MP), and 6-thioguanine are used to treat leukaemia, inflammatory bowel disease (IBD), and autoimmune conditions. Their metabolism is heavily influenced by genetic variations in TPMT (thiopurine S-methyltransferase) and NUDT15 (nudix hydrolase 15). Patients with low or absent TPMT activity accumulate toxic levels of active thioguanine nucleotides, leading to life-threatening myelosuppression. Similarly, NUDT15 variants, particularly prevalent in East Asian and Hispanic populations, impair DNA repair processes, causing severe cytotoxicity even at standard doses. Due to these risks, PGx testing for TPMT and NUDT15 is recommended before initiating thiopurine therapy to guide dose adjustment or alternative treatment choices. Genotype-based dosing has been shown to significantly reduce hospitalization and drug-related adverse effects. These genes exemplify how pharmacogenomics can be life-saving and cost-effective, especially in chronic diseases requiring long-term immunosuppressive therapy.
- **VKORC1 and CYP2C9- Warfarin Dosing:** Warfarin, a commonly used oral anticoagulant, has a narrow therapeutic index and significant inter-individual variability in dosing. Two key genes—VKORC1 (Vitamin K epoxide reductase complex subunit 1) and CYP2C9—affect warfarin's pharmacodynamics and pharmacokinetics, respectively. VKORC1 polymorphisms influence the drug's target sensitivity, with certain variants requiring lower maintenance doses to avoid bleeding risks. Meanwhile, CYP2C9 metabolizes the more potent S-enantiomer of warfarin; patients with CYP2C9 *2 or *3 alleles have reduced clearance and are prone to over-anticoagulation and haemorrhage. Clinical guidelines now recommend genotyping for both genes before initiating warfarin therapy to personalize the initial dose and minimize the risk of adverse events. Algorithms integrating VKORC1 and CYP2C9 status with age, weight, and dietary factors can improve time in therapeutic INR

range. Warfarin pharmacogenetics stands as a model for implementing genetic information into routine prescribing protocols for better patient outcomes. These variations can cause therapeutic failure or toxicity if not accounted for during prescribing.

3.4.2 Applications in Clinical Practice

Pharmacogenomic testing has moved from research settings to real-world clinical practice, becoming a critical tool in personalized medicine. In oncology, genetic profiling of tumours and germline DNA is used to tailor chemotherapy and targeted therapies. For instance, testing for DPYD variants can prevent fluoropyrimidine toxicity, and UGT1A1 genotyping helps dose irinotecan to avoid neutropenia. Pharmacogenomics is also foundational in prescribing tyrosine kinase inhibitors, where EGFR, ALK, and BCR-ABL mutations guide drug selection. In cardiology, pharmacogenomic testing of CYP2C19 variants informs the use of clopidogrel, particularly in patients undergoing percutaneous coronary intervention, as poor metabolizers may not effectively activate the drug. Similarly, VKORC1 and CYP2C9 genotyping optimize warfarin dosing, reducing bleeding risks and improving anticoagulation control. In psychiatry, CYP2D6 and CYP2C19 genotypes are used to personalize antidepressant and antipsychotic therapy, minimizing side effects such as sedation, weight gain, or QT prolongation, and increasing the likelihood of therapeutic response. Genetic variations can also inform dose adjustments or drug selection for SSRIs, TCAs, and mood stabilizers, improving medication adherence and long-term outcomes in mental health care. In infectious diseases, the HLA-B*57:01 allele is screened before initiating abacavir for HIV, as its presence is strongly associated with life-threatening hypersensitivity reactions. This is one of the earliest and most successful examples of mandatory pharmacogenomic testing being implemented in clinical guidelines. Across these therapeutic areas, pharmacogenomic testing reduces adverse drug reactions, enhances drug efficacy, and minimizes the trial-and-error approach to prescribing. It supports proactive treatment planning, improves patient safety, and contributes to better health outcomes. As testing becomes more affordable and widely available, and as electronic health records integrate PGx data into decision support tools, its role in routine clinical care is expected to expand significantly, ultimately transforming the landscape of individualized therapy.

Pharmacogenomic testing is now clinically used to guide treatment in several therapeutic areas:

- **Oncology:** In oncology, pharmacogenomic testing is now integral to treatment planning. Tumour and germline genotyping guide both chemotherapeutic dosing and targeted therapy selection. For example, DPYD variants are screened to reduce fluorouracil toxicity, and UGT1A1 variants influence irinotecan dosing. Molecular profiling of tumours identifies mutations such as EGFR, ALK, KRAS, or BRAF, enabling the selection of appropriate kinase inhibitors. These tests improve efficacy, avoid toxicities, and personalize care. Pharmacogenomics also helps in predicting resistance and monitoring therapy response. It plays a vital role in advancing precision oncology.

- **Cardiology:** In cardiology, pharmacogenomics enhances the safety and effectiveness of antithrombotic therapy. CYP2C19 genotyping identifies poor metabolizers who may not benefit from clopidogrel, enabling the use of alternatives like ticagrelor or prasugrel. For patients on warfarin, VKORC1 and CYP2C9 variants predict dose requirements and bleeding risks. Incorporating these insights into dosing algorithms reduces the trial-and-error approach and shortens time to stable anticoagulation. These strategies are now included in clinical guidelines. Pharmacogenomic testing thus improves outcomes and minimizes adverse events in cardiovascular disease management.
- **Psychiatry:** Psychiatric medications often show variable response and side effects across individuals. Pharmacogenomic testing of CYP2D6 and CYP2C19 helps optimize the selection and dosing of antidepressants (e.g., SSRIs, TCAs) and antipsychotics. For instance, poor metabolizers may require lower doses to prevent toxicity, while ultrarapid metabolizers may need higher doses or different drugs for therapeutic efficacy. Genotyping reduces side effects like sedation, weight gain, or agitation. It also improves adherence by enhancing tolerability and response. Personalized prescribing in psychiatry can significantly improve mental health care outcomes.
- **Infectious Diseases:** In infectious diseases, pharmacogenomics is already a clinical standard in some contexts. For HIV, screening for HLA-B57:01* is mandatory before prescribing abacavir, as carriers have a high risk of severe hypersensitivity reactions. This test has greatly improved the safety of abacavir therapy and is a model of successful genomic integration into clinical care. Other pharmacogenomic applications include predicting response to interferon in hepatitis C and managing tuberculosis drug toxicity. As new drugs emerge, PGx testing will play a growing role in infectious disease treatment customization.

3.4.3 Clinical Implementation and Guidelines

The clinical implementation of pharmacogenomics (PGx) is rapidly advancing, supported by an expanding evidence base, technology integration, and the establishment of practice guidelines. Implementing PGx involves incorporating genetic testing into routine clinical workflows to guide drug selection, dosing, and monitoring—tailoring treatments based on a patient's genetic profile to improve efficacy and minimize harm. Leading organizations like the Clinical Pharmacogenetics Implementation Consortium (CPIC), Dutch Pharmacogenetics Working Group (DPWG), and Pharmacogenomics Knowledgebase (PharmGKB) provide evidence-based guidelines that help clinicians translate genetic information into actionable prescribing decisions. These guidelines assign specific drug-gene pairs into categories with recommended actions, such as dose adjustments or alternative therapies. Clinical decision support tools integrated within electronic health records (EHRs) are facilitating real-time access to PGx insights at the point of care. These systems alert prescribers to genetic contraindications, suggest personalized dosing, and flag potential drug-gene interactions. Pre-emptive testing strategies—where patients' PGx data is collected in advance—are also being adopted in institutions to inform future prescribing without the need for repeated tests. Several healthcare systems and hospitals across the US, Europe, and Asia have launched dedicated PGx implementation programs. For example, Vanderbilt University's PREDICT program and St. Jude's PG4KDS have successfully integrated pharmacogenomic testing into paediatric oncology and adult medicine. These programs demonstrate the feasibility and clinical value of PGx in real-world settings. Regulatory agencies are also recognizing the importance of PGx. The U.S. FDA has included PGx information in drug labels for over 300 drugs, indicating when genetic testing may be necessary or useful. Similarly, the EMA encourages the use of pharmacogenomic data in drug submissions and post-market surveillance. However, successful implementation still faces barriers, including clinician awareness, access to testing, test reimbursement, and data interpretation challenges. Educational initiatives and training for healthcare providers are essential to build confidence and competence in using PGx results.

Overall, with harmonized guidelines, supportive policy frameworks, and digital infrastructure, pharmacogenomics is becoming a vital pillar of evidence-based, personalized clinical care. Several pharmacogenomic guidelines are now available to assist clinicians:

- CPIC (Clinical Pharmacogenetics Implementation Consortium) provides peer-reviewed, evidence-based guidelines.
- DPWG (Dutch Pharmacogenetics Working Group) also publishes drug-gene interaction recommendations.
- FDA labelling: More than 300 drugs now include pharmacogenomic information in their labels.

3.4.4 Pharmacogenomic Testing Technologies

Pharmacogenomic testing technologies have evolved to provide accurate, high-throughput analysis of genetic variants affecting drug response. Techniques such as real-time PCR, microarrays, and next-generation sequencing (NGS) are commonly used to detect single nucleotide polymorphisms (SNPs) and copy number variations in key pharmacognosy. These tests can be performed using blood or saliva samples and are increasingly available through clinical laboratories. Point-of-care genotyping platforms are also emerging to enable rapid decision-making in clinical settings. As these technologies become more affordable and integrated into healthcare systems, their utility in personalized prescribing continues to grow.

Modern PGx tests use technologies like:

- **PCR-Based Genotyping:** Polymerase Chain Reaction (PCR)-based genotyping is a widely used technique for identifying known single nucleotide polymorphisms (SNPs) that affect drug metabolism and response. It is precise, cost-effective, and ideal for testing specific gene variants like CYP2C19 or TPMT. PCR assays can be completed quickly and require minimal sample input, making them suitable for routine clinical use. Variants identified via PCR can inform dosing or drug choice with high reliability. However, PCR is limited to detecting only pre-specified mutations. Despite this, it remains a cornerstone in clinical pharmacogenomics, especially for targeted, single-gene assessments.
- **Microarrays:** Microarray platforms allow for simultaneous genotyping of thousands of known variants across multiple pharmacognosy. These tests are useful for screening populations for common SNPs in genes like CYP2D6, SLCO1B1, or VKORC1. The technology provides a balance between breadth and cost, making it attractive for commercial and academic testing panels. Results from microarrays can guide medication choices across several therapeutic areas, including psychiatry and cardiology. However, microarrays typically miss rare or novel mutations not included in the probe set. Despite this, their multiplex capacity enables efficient population-scale pharmacogenomic profiling.
- **Next-Generation Sequencing (NGS):** NGS allows comprehensive analysis of pharmacognosy by sequencing entire exons, genes, or even the whole genome. It is capable of detecting rare, novel, and complex variants that other technologies might miss, including copy number variants and gene rearrangements. NGS provides high-resolution insights into gene-drug interactions, making it powerful for research and personalized therapy. It is increasingly used in oncology and polygenic risk assessment. However, NGS is costlier and more data-intensive, requiring specialized interpretation infrastructure. Its broader utility is expanding as costs decline and bioinformatics tools improve.

- **Point-of-Care Tests:** Point-of-care (POC) pharmacogenomic tests are emerging tools designed for rapid genotyping at the bedside or clinic. These systems aim to deliver actionable results within minutes to hours, enabling immediate treatment decisions. POC tests are especially valuable in emergency or perioperative settings where timely drug choice is critical. They simplify logistics by eliminating the need for centralized laboratories. Current POC PGx tests are limited to a few high-impact variants, but future developments are expected to expand their scope. Their success depends on balancing speed, accuracy, and ease of use for clinical teams.

3.4.5 Barriers to Widespread Adoption

Despite its promise, the widespread adoption of pharmacogenomics faces multiple barriers spanning technical, clinical, economic, educational, and regulatory domains. A major challenge lies in limited clinician awareness and training; many healthcare providers are unfamiliar with how to interpret PGx results or integrate them into treatment plans. Lack of standardized clinical guidelines for many gene-drug pairs further complicates adoption, leaving physicians uncertain about how to act on test results. Additionally, variability in test availability and quality across regions leads to inconsistent clinical application. From a technical standpoint, incomplete electronic health record (EHR) integration of genomic data hampers efficient access and decision support. Economic concerns also pose a major obstacle: costs of testing can be prohibitive, especially in low-resource settings, and insurance reimbursement is often limited or inconsistent. Moreover, concerns about clinical utility persist for many pharmacogenomic markers that have yet to demonstrate strong, reproducible outcomes across large and diverse populations. Regulatory ambiguity surrounding certain test types—especially laboratory-developed tests (LDTs)—can delay market availability or erode provider confidence. Privacy and data security issues also contribute to hesitation among patients and institutions alike, given the sensitivity of genetic data. Furthermore, most PGx tests focus on single-drug, single-gene interactions, limiting their value in patients taking multiple medications. There's also a shortage of genetic counsellors and specialized personnel, which slows implementation in busy clinical environments. Importantly, population diversity is underrepresented in pharmacogenomic studies, leading to disparities in predictive accuracy and clinical relevance for underrepresented ethnic groups. The lack of harmonization in international regulatory standards complicates global adoption and sharing of PGx data. Finally, fragmentation in healthcare systems, differing stakeholder incentives, and the slow pace of institutional change all contribute to delayed implementation. To unlock the full potential of pharmacogenomics, these multifaceted barriers must be addressed through interdisciplinary collaboration, policy reform, workforce training, and patient engagement.

Despite progress, challenges remain:

- **Cost and Reimbursement:** One of the most significant barriers to PGx adoption is the cost of testing and the lack of consistent reimbursement mechanisms. Many pharmacogenomic tests, especially advanced panels or sequencing-based approaches, are expensive and not routinely covered by public or private insurance providers. This limits patient access, particularly in underfunded healthcare systems or in low- and middle-income countries. Without clear reimbursement pathways, healthcare providers are less likely to order these tests, even when clinically appropriate. Furthermore, inconsistent economic evaluations of test utility have led to varied payer decisions, hindering scalability. Demonstrating cost-effectiveness across large populations remains crucial to securing financial coverage and encouraging routine use.
- **Lack of Clinician Awareness or Training:** A substantial number of healthcare providers are not adequately trained in genetics or pharmacogenomics, which undermines confidence in ordering, interpreting, and acting on test results. Medical education often lacks comprehensive coverage of genomic medicine, and practicing clinicians may not have opportunities for continued learning in this rapidly evolving field. As a result, many providers are hesitant to incorporate PGx testing into routine care, fearing misinterpretation or clinical uncertainty. Without appropriate clinical decision support tools integrated into electronic health records, the complexity of genetic data becomes even more daunting. Building genomic literacy through continuing medical education and integrated training is essential to empower clinicians to utilize PGx effectively.
- **Limited Diversity in Genomic Databases:** Most existing pharmacogenomic databases and studies have been conducted in populations of European ancestry, leading to gaps in understanding genetic variation across global ethnic groups. This lack of representation limits the generalizability and predictive accuracy of PGx tests for diverse populations, contributing to health disparities. Variants that are clinically significant in one population may be rare or absent in another, or vice versa. As a result, certain patient groups may receive inaccurate test results or be excluded from the benefits of personalized therapy. Expanding genetic studies to include diverse populations is critical to ensure equitable and effective implementation of pharmacogenomics in global healthcare systems.
- **Complex Interpretation of Results:** Pharmacogenomic test results can be complex, especially when multiple genes, gene-gene interactions, or environmental factors influence drug response. Many therapeutic decisions

involve polygenic traits or multifactorial pathways, which require more nuanced interpretation than simple single-gene results. Additionally, ambiguous or intermediate phenotypes—such as "intermediate metabolizer" status—can create uncertainty in clinical decision-making. Without standardized interpretation frameworks or real-time support tools, this complexity can lead to either over-reliance or underutilization of test results. Developing clear guidelines, integrated clinical decision support systems, and consensus algorithms is crucial for translating PGx data into actionable, confident prescribing decisions.

3.4.6 Future Prospects

The future of pharmacogenomics holds transformative potential for healthcare, promising a shift from generalized prescribing to highly individualized therapy. As genomic technologies become more accessible and cost-effective, pharmacogenomic testing is expected to become a routine part of clinical decision-making across diverse medical specialties. The integration of next-generation sequencing, artificial intelligence, and real-time data analytics will enhance the accuracy, speed, and utility of genetic insights, allowing clinicians to predict drug response, avoid adverse reactions, and optimize therapeutic efficacy more reliably. Innovations such as point-of-care genetic testing and pharmacogenomic integration into electronic health records will bring these capabilities directly to the bedside, improving timeliness and clinical relevance. Moreover, the rise of polygenic risk scores and multi-gene panels will allow for more complex and comprehensive drug response predictions, moving beyond single-gene assessments. Increased efforts toward the inclusion of underrepresented populations in genomic research will also make pharmacogenomics more equitable and globally applicable. Regulatory frameworks are gradually evolving to support broader implementation, while pharmaceutical companies are increasingly embedding PGx data into drug development pipelines. Educational initiatives targeting clinicians and patients will be key to bridging knowledge gaps and fostering widespread adoption. Ultimately, pharmacogenomics is poised to become a cornerstone of personalized medicine—improving patient outcomes, reducing trial-and-error prescribing, and lowering healthcare costs through smarter, genetically informed treatment choices.

The future of pharmacogenomics is promising:

- Pre-emptive PGx testing may become routine during early life or at first clinical contact.
- Integration with polygenic risk scores will enhance individualized care.
- AI and machine learning will assist in interpreting complex gene-drug-environment interactions.

- Global standardization and population-scale studies will improve test applicability across ethnic groups.

Pharmacogenomics will likely play a pivotal role in preventive medicine and precision pharmacotherapy.

3.5 DIGITAL BIOMARKERS AND WEARABLE INTEGRATION

Digital biomarkers and wearable technologies are transforming the landscape of personalized medicine by enabling continuous, real-time monitoring of physiological and behavioural parameters. Unlike traditional biomarkers, which are often measured through invasive laboratory tests at infrequent intervals, digital biomarkers offer the potential to capture dynamic health data seamlessly during daily life. These biomarkers are collected through a range of digital platforms—including smartphones, smartwatches, fitness bands, rings, and remote sensors—that monitor variables such as heart rate, respiration, glucose levels, activity patterns, sleep cycles, body temperature, and more. As these tools become more sophisticated and ubiquitous, they are providing clinicians and researchers with unprecedented insight into the moment-to-moment physiological and lifestyle contexts that influence health and disease progression. Wearable technologies are particularly valuable in managing chronic conditions like diabetes, cardiovascular disorders, and neurodegenerative diseases, where traditional monitoring methods may fail to capture fluctuations or early warning signs. For example, continuous glucose monitors (CGMs) can alert diabetic patients and their providers to real-time glucose excursions, facilitating timely intervention. Similarly, smartwatches equipped with ECG capabilities can detect arrhythmias such as atrial fibrillation, enabling early diagnosis and potentially preventing stroke. In the mental health arena, subtle shifts in voice tone, typing behaviour, or physical activity can serve as digital indicators of mood disturbances, depression, or cognitive decline.

The integration of digital biomarkers into clinical decision-making supports a more nuanced understanding of patient health, going beyond static metrics to reveal patterns, trends, and anomalies over time. Furthermore, when coupled with genomic and other omics data, digital biomarkers enrich the multidimensional profile needed for truly personalized care. In drug development, digital biomarkers are being used as digital endpoints in clinical trials, improving data collection efficiency, participant adherence, and relevance of trial outcomes. Despite challenges like data privacy, standardization, and regulatory oversight, digital biomarkers are ushering in a new era of connected, proactive, and patient-centred healthcare. As artificial intelligence and big data analytics evolve, the value of these digital signals will only grow, offering powerful tools for prediction, prevention, and precision treatment.

3.5.1 Digital Biomarkers

Digital biomarkers are a new class of health indicators derived from objective; quantifiable physiological and behavioural data collected through digital technologies such as smartphones, wearables, biosensors, and remote monitoring tools. Unlike conventional biomarkers—which often require invasive procedures, lab-based testing, and periodic data collection—digital biomarkers allow for real-time, continuous monitoring in the patient's natural environment. They can capture subtle variations in heart rate, gait, voice, sleep, activity, glucose levels, oxygen saturation, and other physiological signals with minimal burden on the patient. This evolution in data acquisition provides a more holistic and dynamic picture of an individual's health status and disease trajectory. In the context of personalized medicine, digital biomarkers offer an unprecedented opportunity to tailor treatment decisions based on a person's daily physiological responses and lifestyle behaviours. For instance, wearable devices that track heart rate variability or activity levels can help assess stress or fatigue, enabling proactive interventions. In chronic disease management, such as Parkinson's or heart failure, digital biomarkers can detect early signs of symptom worsening before clinical deterioration becomes apparent, allowing for timely therapeutic adjustments. They are also proving useful in remote monitoring of at-risk populations, especially in aging or rural populations with limited access to healthcare infrastructure. Digital biomarkers are increasingly incorporated into clinical trials as endpoints to evaluate drug efficacy, adherence, and patient-reported outcomes in a decentralized or hybrid trial model. Their continuous, real-world data stream enhances the granularity and accuracy of clinical evidence. Importantly, these biomarkers empower patients by giving them more control and visibility over their health metrics, promoting engagement, accountability, and adherence to care plans. However, challenges remain regarding standardization, data interoperability, clinical validation, and regulatory approval pathways. Despite these barriers, the convergence of wearable technology, artificial intelligence, and big data analytics is rapidly advancing the clinical utility of digital biomarkers, making them a vital component of the future of precision health and personalized medicine (Fig. 3).

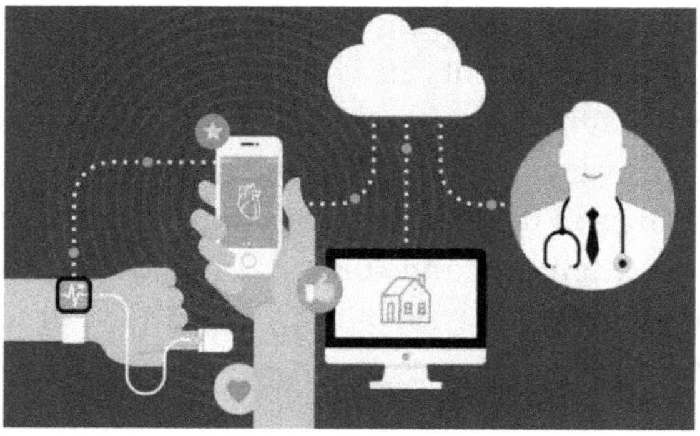

Fig. 3 Digital biomarker

3.5.2 Types of Digital Biomarkers

Digital biomarkers can include a wide range of physiological and behavioural indicators such as:

- Heart rate variability (HRV) and ECG data from smartwatches.
- Activity levels, sleep patterns, and step count from fitness trackers.
- Voice analysis and keystroke dynamics to monitor neurodegenerative conditions.
- Skin temperature, oxygen saturation, and respiration rates from multisensory platforms.

Wearable Devices in Health Monitoring: Wearable health technologies such as the Apple Watch, Fitbit, Oura Ring, and continuous glucose monitors (CGMs) have transformed the landscape of health monitoring by enabling real-time, continuous, and non-invasive collection of physiological data. These devices track a range of biomarkers including heart rate, heart rate variability, body temperature, blood oxygen saturation, sleep patterns, physical activity, and glucose levels. With these data, wearables can provide early warnings for abnormalities such as arrhythmias (e.g., atrial fibrillation), hypoglycaemia or hyperglycaemia, oxygen desaturation, or sleep apnea—all of which are critical indicators of underlying conditions. By offering longitudinal tracking, wearables allow for baseline comparison and trend identification over time, facilitating early disease detection and proactive interventions. In chronic disease management, wearables empower patients by enhancing self-awareness and promoting adherence to lifestyle and treatment regimens. For example, CGMs are revolutionizing diabetes care by providing continuous glucose feedback, helping individuals fine-tune their diet, exercise, and insulin doses in real time. In cardiovascular care, wearables can monitor blood pressure and detect arrhythmic events before they become clinically symptomatic. Sleep tracking features are useful in identifying insomnia, sleep apnea, and fatigue-related disorders, which often go undiagnosed. These technologies are particularly valuable for aging populations or those in rural or underserved areas, as they enable remote monitoring and early escalation of care when needed. Ultimately, wearable devices bridge the gap between daily life and clinical insight, transforming passive patients into active participants in their health journey.

Integration with Personalized Medicine: The integration of wearable-derived digital biomarkers into personalized medicine is redefining how care is delivered. By capturing individualized, real-time physiological signals, clinicians can make dynamic treatment decisions rather than relying solely on periodic clinical assessments. For instance, if a wearable indicates persistent tachycardia or changes in heart rate variability, a clinician may modify beta-blocker therapy or investigate autonomic dysfunction. Similarly, fluctuations in glucose patterns detected by CGMs can inform adjustments to diabetes medications or dietary interventions. These insights help tailor treatment to the patient's current physiological status, rather than waiting for lagging indicators such as lab tests or clinical deterioration. Digital biomarkers from wearables also provide a continuous feedback loop that enables anticipatory care. Subtle deviations in sleep, activity, or heart rate may precede exacerbations in conditions like heart failure, asthma, or depression, prompting pre-emptive therapy modifications. When linked with electronic health records (EHRs), wearable data enriches the patient's longitudinal health profile, offering a comprehensive view that includes genetic predispositions, clinical history, lifestyle patterns, and real-time metrics. This synergy enhances risk stratification, decision-making, and care coordination. Furthermore, the integration of AI and predictive analytics with wearable data may enable clinicians to detect emerging health threats or personalize health interventions even further. Thus, digital biomarkers are central to the evolution of medicine from reactive and episodic to proactive, precise, and personalized.

Applications in Clinical Trials and Drug Development: Digital biomarkers captured through wearable devices are playing an increasingly critical role in the design and execution of clinical trials. Traditional clinical trials are often constrained by infrequent site visits, retrospective data collection, and poor participant retention. Wearables address these limitations by allowing continuous, passive data collection in real-world settings. This not only improves the accuracy and granularity of endpoints such as physical activity, sleep quality, heart rhythm, or glucose control but also enhances patient convenience, leading to better compliance and reduced dropout rates. Pharmaceutical companies now routinely include wearable-based digital biomarkers to monitor drug safety, efficacy, and tolerability throughout the trial duration. Real-time remote monitoring enables more agile trial designs—adaptive trials that can modify protocols based on interim data—and supports decentralized clinical trials (DCTs) where patients participate from home. This is particularly valuable during pandemics or for studies targeting rare diseases or rural populations. Additionally, wearable-derived data can serve as digital endpoints that complement or even replace traditional clinical outcomes, particularly in neurological, metabolic, and cardiovascular research. Regulatory bodies such as the FDA and EMA are increasingly acknowledging the utility of digital biomarkers in regulatory submissions, encouraging sponsors to include them for drug evaluation. Beyond trials, the data can inform post-marketing surveillance, real-world evidence generation, and long-term pharmacovigilance. Thus, wearable-enabled digital biomarkers are enhancing the speed, scalability, and personalization of drug development pipelines.

Challenges in Implementation

Despite their promise, digital biomarkers face challenges including:

- **Data Privacy and Security Concerns:** As digital biomarkers rely on continuous data collection through wearable devices, smartphones, and cloud platforms, they introduce significant privacy and security risks. Sensitive health information—including heart rhythms, activity patterns, location data, and sleep habits—can be vulnerable to hacking, unauthorized sharing, or misuse by third parties such as insurers or employers. Patients may be reluctant to use wearables or share data if they fear breaches of confidentiality. Compliance with regulations like HIPAA, GDPR, and emerging data protection laws is essential but often complex, especially when data flows across borders. Addressing these concerns requires robust encryption, transparent consent processes, clear data ownership policies, and ongoing cybersecurity updates to build and maintain trust in digital health technologies.
- **Standardization of Measurements and Data Formats:** Digital biomarkers today suffer from a lack of standardization across devices, manufacturers, and platforms. Different wearables may measure heart rate, sleep, or activity using proprietary algorithms and sensor technologies, leading to inconsistent results that cannot be reliably compared or aggregated. This variability undermines clinical confidence, limits data interoperability, and complicates integration into electronic health records. Standardized protocols, validated measurement techniques, and common data formats are urgently needed to ensure accuracy, reproducibility, and consistency across digital health tools. Industry-wide collaboration involving device makers, healthcare providers, regulators, and standards organizations will be critical to create universally accepted benchmarks.
- **Regulatory Approval for Clinical Use:** While digital biomarkers hold great promise, they must undergo rigorous evaluation before they can be integrated into routine clinical workflows. Regulatory pathways for digital health tools remain fragmented and evolving, with varying requirements across regions like the US, EU, and Asia. Demonstrating analytical validity, clinical validity, and clinical utility is essential for approval, yet many digital biomarkers lack sufficient high-quality evidence from large-scale trials. Moreover, regulatory frameworks often lag behind rapid technological innovation, creating uncertainty for developers and clinicians. Streamlined guidance, adaptive approval processes, and international regulatory harmonization will be key to accelerating safe and effective deployment of digital biomarkers in clinical care.

- **Data Overload and the Need for Intelligent Interpretation Tools:** Digital biomarkers generate massive amounts of continuous data—often thousands of data points per patient per day—which can quickly overwhelm clinicians and patients if not effectively organized and interpreted. Without intelligent algorithms, visualization tools, or clinical decision support systems, this data deluge risks being ignored or misused, undermining its potential to improve outcomes. Developing advanced analytics, machine learning models, and intuitive dashboards will help extract actionable insights from raw data streams. These tools must be carefully designed to integrate seamlessly into clinical workflows, providing clear, context-sensitive recommendations without contributing to information overload or alert fatigue

4 Chapter

PERSONALIZED THERAPEUTICS

4.0 INTRODUCTION: AN OVERVIEW

Personalized therapeutics represents a paradigm shift in modern medicine, moving beyond the traditional "one-size-fits-all" approach to treatment. Rooted in the principles of individualized care, personalized therapeutics tailors drug therapies to the unique genetic, molecular, environmental, and lifestyle characteristics of each patient. This approach acknowledges the biological diversity among individuals and leverages advanced tools—such as genomic sequencing, transcriptomics, proteomics, metabolomics, and digital health data—to optimize therapeutic decisions. The goal is to enhance efficacy, minimize adverse drug reactions, and improve long-term clinical outcomes across a wide spectrum of diseases, including cancer, cardiovascular disorders, infectious diseases, autoimmune conditions, and psychiatric illnesses. Historically, conventional therapeutics have relied on population averages derived from large clinical trials. While this has produced effective therapies for many, it also revealed wide variability in treatment responses. Some patients respond well to a drug, while others may experience little benefit or even severe side effects. This inter-individual variability is influenced by a host of factors—chief among them being genetic differences, especially single nucleotide polymorphisms (SNPs), gene expression patterns, and copy number variations that affect drug metabolism, transport, and receptor interactions. Personalized therapeutics aims to decode these factors and align therapy accordingly. The field has gained momentum with the rise of pharmacogenomics, which investigates how genetic variation influences drug response. For example, polymorphisms in the CYP450 family of enzymes significantly impact the metabolism of drugs such as warfarin, clopidogrel, antidepressants, and many chemotherapeutic agents. Similarly, genomic profiling of tumours enables oncologists to choose targeted therapies that inhibit specific molecular pathways active in an individual's cancer. Such advances are not only improving survival and quality of life but also reducing the economic burden of trial-and-error prescribing (Fig. 1).

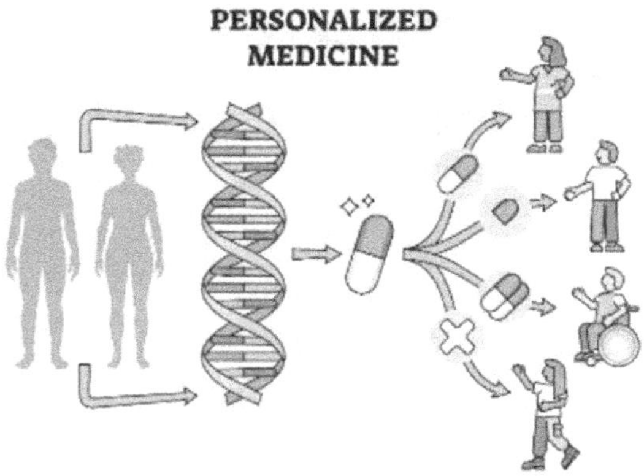

Fig. 1 Personalized Medicine: A Paradigm Shift in Healthcare

Beyond pharmacogenomics, personalized therapeutics integrates multi-omics data to build a comprehensive health profile. Proteomics sheds light on protein expression and modification; metabolomics explores metabolic signatures related to drug action and toxicity; and epigenomics examines gene regulation that might affect therapeutic outcomes. When these datasets are layered and interpreted using advanced computational tools and artificial intelligence (AI), they offer unprecedented insights into disease mechanisms and optimal intervention strategies. This integrative approach is fostering the emergence of systems pharmacology—where drugs are viewed not in isolation but as dynamic modulators of complex biological networks. A critical enabler of personalized therapeutics is the use of biomarkers—measurable indicators of biological state or response to therapy. Predictive biomarkers identify patients likely to respond to a given drug, while prognostic biomarkers provide information about disease progression regardless of treatment. Companion diagnostics, co-developed with specific drugs, are increasingly being employed in clinical practice to stratify patients and guide therapy selection. For instance, the presence of HER2 amplification in breast cancer directs the use of trastuzumab, while EGFR and ALK mutations guide therapy in non-small cell lung cancer. Personalized therapeutics also intersects with digital health innovations. Wearable sensors, mobile apps, and remote monitoring tools provide real-time data on patient physiology, behaviour, and drug adherence. These digital biomarkers, when integrated with molecular data, enable dynamic and responsive therapeutic strategies—such as dosage adjustments based on real-time glucose monitoring or AI-driven alerts for early detection of toxicity. This feedback loop enhances precision, promotes patient engagement, and supports the shift toward preventive, participatory, and proactive healthcare. Despite its promise, personalized therapeutics faces several challenges. Scientific complexities in interpreting omics data, variability in biomarker reproducibility, high costs of personalized interventions, ethical issues around data privacy, and disparities in access to genomic technologies are major hurdles. Furthermore, regulatory frameworks must evolve to accommodate adaptive trial designs, biomarker-driven approvals, and integration of digital evidence. Health systems must also build capacity for data management, clinician education, and patient counselling to implement personalized care effectively. Nonetheless, the trajectory is clear: personalized therapeutics is redefining the future of medicine. It is fostering the transition from reactive treatment to predictive and preventive care, from symptom management to root-cause targeting, and from generic interventions to deeply individualized therapies. In this context, patients are no longer passive recipients of care but active participants in a data-rich, continuously learning healthcare ecosystem. As technologies mature, costs decline, and public awareness grows, personalized therapeutics is poised to become the new standard of care—transforming lives by aligning the right treatment to the right patient at the right time.

4.1 GENETICALLY TARGETED THERAPIES

Genetically targeted therapies are an innovative class of medical treatments precisely tailored to an individual's unique genetic makeup. Unlike traditional approaches that apply standardized treatments to all patients with a particular condition, these therapies take into account the specific genetic mutations, gene expression profiles, or inherited variants that underlie a person's disease. This molecular-level targeting allows for a more accurate and effective intervention, reducing the risk of adverse drug reactions and enhancing therapeutic success. The foundation of genetically targeted therapy lies in the recognition that human diseases—especially cancer, rare genetic disorders, and some chronic illnesses—often arise from or are influenced by identifiable alterations in DNA. These changes can disrupt biological pathways, protein functions, or cell signalling mechanisms, ultimately manifesting as clinical symptoms. By identifying the exact mutation or pathway involved, therapies can be selected or developed that directly counteract the disease process. In cancer treatment, for example, genetically targeted therapies are revolutionizing care. Tumours with specific driver mutations such as EGFR, BRAF, ALK, or KRAS are treated with drugs designed to inhibit the activity of the mutant protein, thereby halting tumour growth. Similarly, in inherited conditions like cystic fibrosis, therapies such as ivacaftor are tailored to improve the function of specific CFTR gene variants. Pharmacogenomics, a key component of this field, studies how genetic differences affect individual responses to drugs, enabling clinicians to predict which patients will benefit from a treatment and which may suffer harm. For example, patients with certain TPMT or NUDT15 variants are at higher risk of toxicity from thiopurines and require dose adjustments.

The rise of genome sequencing technologies and bioinformatics tools has further propelled the feasibility and affordability of genetically targeted approaches.

Gene therapy, RNA-based interventions (such as antisense oligonucleotides and siRNAs), and genome editing techniques like CRISPR-Cas9 are now expanding the scope of treatable conditions. These cutting-edge methods allow not only symptom management but also potential cures by correcting the underlying genetic defects. Immunotherapies, including CAR-T cells, represent another frontier where genetic engineering is used to reprogram the patient's immune cells to recognize and attack specific molecular targets on diseased cells. Genetically targeted therapies hold the promise of transforming the medical landscape, but their implementation requires robust diagnostic infrastructure, skilled interpretation of genetic data, and careful consideration of ethical, regulatory, and cost-related challenges. As we advance toward a future of truly personalized medicine, this section will examine the major dimensions of genetically targeted therapy under structured subheadings—exploring its mechanisms, applications, challenges, and future prospects in a comprehensive and clinically relevant manner.

4.1.1 Concept and Definition

Genetically targeted therapies involve designing or selecting treatments based on a patient's genetic profile. These therapies aim to correct, inhibit, or bypass the effects of disease-causing genes or mutations. Unlike traditional therapies that treat all patients similarly, genetically targeted therapies personalize treatment to maximize efficacy and minimize side effects.

4.1.2 Role of Genomics in Therapy Selection

Genomics plays a pivotal role in modern therapeutic decision-making by enabling the identification of genetic alterations that directly influence disease behaviour and treatment response. Through genomic sequencing—particularly next-generation sequencing (NGS)—clinicians can detect a broad spectrum of genomic abnormalities, including point mutations, insertions, deletions, gene fusions, amplifications, and copy number variations. These alterations often serve as diagnostic markers, prognostic indicators, or predictive biomarkers that guide therapy selection. In oncology, for instance, NGS panels allow for the comprehensive profiling of tumours to uncover actionable mutations such as EGFR, BRAF, PIK3CA, or ALK, which are associated with targeted therapeutic agents. Beyond cancer, genomic insights are increasingly applied in pharmacogenomics to adjust drug types and dosages based on metabolic gene variants—like those in CYP2D6 or CYP2C9. In inherited disorders, whole-exome or whole-genome sequencing facilitates precise molecular diagnoses, which can open pathways to gene-specific therapies. Additionally, genomics assists in stratifying patients for clinical trials, ensuring that only those with the relevant genetic profile are enrolled in studies testing genotype-specific drugs. The integration of genomics into clinical workflows is transforming medicine into a data-driven discipline, allowing for more precise, effective, and individualized therapy decisions.

4.1.3 Monogenic Disorders and Gene Therapy

Monogenic disorders are caused by mutations in a single gene and often present early in life with severe, progressive symptoms. Unlike complex diseases influenced by multiple genes and environmental factors, monogenic diseases offer a clearer target for therapeutic intervention. Gene therapy provides a revolutionary approach to treat these conditions by delivering a functional copy of the defective gene, silencing the mutant gene, or editing the genome directly. Delivery systems typically involve viral vectors such as adeno-associated viruses (AAVs), which are engineered to carry therapeutic genes into the patient's cells. The goal is to restore normal gene function, reduce symptoms, and potentially provide a long-lasting or even curative effect with a single treatment. Advances in molecular biology, vector design, and regulatory approvals have made gene therapy a clinical reality for several monogenic diseases. Examples include:

- **Spinal Muscular Atrophy (SMA):** Spinal Muscular Atrophy is a genetic neuromuscular disorder caused by mutations in the SMN1 gene, leading to progressive muscle wasting and weakness due to motor neuron degeneration. A groundbreaking gene therapy, onasemnogene abeparvovec (marketed as Zolgensma), delivers a functional copy of the SMN1 gene using an AAV9 vector. Administered as a one-time intravenous infusion, it enables sustained production of the survival motor neuron protein, significantly improving motor function and survival outcomes in infants and young children. Early intervention is critical, as it maximizes neuronal rescue before irreversible damage occurs. This therapy represents a landmark in genetic medicine, demonstrating how a single-dose gene replacement can dramatically alter the disease course.
- **Hemophilia:** Hemophilia A and B are bleeding disorders caused by mutations in the genes encoding coagulation factors VIII and IX, respectively. Traditional treatment involves lifelong factor replacement therapy, often complicated by inhibitor development and fluctuating levels. Gene therapy has emerged as a promising alternative, using AAV vectors to deliver functional F8 or F9 genes directly to liver cells, which then produce the missing clotting factor. Clinical trials have shown sustained increases in factor levels, reduced bleeding episodes, and decreased dependence on exogenous factor administration. Some patients have achieved near-normal coagulation levels, suggesting the possibility of long-term disease control or even a functional cure. These therapies mark a significant shift from symptomatic management to genomic correction in haemophilia care.

4.1.4 Somatic Mutations and Targeted Cancer Therapy

Somatic mutations are genetic alterations acquired by cells during a person's lifetime, often playing a key role in the initiation and progression of cancer. These mutations are not inherited but arise spontaneously or due to environmental exposures such as smoking, radiation, or carcinogens. Many cancers are driven by specific somatic mutations that activate oncogenes or disable tumour suppressor genes, leading to uncontrolled cell growth, survival, and metastasis. Targeted cancer therapies are designed to block these molecular abnormalities with high specificity, sparing normal cells and reducing the systemic toxicity associated with conventional chemotherapy. By focusing on the underlying genetic drivers of the tumour, these therapies provide greater precision, improve response rates, and often lead to better quality of life for patients. Therapies directed against these mutations include:

- **EGFR Inhibitors in Non-Small Cell Lung Cancer (NSCLC):** In a subset of NSCLC patients, activating mutations in the EGFR gene drive tumour growth by promoting continuous cell signalling. EGFR tyrosine kinase inhibitors (TKIs), such as erlotinib, gefitinib, afatinib, and osimertinib, selectively block this aberrant signalling pathway. These therapies have significantly improved progression-free survival and symptom control in patients with EGFR-mutated NSCLC. Resistance mechanisms may develop, such as the T790M mutation, for which third-generation TKIs like osimertinib are specifically designed. Routine genomic testing for EGFR mutations is now standard practice in managing advanced lung cancer.
- **BRAF Inhibitors in Melanoma:** Approximately 40–50% of cutaneous melanomas harbour mutations in the BRAF gene, most commonly the V600E mutation. This mutation leads to hyperactivation of the MAPK/ERK signalling pathway, promoting cell proliferation and survival. Targeted therapies such as vemurafenib and dabrafenib specifically inhibit mutant BRAF, causing tumour regression in many patients. These drugs are often used in combination with MEK inhibitors (e.g., trametinib) to enhance efficacy and delay resistance. BRAF-targeted therapy has transformed the prognosis for patients with advanced melanoma, offering rapid and durable responses in selected individuals.
- **PARP Inhibitors in BRCA-Mutated Cancers:** Patients with inherited or somatic mutations in BRCA1 or BRCA2 genes have defective homologous recombination DNA repair pathways, making their tumour cells particularly vulnerable to DNA damage. PARP inhibitors, such as olaparib and niraparib, exploit this vulnerability by blocking the PARP enzyme involved in single-strand DNA repair. This leads to synthetic lethality in BRCA-deficient cells,

causing cancer cell death while sparing normal tissues. PARP inhibitors have become a cornerstone in the treatment of BRCA-mutated breast and ovarian cancers, and their role is expanding into prostate and pancreatic cancers with similar genetic vulnerabilities.

4.1.5 Pharmacogenomics-Guided Drug Selection

Pharmacogenomics is a cornerstone of personalized medicine, focusing on how genetic variations influence an individual's response to drugs. These genetic differences, often in genes coding for drug-metabolizing enzymes, transporters, or drug targets, can profoundly affect how a patient absorbs, metabolizes, distributes, or eliminates medications. By identifying these variants before treatment begins, clinicians can select the most appropriate drug, determine optimal dosing, and avoid potentially serious adverse reactions. This genotype-guided approach minimizes trial-and-error prescribing, enhances drug efficacy, and improves patient safety, especially in treatments with narrow therapeutic indices or high variability in response. Examples include:

- **CYP2C19 Testing Before Prescribing Clopidogrel:** Clopidogrel is an antiplatelet drug that requires metabolic activation by the liver enzyme CYP2C19. Individuals with CYP2C19 loss-of-function alleles (e.g., CYP2C19 *2 or *3) have reduced ability to convert clopidogrel into its active form, resulting in inadequate platelet inhibition and increased risk of cardiovascular events. Pharmacogenomic testing helps identify poor metabolizers who may benefit more from alternative antiplatelet agents like prasugrel or ticagrelor. This testing is especially critical in patients undergoing percutaneous coronary intervention (PCI).
- **TPMT and NUDT15 Genotyping Before Thiopurine Therapy:** Thiopurine drugs such as azathioprine, mercaptopurine, and thioguanine are used to treat autoimmune diseases and leukaemia's. Variants in the TPMT and NUDT15 genes can impair thiopurine metabolism, leading to excessive accumulation of toxic metabolites that cause severe bone marrow suppression. Genotyping these enzymes before initiating therapy allows for dose adjustments or alternative treatments to avoid life-threatening complications. NUDT15 testing is particularly important in Asian populations, where the variant is more prevalent.
- **VKORC1 and CYP2C9 Genotyping to Adjust Warfarin Doses:** Warfarin is an oral anticoagulant with a narrow therapeutic window and significant interindividual variability in dosing requirements. Variants in CYP2C9 affect warfarin metabolism, while polymorphisms in VKORC1 influence sensitivity to the drug. Patients with these variants are at higher risk of bleeding or thrombosis if dosed inappropriately. Genetic testing helps in

personalizing warfarin dosing, improving time in therapeutic range, and reducing adverse events. Some clinical algorithms now integrate genotypic data to guide warfarin initiation and management

4.1.6 CAR-T Cell Therapy

Chimeric Antigen Receptor T-cell (CAR-T) therapy is a groundbreaking form of personalized immunotherapy that reprograms a patient's own immune system to target and eliminate cancer cells. The process begins by extracting T cells from the patient's blood, which are then genetically engineered in the laboratory to express synthetic receptors—called CARs—that recognize specific antigens on the surface of cancer cells. Once modified, these CAR-T cells are expanded and reinfused into the patient, where they seek out and destroy tumour cells with remarkable precision.

CAR-T therapy has demonstrated dramatic success in treating hematological malignancies, particularly relapsed or refractory B-cell acute lymphoblastic leukemia (ALL) and diffuse large B-cell lymphoma (DLBCL). FDA-approved therapies such as tisagenlecleucel and axicabtagene ciloleucel have shown high remission rates in patients with otherwise limited treatment options. This therapy bypasses the limitations of conventional treatments by harnessing the body's own immune system, offering the potential for durable, even curative responses. However, CAR-T therapy is not without challenges. Patients may experience severe side effects such as cytokine release syndrome (CRS) and neurotoxicity, requiring specialized care. Moreover, the manufacturing process is complex, time-consuming, and costly, limiting widespread accessibility. Despite these hurdles, ongoing innovations aim to expand CAR-T applications to solid tumours, improve safety, and develop off-the-shelf allogeneic CAR-T products, potentially transforming cancer treatment across the board.

4.1.7 RNA-Based Therapies

RNA-based therapies offer a novel and precise approach to modulate gene expression by directly targeting RNA transcripts rather than DNA or proteins. These therapies include antisense oligonucleotides (ASOs) and small interfering RNAs (siRNAs), which work by altering splicing patterns, promoting RNA degradation, or blocking translation of specific mRNA sequences. By intervening at the post-transcriptional level, these molecules can downregulate or correct the expression of disease-causing genes with high specificity. RNA-based approaches are particularly valuable for diseases caused by toxic gain-of-function mutations, aberrant splicing, or overactive protein production. These therapies are often delivered systemically or intrathecally and have the advantage of being chemically synthesized and programmable to new targets, accelerating their development pipeline. Examples include:

- **Nusinersen for Spinal Muscular Atrophy (SMA):** Nusinersen is an antisense oligonucleotide designed to treat spinal muscular atrophy (SMA), a genetic disorder caused by mutations in the SMN1 gene. While SMN1 is non-functional in SMA patients, they retain a backup gene, SMN2, which primarily produces a truncated, ineffective protein due to faulty splicing. Nusinersen corrects this splicing defect by binding to a specific intronic region of SMN2 pre-mRNA, promoting the inclusion of exon 7 and thereby restoring production of functional SMN protein. Administered via intrathecal injection, nusinersen has been shown to improve motor function and survival, particularly when initiated early. It marked the first approved disease-modifying therapy for SMA and paved the way for RNA-based treatments in neurogenetic disorders.
- **Inclisiran for Hypercholesterolemia:** Inclisiran is a small interfering RNA (siRNA) that targets the mRNA of the PCSK9 gene, which plays a central role in regulating low-density lipoprotein cholesterol (LDL-C) levels. PCSK9 promotes the degradation of LDL receptors on liver cells, reducing the body's ability to clear cholesterol from the bloodstream. By silencing PCSK9 expression, inclisiran increases LDL receptor availability, enhancing cholesterol clearance and significantly lowering LDL-C levels. Administered as a subcutaneous injection every six months, inclisiran offers a convenient and long-lasting lipid-lowering solution, especially for patients who are statin-intolerant or have familial hypercholesterolemia. Its durability and low dosing frequency make it a promising addition to cardiovascular risk management.

4.1.8 Genome Editing Technologies

Genome editing technologies, particularly CRISPR-Cas9, have revolutionized the landscape of molecular medicine by enabling precise, programmable modifications to the DNA sequence within living cells. These tools can introduce targeted insertions, deletions, or substitutions at specific genomic loci, offering the potential to correct disease-causing mutations at their source. CRISPR-Cas9 operates like molecular scissors, guided by a synthetic RNA sequence that directs the Cas9 enzyme to a precise DNA target, where it induces a double-strand break. The cell's natural repair mechanisms then modify the genome, allowing for correction or inactivation of faulty genes. This transformative technology holds promise for treating a wide range of genetic disorders, particularly monogenic diseases, with increasing success in early-phase clinical trials (Fig. 2).

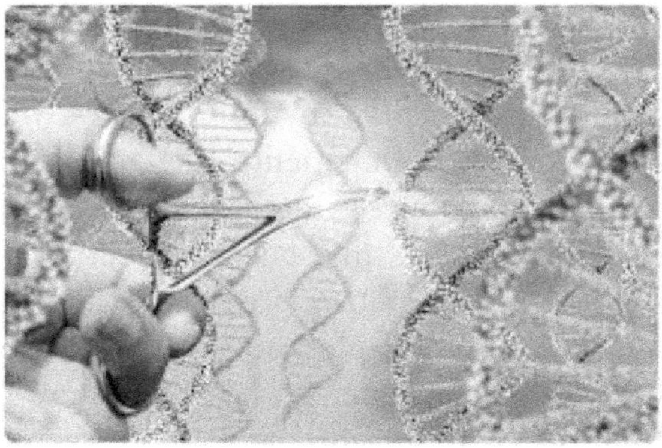

Fig. 2 Types of gene editing

Early clinical applications include:

Treating β-thalassemia and sickle cell disease by editing the BCL11A enhancer.

Ongoing trials for inherited blindness and metabolic disorders.

4.1.9 Companion Diagnostics

Companion diagnostics are specialized laboratory tests developed in parallel with specific genetically targeted therapies to identify patients who are most likely to benefit from a particular drug. These tests detect genetic, molecular, or cellular markers that predict therapeutic response, resistance, or risk of adverse effects. By stratifying patients based on their molecular profile, companion diagnostics ensure that treatments are only administered to those for whom they are safe and effective, thus enhancing precision, improving outcomes, and avoiding unnecessary toxicity or expense. These diagnostics are essential tools in the clinical implementation of personalized medicine and are often required by regulatory agencies for drug approval and use. nIn oncology, companion diagnostics have become a standard component of care. For instance, HER2 testing is mandatory before prescribing trastuzumab in breast cancer, as only tumours that overexpress HER2 are likely to respond. Similarly, EGFR mutation testing is used to guide the use of EGFR inhibitors in lung cancer, and ALK or ROS1 rearrangement tests identify candidates for ALK inhibitors like crizotinib. In other therapeutic areas, testing for HLA-B*57:01 is required before initiating abacavir (to prevent hypersensitivity), and CYP2C9/VKORC1 genotyping is used to optimize warfarin dosing. The integration of companion diagnostics into clinical workflows supports evidence-based decision-making and helps fulfil the promise of delivering the right drug to the right patient at the right time. As genomic and proteomic technologies advance, the development of multiplexed and next-generation sequencing-based diagnostics is expected to expand the utility and accessibility of companion diagnostics across more diseases and therapies. These include:

- **Treating β-Thalassemia and Sickle Cell Disease by Editing the BCL11A Enhancer:** One of the most successful clinical applications of genome editing has been in the treatment of β-thalassemia and sickle cell disease, two inherited blood disorders caused by mutations in the HBB gene, which encodes the β-globin subunit of haemoglobin. Instead of directly correcting the defective gene, researchers use CRISPR-Cas9 to disrupt an enhancer region of the BCL11A gene, a key repressor of fetal haemoglobin (HbF) production. By turning off BCL11A in hematopoietic stem cells, patients begin producing high levels of HbF, which can compensate for the defective adult haemoglobin. Clinical trials have demonstrated that this approach can eliminate the need for blood transfusions or pain crises in most treated patients, offering a potentially curative, one-time therapy.
- **Ongoing Trials for Inherited Blindness and Metabolic Disorders:** CRISPR-based therapies are also being explored for conditions like inherited retinal diseases and rare metabolic disorders. For example, trials are underway to treat Leber congenital amaurosis 10 (LCA10), a form of inherited blindness caused by mutations in the CEP290 gene. In this case, CRISPR components are delivered directly into the retina to correct the faulty gene in situ. Similarly, genome editing is being tested for disorders like phenylketonuria and Gaucher disease, where correcting enzyme deficiencies at the genomic level could restore normal metabolic function. These early trials represent critical milestones, demonstrating both the feasibility and safety of in vivo genome editing and paving the way for broader applications in personalized medicine.

4.1.10 Challenges and Limitations

Despite the transformative potential of genetically targeted therapies, several critical challenges and limitations continue to hinder their widespread implementation and long-term success. These barriers are scientific, economic, ethical, and infrastructural in nature, and addressing them is essential to ensure equitable and effective delivery of personalized treatments.

- **Tumour Heterogeneity Leading to Drug Resistance:** Cancers often consist of multiple subclones with distinct genetic profiles, a phenomenon known as tumour heterogeneity. While targeted therapies may initially be effective against dominant clones, resistant subpopulations can emerge and drive disease relapse. This dynamic evolution of tumours complicates long-term treatment and necessitates ongoing molecular monitoring and combination strategies.
- **Limited Access to Genetic Testing in Resource-Poor Settings:** Access to comprehensive genetic testing remains limited in low- and middle-income

countries due to high costs, lack of infrastructure, and shortage of trained personnel. Without proper diagnostics, patients are unable to benefit from genotype-guided therapies. Bridging this gap requires global investment in testing facilities, training, and affordable technologies.

- **Ethical Concerns Around Gene Editing:** Genome editing technologies like CRISPR-Cas9 raise complex ethical questions, particularly regarding germline modifications that can be inherited by future generations. Concerns about unintended consequences, consent, equity, and the potential for "designer babies" have sparked international debates. Ethical guidelines and oversight are critical to balancing innovation with responsibility.
- **High Cost and Regulatory Hurdles:** Genetically targeted therapies and associated diagnostics are often extremely expensive, limiting affordability and access even in high-income countries. Additionally, navigating regulatory approvals for novel therapies—especially those involving gene editing or cell engineering—is complex and time-consuming. Streamlined regulatory pathways and pricing reforms are essential to scale these innovations sustainably.

4.1.11 Regulatory and Reimbursement Issues

The clinical implementation of genetically targeted therapies is closely tied to regulatory approval and reimbursement decisions, which require rigorous evidence of safety, efficacy, clinical validity, and cost-effectiveness. Regulatory agencies such as the U.S. Food and Drug Administration (FDA) and the European Medicines Agency (EMA) have responded to the complexity and urgency of personalized therapies by establishing accelerated approval pathways. These include designations like "Breakthrough Therapy," "Fast Track," and "Priority Review" in the U.S., which are especially valuable for treatments addressing rare diseases, life-threatening conditions, or unmet medical needs. However, gaining approval still demands robust data from clinical trials, often with biomarker-based patient stratification, which adds layers of design complexity. On the reimbursement side, payers require proof of clinical utility—evidence that the therapy not only works in a controlled setting but also improves patient outcomes and is cost-effective in real-world use. High development costs and specialized delivery methods for many genetically targeted therapies, such as CAR-T cells or gene therapies, lead to exceptionally high price points, posing challenges for insurance coverage and health system budgets. Countries with value-based pricing models or universal healthcare systems often negotiate reimbursement based on outcomes or cost-effectiveness thresholds. For widespread adoption, coordinated efforts between regulators, payers, manufacturers, and healthcare providers are essential to ensure equitable access, sustainability, and responsible innovation.

4.1.12 Future Directions

The future of genetically targeted therapy is poised to become more comprehensive, predictive, and inclusive. Integration of multi-omic data—combining genomic, epigenomic, and transcriptomic profiles—will enable deeper insights into disease mechanisms and personalized treatment strategies. Artificial intelligence (AI) will enhance this process by analysing complex datasets to predict optimal therapies and resistance patterns. The scope of targeted therapies is also expanding beyond rare and cancerous conditions to include common chronic diseases like diabetes and hypertension Furthermore, large-scale genomic studies focused on diverse populations will drive the development of population-specific therapies, address current inequities and improve global healthcare outcomes. The future of genetically targeted therapy includes:

- Multi-omic integration (genomic + epigenomic + transcriptomic profiling).
- AI-based prediction models for therapy selection.
- Expansion into common chronic diseases (e.g., diabetes, hypertension).
- Population-specific therapy development using large-scale genomic datasets.

4.2 IMMUNOTHERAPIES AND PERSONALIZED ONCOLOGY

Immunotherapies have revolutionized cancer treatment by harnessing the body's immune system to recognize and eliminate tumour cells. Unlike traditional chemotherapy, which targets rapidly dividing cells indiscriminately, immunotherapy offers a more selective and dynamic approach. Personalized oncology integrates immunotherapy with molecular profiling to identify which patients are most likely to benefit from treatments such as immune checkpoint inhibitors (e.g., anti-PD-1/PD-L1, CTLA-4 inhibitors), cancer vaccines, and adoptive cell therapies including CAR-T cells. Biomarkers such as tumour mutational burden (TMB), PD-L1 expression, and microsatellite instability (MSI) guide the selection and intensity of immune-based treatments. Furthermore, neoantigen prediction from tumour sequencing allows for the development of patient-specific cancer vaccines. Despite remarkable success in malignancies like melanoma, lung cancer, and lymphoma, not all patients respond. Personalized immunotherapy aims to overcome this limitation by tailoring immune interventions to the tumour's molecular and immunologic landscape, thereby enhancing efficacy and reducing immune-related adverse events.

4.2.1 Distinction from Chemotherapy

Traditional chemotherapy acts by killing all rapidly dividing cells, including cancerous and some healthy cells, which often leads to significant side effects. Immunotherapy, on the other hand, is more selective—it modulates immune pathways and leverages the body's natural defence mechanisms. This results in a different side-effect profile and, in many cases, better tolerability.

4.2.2 Role of Molecular Profiling in Personalized Oncology

Molecular profiling uses genomic, transcriptomic, and proteomic tools to identify unique tumor characteristics. These include somatic mutations, gene expression patterns, and immune markers that can predict response to immunotherapy. Personalized oncology uses this data to match each patient with the most effective and least toxic immune-based treatment.

4.2.3 Immune Checkpoint Inhibitors

Checkpoint inhibitors work by blocking proteins that suppress immune responses, such as PD-1, PD-L1, and CTLA-4. These proteins normally prevent overactivation of T-cells, but in cancer, they are exploited by tumour cells to escape immune detection. Inhibiting these checkpoints "releases the brakes" on the immune system, allowing T-cells to attack tumours effectively. Drugs like pembrolizumab (anti-PD-1) and ipilimumab (anti-CTLA-4) have shown efficacy in melanoma, NSCLC, and RCC.

4.2.4 Cancer Vaccines and Neoantigen Targeting

Cancer vaccines aim to train the immune system to recognize and destroy cancer cells. Personalized cancer vaccines are designed based on neoantigens, which are novel proteins formed due to tumour-specific mutations. By sequencing a patient's tumour and identifying these neoantigens, individualized vaccines can be developed to generate a precise immune attack.

4.2.5 Adoptive Cell Therapies (ACT)

ACT involves extracting immune cells from a patient, modifying or expanding them ex vivo, and reinfusing them to enhance their anti-tumour activity. A prominent example is CAR-T cell therapy, where T-cells are genetically engineered to express receptors targeting specific cancer antigens like CD19 in B-cell leukaemia's and lymphomas. This has led to remarkable remission rates in certain hematologic cancers.

4.2.6 Predictive Biomarkers in Immunotherapy

The success of immunotherapy often depends on certain biomarkers:

- **Tumour Mutational Burden (TMB):** High TMB increases the likelihood of neoantigen formation, improving immunotherapy response.
- **PD-L1 Expression:** Higher expression correlates with better response to PD-1/PD-L1 inhibitors in some cancers.

- **Microsatellite Instability (MSI):** MSI-high status often indicates a favourable response to checkpoint inhibitors, especially in colorectal and endometrial cancers.

4.2.7 Challenges in Immunotherapy

Despite its promise, not all patients respond to immunotherapy. Resistance can arise due to:

- Immunosuppressive tumour microenvironment.
- Low neoantigen load.
- Defective antigen presentation machinery.
- Genetic mutations that affect immune signalling pathways.

4.3 GENE THERAPY AND GENOME EDITING (CRISPR/CAS9)

Gene therapy and genome editing represent transformative approaches to treating inherited and acquired diseases by addressing the root genetic cause rather than managing symptoms. Gene therapies typically involve delivering a functional copy of a defective gene using viral vectors (like AAV or lentivirus), while genome editing—exemplified by CRISPR/Cas9—allows precise, targeted changes to the DNA sequence. These tools have shown success in treating monogenic diseases such as spinal muscular atrophy, β-thalassemia, and sickle cell disease, and hold promise for polygenic disorders and certain cancers. CRISPR-based therapies are under clinical evaluation for correcting gene mutations, disrupting pathogenic genes, or enhancing immune cell function. Genome editing can also be ex vivo, modifying a patient's stem or immune cells outside the body before reinfusion, reducing off-target effects. Despite ethical and technical challenges—like off-target edits, delivery limitations, and regulatory oversight—the potential for durable, even curative outcomes makes gene editing a cornerstone of future precision medicine.

4.3.1 A Paradigm Shift in Medicine

Gene therapy and genome editing have revolutionized biomedical science by shifting the therapeutic paradigm from symptom control to genetic correction. These technologies offer the possibility of one-time, potentially curative treatments, particularly for genetic diseases that were previously considered untreatable or chronic.

4.3.2 Gene Therapy: Replacing Faulty Genes

Gene therapy typically involves delivering a functional version of a mutated gene to compensate for loss of function. This is often achieved using viral vectors such as:

- Adeno-Associated Virus (AAV): Known for stable, long-term gene expression with low immunogenicity.
- Lentivirus: Capable of integrating into host DNA, useful for long-term expression in dividing cells.

Applications include:

- Spinal Muscular Atrophy (SMA) treated with onasemnogene abeparvovec (Zolgensma), delivering SMN1.
- Haemophilia A and B, by delivering clotting factor VIII or IX genes.

4.3.3 Genome Editing: Direct Modification of DNA

Genome editing allows for precise, targeted alterations of the genetic code. The CRISPR/Cas9 system, adapted from bacterial immune defenses, has emerged as the leading genome editing tool. It uses a guide RNA to direct the Cas9 enzyme to a specific DNA sequence, where it can:

- Cut out disease-causing mutations.
- Insert healthy gene sequences.
- Knock down gene expression.

4.3.4 CRISPR/Cas9 in Clinical Medicine

CRISPR-based therapies are in clinical trials for:

- β-thalassemia and Sickle Cell Disease: By disabling the BCL11A gene, foetal haemoglobin production is reactivated.
- Leukaemia and Lymphoma: CRISPR-engineered T cells enhance immune response.
- Inherited blindness: Such as editing the CEP290 gene in Leber congenital amaurosis.

4.3.5 Ex Vivo vs. In Vivo Editing

- **Ex vivo editing:** Cells (e.g., hematopoietic stem cells or T cells) are removed from the body, edited in the lab, and reinfused into the patient. This approach enhances control and reduces unintended systemic effects.
- **In vivo editing:** The genome editing tool is delivered directly into the patient, often through viral vectors or lipid nanoparticles. This method is more technically challenging but enables treatment of tissues not easily accessed ex vivo.

4.3.6 Targeting Monogenic and Polygenic Diseases

While most current applications target monogenic disorders like SMA, SCID, and sickle cell disease, research is expanding to:

- Polygenic disorders (e.g., cardiovascular disease, type 2 diabetes) by modulating gene networks.
- Cancer, through gene editing to engineer immune cells for targeted therapy.

4.3.7 Technical and Ethical Challenges

Major challenges include:

- **Off-target effects:** Unintended edits that could cause harmful mutations.
- **Delivery systems:** Ensuring the editing tool reaches the right cells without degradation or immune reactions.
- **Durability:** Some gene therapies may require re-administration if expression wanes over time.
- **Ethics:** Concerns about germline editing, equitable access, and long-term safety.

4.3.8 Regulatory Landscape

Gene editing therapies face stringent regulatory oversight due to their irreversible nature. Agencies like the FDA and EMA require extensive preclinical data and robust safety mechanisms. Ethical approval and post-treatment surveillance are mandatory, especially for first-in-human studies.

4.3.9 Future Prospects

Future advancements will focus on:

- Base editing and prime editing, which allow even more precise DNA changes without double-strand breaks.
- Non-viral delivery methods, such as nanoparticles or electroporation.
- Scalable manufacturing for broader clinical access.
- Multi-gene modulation using CRISPR multiplexing techniques.

4.4 MRNA THERAPEUTICS AND INDIVIDUALIZED VACCINES

mRNA therapeutics have gained global prominence, especially after the rapid development and deployment of COVID-19 vaccines. These therapies use synthetic messenger RNA to instruct cells to produce specific proteins that trigger immune responses or correct molecular defects. The platform is adaptable, scalable, and can be customized quickly based on a patient's molecular profile, making it ideal for personalized applications. In oncology, individualized mRNA cancer vaccines are being developed using tumour-specific neoantigens identified from the patient's tumour sequencing. These vaccines train the immune system to recognize and destroy cancer cells expressing these unique markers. Beyond vaccines, mRNA is being explored for treating genetic diseases, enzyme deficiencies, and autoimmune conditions by replacing or modulating dysfunctional proteins. Its non-integrative nature avoids the risk of insertional mutagenesis seen in some gene therapies. Continued advancements in lipid nanoparticle delivery systems and stability enhancement are expanding the therapeutic potential of mRNA technology across various disease domains.

4.4.1 The Rise of mRNA Therapeutics

Messenger RNA (mRNA) therapeutics have emerged as a revolutionary platform in modern medicine, gaining international recognition with the success of mRNA-based COVID-19 vaccines. Unlike traditional vaccines or protein-based drugs, mRNA therapies instruct the body's own cells to produce therapeutic proteins, enabling rapid, flexible, and highly targeted treatment options.

4.4.2 Mechanism of Action

mRNA therapeutics involve delivering synthetic mRNA sequences into the body, where cellular machinery translates them into functional proteins. These proteins can:

- Stimulate immune responses (e.g., vaccines).
- Replace missing or defective proteins (e.g., enzyme deficiencies).
- Modulate disease pathways (e.g., suppress autoimmune reactions).

The temporary and non-integrative nature of mRNA avoids permanent genetic alterations, reducing long-term safety concerns.

4.4.3 COVID-19 as a Proof-of-Concept

The global rollout of mRNA vaccines for SARS-CoV-2 (by Pfizer-BioNTech and Moderna) demonstrated the technology's rapid development cycle, efficacy, and safety. This success validated the scalability, adaptability, and potential of mRNA platforms for broader clinical use.

4.4.4 Personalized Cancer Vaccines

In oncology, mRNA is being used to develop individualized cancer vaccines based on each patient's unique tumour profile. Steps include:

- Sequencing the patient's tumour to identify neoantigens (mutated tumour-specific proteins).
- Designing mRNA sequences encoding these neoantigens.
- Injecting the vaccine to train the immune system to detect and destroy tumour cells expressing these antigens.

Such patient-specific vaccines are currently being tested in melanoma, glioblastoma, and lung cancers.

4.4.5 Beyond Oncology- Broader Therapeutic Applications: The utility of mRNA extends to:

- **Genetic diseases (e.g., cystic fibrosis, urea cycle disorders):** by supplying mRNA encoding functional versions of deficient proteins.
- **Enzyme replacement therapy:** avoiding repeated protein infusions.
- **Autoimmune diseases:** modulating immune response through tolerogenic proteins or antigens.

4.4.6 Advantages of mRNA Therapeutics

mRNA therapeutics offer rapid design and manufacturing, making them ideal for timely responses to emerging diseases. Their scalability allows cost-effective production across diverse applications. Because mRNA does not integrate into the genome, it presents a favourable safety profile with minimal long-term risks. Additionally, the technology supports high customizability, enabling treatments tailored to individual genetic and molecular profiles. This versatility positions mRNA as a key tool in personalized medicine.

- **Speed and Flexibility:** mRNA sequences can be designed and manufactured quickly.
- **Scalability:** Once delivery systems are optimized, production is cost-effective and adaptable to various targets.
- **Safety:** Non-integrative, transient expression reduces the risk of insertional mutagenesis or permanent off-target effects.
- **Customizability:** Enables personalized treatment tailored to individual genomic or proteomic data.

4.4.7 Delivery Systems and Stability Challenges

A major challenge in mRNA therapeutics is the effective and safe delivery of fragile mRNA molecules into target cells. Lipid nanoparticles (LNPs) are the most widely used carriers, encapsulating mRNA to facilitate cellular uptake and endosomal escape. However, mRNA is inherently unstable and prone to rapid degradation by extracellular and intracellular nucleases, which can severely limit its therapeutic window. Additionally, unmodified mRNA can trigger strong innate immune responses, potentially reduce efficacy and cause inflammation. To address these issues, scientists have developed chemically modified nucleosides that enhance mRNA stability, improve translation efficiency, and reduce immunogenicity. Advances in LNP formulation—including ionizable lipids, polyethylene glycol (PEG) coatings, and optimized particle size—are significantly improving delivery precision, biodistribution, and tolerability. These innovations are critical to realizing the full potential of mRNA technology across diverse therapeutic areas, from infectious disease vaccines to personalized cancer immunotherapy and rare genetic disorders.

Key technical hurdles include:

- Ensuring efficient delivery into cells, typically through lipid nanoparticles (LNPs).
- Protecting mRNA from rapid degradation by nucleases.
- Enhancing translation efficiency and reducing innate immune activation.

Recent innovations in LNP formulation and mRNA chemistry (e.g., modified nucleosides) are overcoming these limitations, improving safety and efficacy.

4.4.8 Regulatory and Manufacturing Considerations

Regulatory pathways for mRNA therapies are still evolving, but lessons from COVID-19 have prompted fast-tracking mechanisms. Manufacturing challenges—such as ensuring purity, sterility, and quality control of RNA formulations—are being addressed through standardization and automation.

4.4.9 Future Directions

The future of mRNA technology is expanding rapidly, driven by innovations that promise broader applications and improved therapeutic outcomes. Self-amplifying RNA (saRNA) platforms are being developed to boost protein expression from lower doses, enhancing potency while reducing costs. In oncology, multiepitope cancer vaccines aim to target multiple tumour-associated antigens simultaneously, improving immune recognition and reducing the risk of escape mutations. mRNA cocktails are also emerging to address polygenic or multifactorial diseases like cardiovascular and neurodegenerative disorders by encoding multiple therapeutic targets within a single treatment. Integration with artificial intelligence (AI) is accelerating personalized therapy design by analysing multi-omic datasets—genomic, proteomic, and transcriptomic—to predict optimal antigen targets or therapeutic proteins. These advancements are positioning mRNA therapeutics as a flexible, data-driven cornerstone of future personalized medicine.

Advances in mRNA technology are moving toward:

- Self-amplifying RNA (saRNA) platforms for stronger effects at lower doses.
- Multiepitope vaccines targeting various stages of tumour progression.
- mRNA cocktails for polygenic or multifactorial diseases.
- Integration with AI to optimize vaccine and therapy design using omic data.

4.5 DRUG REPURPOSING BASED ON PATIENT PROFILES

Drug repurposing, or repositioning, involves identifying new therapeutic uses for existing drugs based on a patient's genetic, proteomic, or phenotypic profile. This approach offers a cost-effective and time-efficient path to personalized medicine, as repurposed drugs have already passed major safety trials. With the help of bioinformatics, AI, and multi-omic data integration, researchers can match existing drugs to off-label indications where molecular mechanisms overlap. For instance, cancer patients with specific mutations may benefit from drugs originally developed for unrelated conditions that target the same pathway. Additionally, pharmacogenomic profiling can reveal which patients might respond to repurposed drugs with minimal toxicity. This strategy is particularly valuable for rare diseases and in resource-limited settings were access to novel, expensive treatments may be restricted. By leveraging existing pharmacological tools in a precision-guided manner, drug repurposing enhances therapeutic options while reducing development risk and cost.

4.5.1 Concept and Rationale

Drug repurposing involves finding new therapeutic applications for existing drugs outside their original approved indications. This strategy capitalizes on prior knowledge of a drug's safety, pharmacodynamics, and pharmacokinetics, drastically reducing time and cost compared to developing new drugs from scratch. Personalized medicine enhances this approach by aligning drug mechanisms with individual patient profiles.

4.5.2 Integration with Patient Profiles

Modern repurposing efforts are increasingly guided by genetic, proteomic, and phenotypic data. By analysing a patient's unique molecular signature—such as gene mutations, protein expression levels, or metabolic patterns—clinicians can identify repurposed drugs that are likely to be effective. This personalization improves treatment precision and minimizes the risk of adverse effects.

4.5.3 Role of Bioinformatics and Artificial Intelligence

Bioinformatics tools and AI-driven platforms mine vast biomedical databases to uncover molecular overlaps between diseases and drug action profiles. Algorithms analyse drug-target interactions, gene expression networks, and signalling pathways to identify potential off-label uses that match the molecular basis of a patient's disease.

4.5.4 Application in Oncology

Cancer treatment has seen major advances through drug repurposing. For example, drugs developed for inflammatory diseases or metabolic syndromes have been redirected to target cancers with shared molecular pathways, such as PI3K/Akt/mTOR or JAK-STAT signalling. Mutation-specific targeting allows for highly individualized regimens using already-approved medications.

4.5.5 Pharmacogenomics-Guided Repurposing

Pharmacogenomic data enables prediction of individual responses to repurposed drugs. For instance, a patient with a CYP2D6 poor metabolizer genotype might avoid drugs that require that pathway, while benefiting from alternatives previously approved for other uses. This genetic tailoring increases therapeutic efficacy and safety.

4.5.6 Benefits for Rare and Neglected Diseases

Rare diseases often lack dedicated drug development due to small market size. Drug repurposing provides an efficient solution by identifying existing agents with relevant biological activity. This is especially critical in low-income regions or for ultra-rare conditions where cost and accessibility are major barriers.

4.5.7 Economic and Regulatory Advantages

Repurposed drugs bypass early-phase safety trials, speeding their path to market. Regulatory agencies like the FDA and EMA have created frameworks to fast-track such applications, especially when addressing unmet clinical needs. This reduces both development timelines and financial risk for pharmaceutical companies.

5 Chapter DATA SCIENCE AND AI IN PERSONALIZED MEDICINE

5.0 INTRODUCTION: AN OVERVIEW

The integration of data science and artificial intelligence (AI) into personalized medicine marks a transformative shift in modern healthcare. As genomic sequencing, wearable devices, electronic health records (EHRs), and other technologies generate vast volumes of complex and heterogeneous data, conventional analytical tools have proven inadequate for deriving clinically actionable insights. Data science, encompassing techniques such as machine learning, statistical modelling, data mining, and pattern recognition, provides the computational power and methodological framework to manage, interpret, and visualize multi-dimensional data across diverse populations. AI, particularly through deep learning and natural language processing (NLP), can identify hidden patterns in genetic, epigenetic, proteomic, metabolomic, clinical, lifestyle, and environmental data that are often imperceptible to human experts. This convergence of technologies allows for the construction of predictive models capable of forecasting disease risk, treatment response, drug toxicity, and patient outcomes at an individualized level. One of the most significant impacts of AI and data science in personalized medicine lies in the realm of diagnosis and prognosis. Algorithms can analyse imaging data (radiomics), histopathology slides (digital pathology), and lab reports to detect early signs of disease, classify subtypes, and estimate progression more accurately than conventional methods. In oncology, AI helps in stratifying patients based on tumour genomics and guides selection of targeted therapies, immunotherapies, or clinical trial enrolment. In pharmacogenomics, AI models can predict drug metabolism and adverse reactions by integrating genomic variants with demographic and clinical data, optimizing dosage and therapeutic choices. Moreover, data-driven insights from AI help decipher polygenic risk scores and gene-environment interactions, enabling personalized prevention strategies for common diseases like diabetes, cardiovascular disorders, and Alzheimer's disease.

Data science also enables the development of digital twins—virtual replicas of individual patients—that simulate disease trajectories and test different treatment strategies in silico. These predictive models offer a risk-free environment for physicians to experiment with interventions before applying them to real patients. In public health and epidemiology, AI-based analytics facilitate the tracking of disease outbreaks, identification of vulnerable subgroups, and allocation of healthcare resources based on precision risk assessments. Moreover, wearable devices and mobile health apps powered by AI collect real-time physiological data (e.g., heart rate, glucose levels, sleep cycles), enabling continuous monitoring and early detection of anomalies. When combined with behavioural and lifestyle data, such tools support personalized wellness programs and chronic disease management. However, the widespread adoption of AI in personalized medicine presents notable challenges. These include data privacy and security, especially when dealing with sensitive genomic and health information; algorithmic bias, which can reinforce existing healthcare disparities; and lack of transparency, as many AI models operate as "black boxes" with limited interpretability. Furthermore, integration into clinical workflows remains a bottleneck, requiring robust validation, regulatory approval, clinician training, and ethical oversight. Interdisciplinary collaboration between data scientists, clinicians, bioinformaticians, ethicists, and policymakers is essential to ensure that AI tools are both scientifically rigorous and socially responsible. Data science and AI are not merely augmenting personalized medicine—they are foundational to its future. By enabling the transition from descriptive to predictive and prescriptive healthcare, these technologies offer unprecedented opportunities to shift the clinical paradigm from reactive treatment to proactive, precise, and preventive care. As computational power, data accessibility, and algorithmic sophistication continue to evolve, the vision of truly individualized medicine—where every decision is informed by deep, data-driven understanding of the person—moves from aspiration to clinical reality (Fig. 1).

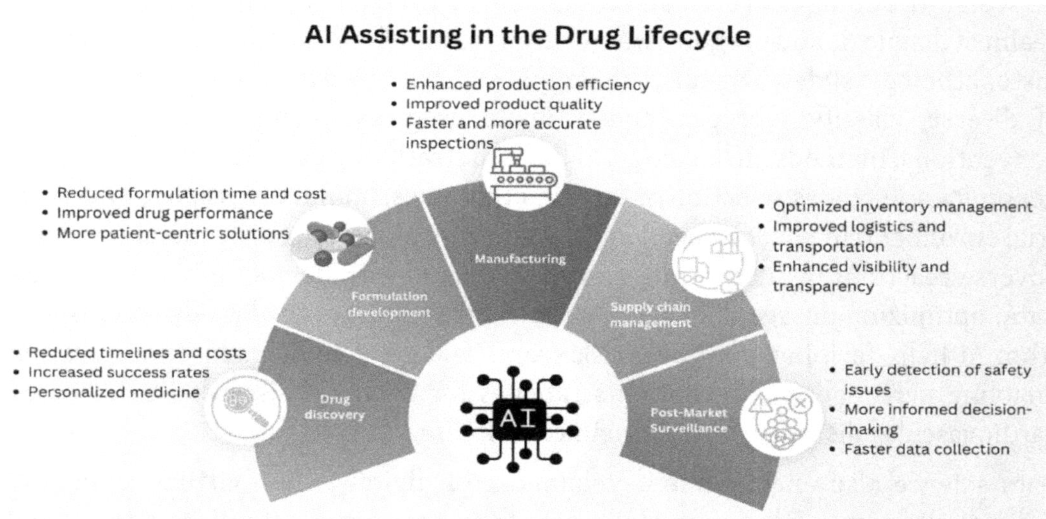

Fig. 1 AI Assisting in the Drug Lifecycle

5.1 BIG DATA IN HEALTH: EHRS, OMICS, AND REAL-WORLD DATA

5.1.1 Introduction to Big Data in Health

Big data in healthcare refers to the massive volume of complex, diverse, and high-velocity datasets generated from various sources such as genomics, clinical practice, wearable sensors, and patient behaviours. These datasets are characterized by the "5 Vs": volume, variety, velocity, veracity, and value. Their integration is central to personalized medicine, enabling insights into disease mechanisms, drug responses, and population health trends that were previously inaccessible. The ability to analyse and extract meaningful patterns from big data is revolutionizing how we diagnose, treat, and prevent diseases.

5.1.2 Electronic Health Records (EHRs)

Electronic Health Records (EHRs) serve as comprehensive digital repositories of patient health information, offering a longitudinal view of an individual's medical history. They encompass structured data such as diagnoses, medication lists, lab results, radiology images, and vital signs, as well as unstructured data like clinical notes and discharge summaries. EHRs improve clinical decision-making by providing real-time access to patient data, reducing duplication of tests, and enabling better care coordination across providers. In personalized medicine, EHRs help link clinical phenotypes with genomic or molecular profiles, supporting predictive analytics and tailored treatment plans. Integration with decision support tools enables risk stratification and alerts for adverse drug interactions. When combined with machine learning, EHRs can uncover hidden patterns to predict disease trajectories or treatment outcomes. However, challenges like interoperability between systems, data standardization, and privacy concerns remain significant. Despite these, EHRs are a foundational asset in leveraging big data for precision healthcare. They form a foundational component of health-related big data. EHRs enable:

- **Population-wide analysis of disease trends, treatment efficacy, and health outcomes:** Big data from EHRs allows researchers and clinicians to study large populations over time, revealing patterns in disease incidence, progression, and response to treatment. This population-scale insight helps identify disparities in healthcare delivery, evaluate real-world effectiveness of interventions, and guide policy-making. For example, trends in diabetes or cancer survival can be monitored across demographics or regions. Such analyses are crucial for public health surveillance, optimizing resource allocation, and designing preventive strategies. They also enable benchmarking across institutions, promoting evidence-based practice improvements.

- **Machine learning applications to predict disease risk, hospital readmissions, or optimal treatment pathways:** Machine learning algorithms trained on EHR and omics data can predict individual patient outcomes such as disease onset, complications, or readmission risks. These predictive models help clinicians intervene earlier, improving patient care and reducing costs. For instance, algorithms can forecast sepsis risk in hospitalized patients or recommend chemotherapy regimens based on genetic profiles. They also support clinical decision-making by identifying personalized treatment strategies with higher success rates. As models learn from continuously updated data, their accuracy and utility improve over time.
- **Natural Language Processing (NLP) to extract unstructured data from clinical notes and discharge summaries:** LP enables the analysis of narrative text in EHRs—such as doctor's notes, pathology reports, or discharge summaries—which often contain vital clinical information not captured in structured fields. By converting unstructured language into computable data, NLP facilitates richer and more accurate patient profiling. For example, it can detect undocumented adverse drug reactions, patient-reported symptoms, or social determinants of health. NLP enhances data completeness and depth, feeding downstream analytics or AI models with valuable insights. This improves both clinical care and research applications.

5.1.3 Omics Data (Genomics, Transcriptomics, Proteomics, Metabolomics)

Omics data offer comprehensive insights into the molecular mechanisms underlying health and disease by examining biological systems at various levels. Genomics reveals DNA-level variations such as SNPs or structural mutations, while transcriptomics studies RNA expression patterns that reflect gene activity. Proteomics analyses the structure, function, and interactions of proteins, the key effectors of cellular processes. Metabolomics focuses on metabolic products, offering a dynamic snapshot of physiological states. Together, these datasets create a holistic picture of the individual's biology. When integrated, they improve disease prediction, diagnosis, and personalized treatment strategies. This multi-omic approach is foundational to precision medicine. Key components include:

- **Genomics:** DNA sequencing data to identify variants associated with disease risk or drug response.
- **Transcriptomics:** RNA expression profiles to understand gene activity in specific conditions or tissues.
- **Proteomics:** Analysis of protein abundance, structure, and function for identifying disease biomarkers.

- **Metabolomics:** Profiling small molecules and metabolites that reflect cellular processes and physiological status. Omics technologies generate vast datasets that require sophisticated bioinformatics tools for storage, normalization, integration, and interpretation. Their value in personalized medicine lies in uncovering patient-specific molecular signatures that guide precision therapies.

5.1.4 Real-World Data (RWD)

Real-world data (RWD) are collected from sources such as electronic health records, insurance claims, patient registries, and wearable devices, offering insights beyond the controlled environments of clinical trials. These data capture the diversity of patient populations, treatment patterns, and health outcomes in everyday settings. RWD helps identify real-world effectiveness, safety signals, and unmet medical needs. It plays a critical role in health economics, regulatory decisions, and personalized care strategies. By reflecting true patient experiences, RWD complements clinical trial findings and enhances evidence-based medicine.

Sources include:

- Claims and billing data from insurance providers.
- Data from wearable devices (e.g., fitness trackers, continuous glucose monitors).
- Mobile health apps and patient-reported outcomes.
- Registries and biobanks tracking large cohorts over time. RWD helps evaluate treatment effectiveness in diverse populations, identify rare adverse events, and support regulatory decision-making. It is increasingly used to design real-world evidence (RWE) studies and to validate findings from randomized controlled trials in practical, real-life settings.

5.1.5 Integration and Interoperability

A major challenge and opportunity in big data-driven health is data integration across EHRs, omics platforms, and RWD sources. Achieving interoperability enables comprehensive patient profiles and allows cross-institutional studies. Standards such as HL7 FHIR, OMOP, and GA4GH frameworks support structured data exchange. Integration facilitates multi-omic analyses, linking molecular data to clinical phenotypes, and drives systems biology approaches to understanding complex diseases.

5.1.6 Ethical and Privacy Considerations

The integration of big data into healthcare brings significant ethical and privacy challenges that demand careful consideration. As health data are increasingly used beyond their original purpose, issues such as informed consent, re-identification risks, and data ownership have come to the forefront. There is growing concern about algorithmic bias and fairness, especially when datasets lack representation from diverse populations. Vulnerable groups, including indigenous communities, face heightened risks related to data misuse and sovereignty. To address these challenges, robust governance frameworks and privacy-preserving technologies like federated learning and differential privacy are being developed. Ensuring ethical data use is essential for building trust in digital health systems.

The use of big data in health raises critical ethical issues, including:

- Informed consent for secondary data use.
- De-identification and re-identification risks.
- Bias and fairness, especially when datasets are not representative of diverse populations.
- Ownership and data sovereignty, particularly with indigenous or marginalized groups. Governance frameworks and secure computing environments (e.g., federated learning, differential privacy) are being developed to address these concerns.

5.1.7 Impact on Personalized Medicine

Big data has transformed personalized medicine by enabling precision at scale through the integration of electronic health records (EHRs), omics data, and real-world evidence. This holistic approach allows clinicians to predict disease risks early, customize treatments based on individual biological and lifestyle profiles, and monitor responses in real time. Continuous feedback from patient data supports dynamic, adaptive interventions that evolve with the patient's condition. As a result, healthcare is shifting from reactive to proactive, from broad-based to individualized, and from occasional interventions to continuous, data-informed care.

Big data enables precision at scale. By combining EHRs, omics, and RWD, clinicians can:

- Predict disease risk before symptoms appear.
- Tailor treatment based on genetic, clinical, and behavioural factors.
- Monitor therapeutic response continuously.
- Adapt interventions dynamically in response to patient data. This data-driven paradigm shifts medicine from reactive to proactive, from generalized to individualized, and from episodic to continuous care.

5.2 MACHINE LEARNING FOR RISK PREDICTION AND TREATMENT OPTIMIZATION

Machine learning (ML), a dynamic subfield of artificial intelligence, is revolutionizing healthcare by empowering data-driven, predictive, and personalized decision-making. Unlike traditional statistical methods, ML algorithms are designed to learn from complex, high-dimensional datasets without explicit programming, making them well-suited for the intricacies of biological systems. In the realm of personalized medicine, ML harnesses diverse data sources—including electronic health records, genomic profiles, imaging, wearable sensor data, and patient-reported outcomes—to identify patterns and associations that might elude human analysis. This enables the early detection of disease, prediction of individual risk trajectories, and precise tailoring of therapeutic strategies. Whether through classifying disease subtypes, predicting treatment response, or optimizing medication dosing, ML is reshaping clinical workflows and medical research. Moreover, its ability to continuously improve with new data facilitates adaptive care models that evolve in real time. As the volume and complexity of healthcare data grow, ML stands at the forefront of enabling proactive, individualized, and efficient healthcare delivery.

5.2.1 Machine Learning in Healthcare

Machine learning involves training algorithms to learn from data and make predictions or decisions without being explicitly programmed. In healthcare, ML utilizes diverse datasets—ranging from genomic sequences to clinical notes—to identify patterns, trends, and predictive markers. Its adaptability makes it ideal for dynamic and complex biological systems.

5.2.2 Risk Prediction and Early Detection

ML models can analyse longitudinal data from electronic health records (EHRs), genomics, and lifestyle variables to predict an individual's risk of developing diseases before symptoms arise. For example, ML-based polygenic risk scores can estimate the likelihood of conditions like diabetes, cardiovascular disease, or cancer. Predictive tools allow for earlier screening, preventive strategies, and lifestyle modifications.

5.2.3 Stratification and Phenotyping

Machine learning aids in the stratification of patients into subgroups based on disease severity, genetic makeup, or treatment response. Unsupervised algorithms like clustering can uncover hidden phenotypes within diseases—such as identifying distinct subtypes of asthma or depression—which may respond differently to treatments. This enhances diagnostic precision and therapeutic targeting.

5.2.4 Treatment Optimization and Decision Support

ML algorithms can analyse patient-specific data to recommend optimal therapies, dosages, or interventions. For instance, supervised learning models can predict which chemotherapy protocol is most likely to succeed for a cancer patient based on tumour genomics. Clinical decision support systems (CDSS) powered by ML assist physicians in real-time, minimizing trial-and-error in treatment selection.

5.2.5 Adaptive Learning and Continuous Improvement

Unlike static models, some machine learning systems are designed to continuously learn from new patient data. This allows models to adapt to changing populations, medical practices, or emerging health threats. Reinforcement learning approaches can optimize treatment sequences, as seen in personalized radiotherapy schedules or chronic disease management plans.

5.2.6 Integration with Multimodal Data

ML is uniquely capable of integrating and interpreting diverse data types—structured (lab values), semi-structured (EHRs), and unstructured (imaging, clinician notes). This multimodal integration provides a comprehensive view of patient health, facilitating holistic risk assessment and personalized care plans.

5.2.7 Examples and Case Studies:

- **Cardiology:** ML predicts heart failure readmission risk using EHR and wearable data.
- **Oncology:** ML-driven tumour classification based on histopathological and genomic features improves treatment precision.
- **Psychiatry:** Predictive models identify individuals at risk of developing schizophrenia or depression based on early-life data and neuroimaging.

5.2.8 Challenges and Limitations

While promising, ML in healthcare faces challenges such as data quality, algorithmic bias, model interpretability, and generalizability across populations. Models trained on non-representative data may produce skewed results, raising concerns about fairness and equity.

5.2.9 Ethical and Regulatory Considerations

Use of ML in risk prediction and treatment selection raises ethical issues, including transparency, accountability, and informed consent. Regulatory agencies like the FDA are working toward frameworks for approving and monitoring AI-based clinical tools to ensure patient safety (Table-1).

Table:1 Concise summary of Machine Learning for Risk Prediction and Treatment Optimization

S.No.	Title	Summary
1	Machine Learning in Healthcare	ML learns from health data (genomics, clinical notes, etc.) to detect patterns and make informed predictions, ideal for complex biological systems.
2	Risk Prediction and Early Detection	ML predicts disease risk from EHRs, genomics, and lifestyle data, enabling early screening and preventive care.
3	Stratification and Phenotyping	ML groups patients into subtypes based on disease traits, improving diagnosis and treatment targeting.
4	Treatment Optimization and Decision Support	ML personalizes therapy by recommending optimal drugs and doses using patient-specific data; supports clinicians via CDSS.
5	Adaptive Learning and Continuous Improvement	ML models evolve over time with new data, adapting to changing populations and treatment trends through reinforcement learning.
6	Integration with Multimodal Data	ML integrates structured, semi-structured, and unstructured data for comprehensive health assessments.
7	Examples and Case Studies	Cardiology, oncology, and psychiatry show real-world ML use for risk prediction, tumour classification, and mental health assessment.
8	Challenges and Limitations	Issues include data bias, poor generalizability, and lack of interpretability, which can affect model reliability and fairness.
9	Ethical and Regulatory Considerations	Ethical concerns include consent, bias, and transparency; regulatory bodies are establishing guidelines for safe ML adoption in healthcare.

5.3 DECISION SUPPORT SYSTEMS IN CLINICAL SETTINGS

Clinical Decision Support Systems (CDSS) are intelligent digital platforms that assist healthcare professionals in making accurate, timely, and evidence-based clinical decisions. By integrating patient-specific information—such as laboratory results, imaging data, genomics, and medical history—with established clinical guidelines and real-time analytics, CDSS provide actionable insights at the point of care. These systems support a range of functions, from diagnostic suggestions and drug interaction alerts to risk stratification and treatment optimization. In the context of personalized medicine, CDSS play a critical role in translating complex data into individualized care plans, minimizing trial-and-error approaches, and improving therapeutic outcomes. They also reduce clinician burden by streamlining workflows and enhancing consistency in decision-making. As healthcare shifts toward precision, prevention, and value-based care, CDSS are emerging as essential components of digital health infrastructure, fostering safer, more effective, and patient-centred practices.

5.3.1 Components of a CDSS

A typical CDSS includes:

- **Knowledge Base:** A repository of clinical guidelines, protocols, and medical literature.
- **Inference Engine:** The logic processor that applies rules or algorithms to patient data.
- **User Interface:** The platform through which clinicians interact with the system (e.g., dashboards, alerts, recommendations).

5.3.2 Types of CDSS

- **Rule-Based Systems:** Rule-based systems are among the earliest forms of CDSS and operate using predefined IF-THEN logic. These systems apply established clinical guidelines or expert knowledge to generate alerts or recommendations. For example, they may trigger an alert if a patient is prescribed two medications known to interact adversely. Rule-based CDSS are straightforward to design, easy to interpret, and reliable when the clinical scenarios are well understood. They are particularly effective for tasks like drug allergy checks, dosage adjustments, and protocol compliance reminders. However, their rigidity limits adaptability in complex or novel clinical situations. Since they do not learn from new data, they require constant manual updates to stay current with evolving medical knowledge.
- **Machine Learning-Based Systems:** Machine learning-based CDSS represent a more advanced and adaptive class of systems that learn patterns from large volumes of clinical data. These tools can identify subtle, non-linear relationships that human clinicians or rule-based systems may miss. For example, ML models can predict the onset of sepsis or the likelihood of hospital readmission by analysing trends across a patient's vitals, lab values, and historical data. They can continuously improve their performance with new data, making them highly scalable and robust in dynamic clinical environments. Their predictive capabilities support proactive interventions, enabling early diagnosis and targeted treatment. However, challenges remain in interpretability, bias mitigation, and integration into clinical workflows.
- **Diagnostic Aids:** Diagnostic aid systems assist clinicians in identifying potential diseases based on input symptoms, patient history, and diagnostic test results. They use decision trees, Bayesian reasoning, or AI algorithms to

generate ranked differential diagnoses. Such tools are especially useful in complex or rare cases where diagnostic uncertainty is high. By suggesting overlooked possibilities, diagnostic aids can reduce diagnostic errors and support less-experienced practitioners. Some systems also integrate imaging or pathology data to enhance diagnostic accuracy. While not intended to replace clinical judgment, they augment physician decision-making by ensuring that critical possibilities are considered. These systems are becoming increasingly valuable in emergency and primary care settings.

- **Therapeutic Advisors:** Therapeutic advisor systems recommend personalized treatment plans by analysing patient-specific data such as genetic information, disease subtypes, comorbidities, and drug response profiles. For instance, they can suggest targeted cancer therapies based on tumour genomics or optimize anticoagulant dosing based on pharmacogenomic markers. These systems synthesize evidence-based guidelines, clinical trial data, and real-world evidence to tailor interventions to individual needs. They support shared decision-making by presenting benefits, risks, and alternatives in a structured format. Therapeutic advisors are essential in personalized medicine, where treatment efficacy and safety can vary widely across patients. Their ability to deliver context-sensitive recommendations significantly enhances treatment precision and patient outcomes.

5.3.3 Integration with Electronic Health Records (EHRs)

Modern Clinical Decision Support Systems (CDSS) are increasingly embedded within Electronic Health Record (EHR) platforms, creating a unified ecosystem for data-driven clinical care. This integration enables real-time access to a patient's comprehensive health profile—including lab test results, medication history, allergies, vital signs, imaging reports, and clinician notes. By operating within the same digital environment that providers use daily, CDSS can deliver context-aware alerts, reminders, and recommendations precisely when and where they are needed. This reduces the need for clinicians to switch between systems, enhancing workflow efficiency and reducing cognitive load. For example, a CDSS can automatically flag a high-risk drug interaction as a prescription is being written or suggest a diagnostic test based on abnormal lab trends. Seamless integration also supports longitudinal monitoring, enabling better tracking of disease progression and response to treatment. Ultimately, embedding CDSS within EHRs strengthens clinical decision-making, reduces medical errors, and enhances the quality and safety of patient care.

5.3.4 Applications in Personalized Medicine

Clinical Decision Support Systems (CDSS) are central to the implementation of personalized medicine by enabling care that is precisely tailored to an individual's unique genetic, clinical, and lifestyle characteristics. One key application is genomic decision support, where CDSS integrates pharmacogenomic data to guide drug selection and dosing, helping avoid adverse reactions and enhance therapeutic efficacy. In oncology, CDSS can match patients with targeted therapies based on tumour biomarkers, histopathological data, and molecular profiling, ensuring the most effective treatment for their cancer subtype. For chronic disease management, CDSS leverages real-time patient monitoring data—such as glucose levels, blood pressure, and physical activity—from wearables or remote sensors to recommend lifestyle interventions, medication changes, or follow-up testing. These systems synthesize vast amounts of individual-level data to deliver insights at the point of care, promoting early interventions, improving outcomes, and reducing unnecessary treatments. By supporting truly data-driven decisions, CDSS are transforming healthcare from reactive to proactive, and from standardized to deeply personalized.

5.3.5 Benefits of CDSS

Clinical Decision Support Systems (CDSS) offer a wide array of benefits that significantly improve the quality, safety, and efficiency of healthcare delivery. One of the primary advantages is their ability to enhance diagnostic accuracy by providing evidence-based suggestions, cross-referencing patient data, and highlighting potential errors or oversights. This helps in reducing misdiagnoses and ensuring that critical conditions are identified promptly. CDSS also play a vital role in reinforcing adherence to clinical guidelines and standard treatment protocols, thereby promoting consistent and high-quality care across different providers and settings. By continuously analysing patient data, CDSS can support the early detection of adverse drug reactions, deteriorating vitals, or complications, allowing for timely interventions. These systems contribute to better patient outcomes by ensuring personalized, data-informed decisions that align with current best practices. Additionally, CDSS alleviate the cognitive burden on clinicians by filtering relevant information and reducing information overload, which minimizes decision fatigue. They streamline clinical workflows, save time, and foster greater clinician confidence. Collectively, these benefits contribute to higher patient satisfaction, improved operational efficiency, and a more proactive, patient-centred approach to care.

5.3.6 Real-World Examples

Several advanced Clinical Decision Support Systems are already in use, demonstrating the real-world potential of data-driven healthcare. IBM Watson for

Oncology is a leading example that uses artificial intelligence to analyse a patient's clinical, genetic, and diagnostic data, comparing it with vast medical literature to recommend personalized cancer treatments. It helps oncologists identify the most suitable therapy options based on tumour characteristics and global treatment guidelines. Another widely adopted tool is Epic's Best Practice Advisory, which is integrated into the Epic EHR system. It provides real-time alerts and clinical recommendations for high-risk patients, such as flagging abnormal vital signs or lab values that meet predefined thresholds, ensuring prompt intervention. MedWise CDSS is specifically focused on pharmacotherapy and uses advanced pharmacokinetic modelling to predict and prevent adverse drug interactions, especially in polypharmacy cases. By assessing how drugs interact within an individual's system, it helps optimize medication regimens and safeguard patient safety. These examples reflect how CDSS is actively enhancing personalized care, clinical efficiency, and patient safety across diverse healthcare settings.

5.3.7 Limitations and Challenges

- **Alert Fatigue:** Alert fatigue occurs when clinicians are overwhelmed by frequent, repetitive, or low-value notifications generated by CDSS. When systems issue excessive alerts—many of which may be clinically irrelevant or redundant—healthcare providers may become desensitized, leading to important alerts being ignored or overridden. This undermines the system's intent to improve safety and may increase the risk of missed diagnoses or medication errors. The balance between sensitivity and specificity is critical to maintaining the utility of alerts. Customizable alert thresholds, context-aware notifications, and tiered alert systems can help mitigate fatigue. Without proper alert management, even well-designed CDSS may become counterproductive.
- **Data Quality:** The effectiveness of any CDSS depends heavily on the quality of the data it processes. Incomplete, outdated, or incorrect data—whether from electronic health records, lab reports, or user input—can significantly compromise the accuracy of recommendations. For instance, missing allergy information might lead to inappropriate drug suggestions. Additionally, variability in documentation practices and coding standards further complicates data reliability. CDSS must be supported by robust data governance, validation protocols, and real-time updating mechanisms. High-quality, standardized, and interoperable data are foundational to ensuring the system produces safe and clinically relevant outcomes.
- **Interoperability:** Interoperability refers to the ability of CDSS to integrate and function seamlessly across different health information systems, devices, and platforms. In reality, many healthcare settings

use heterogeneous technologies that lack standardized interfaces or data formats. This makes integration challenging and may limit the CDSS's ability to access comprehensive patient information. Without full interoperability, the system's recommendations may be based on partial data, reducing accuracy and clinical value. Efforts like HL7 FHIR (Fast Healthcare Interoperability Resources) aim to address these gaps, but widespread adoption remains a work in progress. True interoperability is essential for scalable and effective CDSS implementation.

- **Usability Issues:** Poorly designed user interfaces can hinder the adoption and effectiveness of CDSS tools. If the system is unintuitive, cluttered, or difficult to navigate, clinicians may resist its use or misuse its recommendations. Usability issues can also disrupt workflow efficiency, increasing time per patient and contributing to clinician burnout. A successful CDSS must align with the natural clinical workflow, offer intuitive navigation, and present insights clearly and concisely. Involving end-users—physicians, nurses, and other care providers—in the design and testing phases can greatly improve usability. A well-designed interface is critical for clinician acceptance, trust, and sustained use in daily practice.

5.3.8 Ethical and Legal Considerations:

The integration of Clinical Decision Support Systems (CDSS) into clinical practice raises a complex set of ethical and legal challenges that must be addressed to ensure responsible use. One of the foremost concerns is liability—when clinicians rely on CDSS recommendations, determining who is accountable in the event of an adverse outcome becomes murky. While physicians are ultimately responsible for clinical decisions, the growing reliance on algorithm-driven suggestions creates potential legal ambiguity, especially if the recommendation contradicts human judgment or accepted guidelines.

Another major concern is data privacy. CDSS depend on sensitive patient information, including genetic, behavioural, and clinical data, to function effectively. Ensuring that this data is collected, stored, and processed securely—while complying with laws such as HIPAA, GDPR, and emerging national privacy frameworks—is crucial. Improper handling or breaches of data can have serious legal and reputational consequences. Transparency and explainability are also ethical imperatives. Many advanced CDSS, especially those using machine learning, operate as "black boxes" with limited insight into how decisions are made. This lack of interpretability undermines trust and makes it difficult for clinicians to justify decisions to patients or regulators. Clear documentation, validation studies, and explainable AI techniques are essential to foster clinician confidence and support patient-centred care.

Further, bias and fairness must be addressed. If the training data for CDSS is skewed or non-representative, it can lead to biased recommendations, potentially exacerbating health disparities. Ethical implementation requires continuous evaluation to ensure equity across gender, ethnicity, and socioeconomic groups.

5.4 DIGITAL TWINS AND SIMULATION MODELS

Digital twins and simulation models are cutting-edge technologies revolutionizing personalized medicine. By creating dynamic, virtual replicas of individuals or biological systems, these tools allow for testing, prediction, and optimization of health interventions in a risk-free digital environment.

A digital twin is a virtual model of a real-world system—in healthcare, it typically represents a patient's physiology, anatomy, or disease trajectory. It is continuously updated with real-time data from sensors, wearables, electronic health records (EHRs), and other health sources, enabling a living, evolving digital representation of the individual.

5.4.1 Concept of Simulation Models

Simulation models are powerful computational tools designed to replicate biological systems, disease dynamics, and healthcare delivery processes in a virtual environment. By mathematically modelling physiological mechanisms or patient pathways, these simulations provide a safe, controlled space for testing hypotheses, predicting outcomes, and evaluating medical interventions without exposing real patients to risk. They can be individual-specific, incorporating personal data such as genetics, comorbidities, and treatment history, or population-based, reflecting broader demographic or epidemiological patterns. These models are widely used for exploring disease progression, forecasting outbreaks, optimizing resource allocation, and designing public health strategies. In clinical research, simulation enables virtual trials, drug dosing optimization, and procedural planning. It also aids in medical education and policy-making by visualizing complex scenarios. The adaptability and scalability of simulation models make them indispensable in personalized medicine, where dynamic prediction and iterative testing are essential. With continual improvements in data integration and computing power, simulation models are becoming increasingly accurate, interactive, and impactful in both clinical and research settings

5.4.2 Construction of a Digital Twin in Healthcare

- **Data Collection:** Digital twin models rely on the aggregation of multimodal data to accurately represent individual health status. This includes genomic information that reflects inherited traits, proteomic and metabolomic profiles that capture real-time physiological changes, and clinical data from electronic health records. Imaging studies like MRIs or CT scans offer anatomical context, while wearable devices and lifestyle inputs (diet, sleep, physical activity) provide continuous, real-world updates. The integration of these diverse data types creates a holistic and dynamic representation of the patient's health. This comprehensive input is foundational for accurate modeming and prediction.

- **Modelling and Algorithms:** To construct and operate a digital twin, advanced computational models are developed using artificial intelligence, systems biology, and machine learning techniques. These algorithms simulate biological functions such as metabolism, immune responses, and organ interactions under different scenarios. Mechanistic models can replicate physiological pathways, while data-driven models identify trends and make predictions. By incorporating feedback loops and adaptive mechanisms, these algorithms allow simulations to evolve over time. The goal is to create a virtual replica that mimics the complexity and variability of human biology, enabling predictive and personalized medicine applications.
- **Personalization:** Unlike static models, digital twins are customized to the individual, reflecting their unique genetic makeup, disease history, comorbidities, and treatment responses. This personalization allows simulations to accurately predict how a specific patient will respond to medications, interventions, or disease progression. Personalization is achieved by fine-tuning model parameters based on individual health records, lab data, and genetic profiles. The resulting digital twin can be used to test virtual interventions before applying them in the real world. Such individualized modelling ensures tailored healthcare strategies that reduce trial-and-error approaches and improve clinical outcomes.
- **Real-Time Updating:** A core feature of digital twins is their ability to update in real-time as new data becomes available. Inputs such as lab test results, imaging updates, sensor data from wearable devices, and clinical observations continuously refine the model. This dynamic updating allows the digital twin to remain aligned with the patient's current health status. As a result, the twin becomes more accurate and predictive over time, enabling ongoing monitoring, proactive care, and timely intervention. This real-time adaptability transforms healthcare from episodic treatment to continuous management, improving precision and responsiveness in patient care.

5.4.3 Applications in Personalized Medicine

- **Treatment Simulation:** Digital twins allow clinicians to simulate treatment strategies on a virtual replica of the patient before applying them in real life. By testing various therapeutic options—including drug combinations, dosages, and sequences—in silico, doctors can identify the most effective and least harmful regimen. This minimizes the risks associated with trial-and-error in treatment planning. It is especially valuable in oncology, cardiology, and autoimmune disorders where personalized therapy selection is critical. Treatment simulation helps optimize outcomes and reduce adverse effects in a highly individualized manner.

- **Disease Progression Modelling:** Digital twins can predict how a patient's disease will progress over time under different conditions, such as untreated states, lifestyle changes, or varying treatment regimens. These models simulate biological and environmental interactions, providing forecasts for disease trajectories. For chronic illnesses like diabetes or neurodegenerative diseases, this helps clinicians anticipate complications and intervene early. By modelling these outcomes, care teams can plan personalized long-term strategies that adapt to patient-specific risk factors, improving both prognosis and quality of life.
- **Surgical Planning:** Anatomical digital twins created from imaging data (e.g., CT or MRI scans) allow surgeons to rehearse procedures virtually. These simulations help visualize patient-specific anatomy, assess surgical challenges, and test different techniques before entering the operating room. This level of preparation enhances precision, reduces intraoperative surprises, and can lower surgical risks. In complex procedures like cardiac surgery, organ transplants, or tumour excisions, digital twins optimize planning and predict patient-specific outcomes, contributing to safer and more efficient interventions.
- **Drug Development:** Pharmaceutical companies use digital twin technology to create virtual patient populations for simulating drug effects, side effects, and trial outcomes. This approach accelerates the preclinical and clinical trial phases by enabling in silico testing before or alongside real-world trials. Digital twins help identify suitable patient subgroups for targeted therapies, optimize trial design, and reduce cost and time. They also provide insights into long-term safety and efficacy, enhancing precision drug development and improving the success rate of therapeutic innovations in personalized medicine.

5.4.4 Use Cases and Examples

- **Cardiology:** Digital twins in cardiology involve building patient-specific heart models using imaging data, electrophysiology, and hemodynamic parameters. These models simulate cardiac function under various conditions—such as exercise, medication, or surgical intervention.

Clinicians can assess how a heart would respond to stents, ablations, or valve replacements before performing the actual procedure. By predicting arrhythmia risk or heart failure progression, digital twins support safer, more tailored interventions. This technology is especially valuable in complex congenital heart disease or personalized device implantation planning.

- **Oncology:** In oncology, digital twins model tumour growth dynamics by incorporating molecular, histological, and genomic data from individual patients. These models simulate how different chemotherapy or immunotherapy regimens might impact tumour size, spread, or resistance. Clinicians can test multiple therapeutic combinations in silico to identify the most promising personalized regimen. By predicting treatment efficacy and potential side effects, digital twins reduce trial-and-error approaches in cancer care. They also aid in designing adaptive protocols that evolve with the tumour's molecular changes.
- **Diabetes Management:** Digital twin models of glucose-insulin interactions help optimize insulin therapy in patients with Type 1 and Type 2 diabetes. These models incorporate real-time data from continuous glucose monitors (CGMs), dietary intake, physical activity, and stress levels. They simulate blood glucose responses to various insulin doses and schedules, enabling clinicians to fine-tune personalized treatment plans. Over time, these dynamic models can adapt and offer real-time insulin dosing recommendations, improving glycaemic control and reducing the risk of hypo- or hyperglycaemia.
- **Organ Transplant:** Digital twins in transplant medicine simulate immune system responses to donor organs by integrating data on HLA matching, immunosuppressive drug levels, and immune profiling. These models can predict the likelihood of organ rejection or graft-versus-host disease under different therapeutic regimens. By virtually testing immunosuppressive strategies, clinicians can personalize post-transplant care, reduce complications, and extend graft survival. This approach is especially useful in high-risk or sensitized patients, where immune response prediction is critical to transplant success.

5.4.5 Benefits of Digital Twins and Simulation

Digital twins and simulation models offer transformative benefits in healthcare by creating a virtual mirror of the patient or biological process, enabling safe and efficient experimentation. Clinicians can simulate multiple treatment strategies without any real-world risk, helping to identify the most effective and least harmful options before actual intervention. This ability to "test before treating" significantly reduces the reliance on trial-and-error methods, cutting down the time and cost involved in personalized care. Since digital twins are constructed from multimodal data—genomic, physiological, behavioural—they reflect the unique biological makeup of an individual, making treatment planning more accurate and relevant. Predictive simulations assist in early detection of complications, disease progression, or therapy failure, supporting proactive clinical decision-making. These tools are especially beneficial in high-risk scenarios, such as complex surgeries or drug trials, where precision is paramount. Furthermore, digital twins serve as powerful educational tools, allowing healthcare professionals to train in realistic, patient-specific environments. As they evolve, digital twin systems will not only augment clinical workflows but also redefine standards of safety, personalization, and cost-effectiveness in modern medicine.

5.4.6 Challenges and Limitations

- **Data Requirements:** The effectiveness of digital twins relies heavily on access to high-quality, multimodal datasets. These include genomic sequences, imaging results, electronic health records, sensor data, and lifestyle factors. Data must be comprehensive, longitudinal, and consistently updated to maintain model relevance. Missing, noisy, or biased data can compromise model performance and result in inaccurate simulations. Moreover, standardization across diverse data sources is a challenge, especially when integrating structured and unstructured formats. Secure data sharing protocols and interoperable platforms are essential for scaling digital twin applications.
- **Model Complexity:** Biological systems are highly nonlinear, adaptive, and multi-scale, involving complex interactions among genes, proteins, cells, and organs. Capturing these dynamics accurately in a computational model is a significant challenge. Simplifications or assumptions in modelling may limit real-world applicability or reduce predictive precision. Variability across individuals due to genetics, environment, and lifestyle further complicates modelling. A delicate balance is required between creating detailed, biologically accurate models and ensuring computational feasibility. Robust, domain-specific ontologies and systems biology frameworks are vital for managing this complexity.
- **Computational Demands:** Running digital twin models requires substantial computing power, particularly for real-time simulations or high-resolution anatomical models. Tasks like integrating big data, performing multi-variable simulations, and updating models dynamically demand advanced infrastructure, including GPUs, high-performance computing clusters,

and cloud platforms. Latency and processing time can hinder clinical applicability in fast-paced settings. Moreover, ensuring data security and compliance during computation adds another layer of complexity. Efficient algorithms and scalable architecture are critical to manage resource usage without compromising model performance.

- **Validation:** Before digital twins can be deployed clinically, their accuracy, safety, and reliability must be thoroughly validated. This involves benchmarking predictions against real patient outcomes across diverse cohorts. Lack of validation could lead to incorrect treatment decisions, compromising patient safety. Regulatory bodies require rigorous testing and documentation to approve such models for clinical use. Furthermore, validation must be an ongoing process, as models need to adapt to new data and medical advancements. Establishing robust validation frameworks and clinical trial protocols is essential for widespread adoption.

5.4.7 Ethical and Regulatory Considerations

The integration of digital twins into personalized medicine introduces profound ethical and regulatory challenges that must be addressed to ensure safe, equitable, and responsible use. One of the central concerns revolves around data ownership—patients contribute vast amounts of sensitive biological and behavioural data, yet questions persist about who owns, controls, and profits from that information. Informed consent becomes more complex, as individuals may not fully understand the long-term implications of sharing data used to construct and update their digital replica. Moreover, as digital twins evolve to resemble a person's biological and clinical profile more closely, the concept of digital identity—a computational reflection of the self—raises new ethical dilemmas regarding autonomy, privacy, and dignity. Another major concern is transparency. Clinical decisions informed by digital twins must be explainable to both clinicians and patients to maintain trust and ensure accountability. "Black-box" algorithms that simulate or predict health outcomes without clear reasoning can undermine patient confidence and complicate clinical liability. There is also the issue of bias; if digital twins are trained on non-representative data, they may yield unequal results across populations, exacerbating health disparities rather than mitigating them.

To address these concerns, regulatory frameworks are emerging. Bodies like the FDA and EMA are beginning to develop guidelines for validation, reliability, and clinical safety of digital twin applications in healthcare. These include requirements for rigorous testing, performance benchmarks, and post-deployment monitoring. Yet, current standards are still evolving, and a global consensus is lacking. Collaborative efforts among technologists, ethicists, clinicians, regulators, and patient advocates will be essential to create policies that balance innovation with ethical integrity and public trust.

5.5 FEDERATED LEARNING AND DATA PRIVACY IN AI

As artificial intelligence (AI) becomes increasingly central to healthcare, ensuring patient data privacy while enabling collaborative model training has emerged as a critical challenge. Federated learning (FL) addresses this issue by allowing AI models to learn from distributed data sources without transferring sensitive data. This approach safeguards privacy while unlocking the full potential of AI in personalized medicine.

5.5.1 Why Privacy Matters in Healthcare AI

Privacy is a cornerstone of ethical healthcare, and its importance becomes even more critical in the era of artificial intelligence. Healthcare data—including medical histories, genetic profiles, mental health records, and lifestyle patterns—are among the most personal and sensitive forms of information. When centralized AI systems aggregate data from multiple institutions or patients into a single location for training, they create vulnerabilities. Data breaches, accidental exposure, or unauthorized access can compromise patient confidentiality and lead to serious consequences such as identity theft, insurance discrimination, or social stigma. Moreover, centralized models may violate privacy regulations like HIPAA (in the U.S.) and GDPR (in the EU), which require strict control over how patient data is collected, stored, and shared. Patients may also lose trust in healthcare institutions that rely on opaque or insecure digital systems, reducing their willingness to participate in AI-driven initiatives that could benefit public health. In this context, federated learning emerges as a promising solution. It allows AI models to be trained locally on decentralized data, ensuring that raw patient information never leaves its source. Only model updates, not the data itself, are shared—thus preserving privacy while still enabling collaboration across hospitals, research centres, and countries. This privacy-centric approach helps healthcare AI remain compliant, trustworthy, and ethically sound in its pursuit of innovation.

5.5.2 How Federated Learning Works

- **Step 1: Model Initialization and Distribution:** The process begins with the initialization of a global machine learning model, typically on a secure central server. This base model contains generalized parameters and is not yet tailored to specific healthcare data. The server then securely distributes this model to participating nodes, such as hospitals or research institutions. These nodes act independently and retain their local patient data. This decentralization ensures that sensitive information remains protected at the source.

- **Step 2: Local Training on Private Data:** Each participating node receives the global model and trains it using its own locally stored patient data. The model learns from patterns unique to that institution's population—whether in genomics, clinical records, or imaging. Importantly, this training is done without ever transmitting patient data outside the local system. This step ensures model relevance while upholding privacy regulations and institutional autonomy.
- **Step 3: Encrypted Sharing of Model Updates:** After local training, each node generates model updates—such as weight adjustments or gradients—that reflect new learning from their data. These updates are then encrypted to safeguard against interception or tampering during transfer. Only the encrypted model parameters, not the raw data, are sent to the central server. This preserves data privacy while still contributing valuable insights.
- **Step 4: Aggregation and Improvement of the Global Model:**T he central server collects the encrypted updates from all participating nodes and uses secure aggregation algorithms to combine them. This results in a more accurate and generalizable global model that incorporates learning from multiple sources without violating data privacy. Federated averaging is a common method used here to balance contributions from different nodes.
- **Step 5: Iterative Learning and Model Refinement:** Once aggregated, the improved global model is redistributed to the nodes for another round of localized training. This iterative cycle continues over multiple rounds, allowing the model to progressively improve in accuracy and robustness. Over time, the system builds a powerful, privacy-preserving AI that is both globally informed and locally adapted—ideal for real-world healthcare applications.

5.5.3 Applications in Personalized Medicine

- **Multi-Institutional Genomic Research:** Genomic data are among the most sensitive and high-dimensional forms of medical information. Federated learning enables multiple hospitals and research centres to collaboratively train models on this data without ever sharing the actual DNA sequences. This approach preserves patient privacy while still allowing institutions to build powerful predictive models for disease risk, drug response, or trait heritability. Federated frameworks ensure compliance with ethical and legal standards, including data sovereignty and consent. Moreover, it allows global collaboration in precision medicine initiatives. As a result, breakthroughs can emerge faster and more equitably across populations.

- **Rare Disease Modelling:** Rare diseases often suffer from data scarcity due to their low prevalence. Federated learning addresses this challenge by aggregating learnings from distributed patient datasets across different geographic and institutional boundaries. Instead of pooling the raw data, each centre trains on its local cases, and model updates are combined to improve overall performance. This allows for the development of more accurate diagnostic tools and therapeutic insights, even when each site has only a few relevant cases. It accelerates the pace of discovery and supports global rare disease registries without breaching confidentiality.
- **Medical Imaging:** High-resolution medical images—like MRIs, CT scans, and digital pathology slides—contain valuable diagnostic signals but are often stored in siloed databases. Federated learning enables the training of advanced image classification and segmentation models across these silos while maintaining local control over sensitive image data. Hospitals contribute to a shared model without uploading their proprietary data, reducing legal and ethical barriers. This results in more generalized and robust AI models capable of detecting diseases like cancer, stroke, or COVID-19 across diverse imaging modalities and patient populations. It also mitigates bias caused by training on a single source.

Table 2 Concise summary of the application of personalised medicine

Application	Description	Key Benefits
Multi-Institutional Genomic Research	Uses federated learning to train predictive models across hospitals without sharing raw genomic data.	Preserves privacy, ensures compliance, supports global collaboration, accelerates breakthroughs.
Rare Disease Modelling	Aggregates model updates from rare disease cases across institutions without pooling raw data.	Improves diagnostic accuracy, speeds up discovery, enables global registries, protects confidentiality.
Medical Imaging	Trains image analysis models (MRI, CT, pathology) across hospitals while keeping images local.	Reduces bias, improves generalization, maintains legal/ ethical compliance, enables cross-population accuracy.
Wearable Device Analytics	Trains AI models on edge devices using user data (heart rate, sleep, glucose) without cloud uploads.	Enhances privacy, aligns with GDPR, allows real-time monitoring, reduces data leakage risk.

- **Wearable Device Analytics:** Wearable devices generate continuous streams of health data, including heart rate, sleep patterns, glucose levels, and physical activity. Traditional AI requires uploading this data to cloud servers, risking user privacy. Federated learning offers a privacy-first alternative by allowing models to be trained directly on users' smartphones, smartwatches, or other edge devices. These devices compute updates locally and only send encrypted summaries to improve the global model. This method reduces data leakage risks, aligns with privacy regulations like GDPR, and empowers users to retain control over their health data. It's particularly valuable for real-time health monitoring and early anomaly detection (Table 2).

5.5.4 Benefits of Federated Learning

- **Data Sovereignty:** Federated learning supports data sovereignty by allowing institutions to retain full control over their datasets. Hospitals, research centres, and clinics can participate in model training without transferring their sensitive information to centralized servers. This decentralized approach respects local governance policies and legal constraints. It ensures that institutions manage access, usage, and storage in alignment with their internal protocols. As a result, data security and institutional autonomy are preserved.
- **Enhanced Privacy:** One of the core strengths of federated learning is that raw patient data never leaves the local source. Only encrypted model updates (e.g., gradients or weights) are shared, drastically reducing the risk of data breaches or unauthorized access. This approach complies with global privacy regulations such as HIPAA, GDPR, and India's DPDP Act. It builds patient trust in AI-driven healthcare systems. Overall, it enables safe, large-scale AI development without compromising individual confidentiality.
- **Improved Collaboration:** Federated learning creates a secure framework for collaboration across hospitals, laboratories, and research institutions. It enables joint model development on diverse datasets while keeping proprietary or sensitive information confidential. This fosters greater scientific exchange and accelerates breakthroughs in diagnostics and therapeutics. Institutions that may not have large datasets alone can still contribute to high-impact research. It promotes democratization of AI benefits across healthcare systems.
- **Bias Reduction:** Centralized models often reflect the biases of limited or non-representative datasets. Federated learning incorporates data from diverse populations and clinical settings, leading to more balanced and generalizable models. By training across multiple nodes, it helps capture variations in demographics, genetics, geography, and clinical practice. This reduces the likelihood of performance disparities in underrepresented groups. In personalized medicine, it ensures equitable model accuracy across patient populations.

- **Scalability:** Federated learning is inherently scalable, making it well-suited for both large cloud-based systems and distributed edge devices like smartphones and wearables. Its architecture supports dynamic inclusion of new nodes without the need for centralized reconfiguration. This flexibility allows real-time learning at the point of care while keeping infrastructure costs low. Moreover, it facilitates global health monitoring and personalized recommendations without centralizing vast amounts of data.

5.5.5. Challenges and Limitations

- **System Heterogeneity:** In federated learning, participating nodes (such as hospitals, labs, or personal devices) often differ in terms of computing power, storage capacity, and data quality. This heterogeneity can lead to unequal contributions to model training and may cause slower convergence or biased outcomes. For example, a node with outdated hardware may struggle to process large models or handle real-time updates. Additionally, inconsistent data formats and quality across institutions can complicate model harmonization and reduce accuracy.
- **Communication Overhead:** Federated learning involves frequent and sometimes large-scale transmission of model parameters (e.g., weights or gradients) between central servers and decentralized nodes. This can strain existing communication networks, especially in regions with limited bandwidth or unreliable connectivity. Synchronizing updates across multiple institutions or edge devices may increase latency and delay training cycles. Efficient communication protocols and compression techniques are necessary to manage this overhead and ensure smooth performance.
- **Security Risks:** Although federated learning keeps raw data localized, it still involves sharing model updates—which may unintentionally expose sensitive patterns through inference attacks. Adversaries could potentially reconstruct patient information by analysing gradients or model behaviour over time. Without proper encryption, differential privacy, or secure multiparty computation (SMPC), these vulnerabilities pose real threats. Ensuring rigorous security standards during aggregation and communication phases is essential to safeguard data privacy.
- **Complex Implementation:** Deploying a federated learning system is technically demanding. It requires specialized infrastructure, such as secure aggregators, client-server synchronization protocols, and privacy-preserving technologies like homomorphic encryption. Additionally, coordinating between multiple stakeholders—each with distinct regulations, IT systems, and expertise—can be challenging. The need for

continuous monitoring, model validation, and legal compliance further increases operational complexity, especially in large-scale healthcare environments.

5.5.6 Real-World Examples

- **Google & Apple:** Google and Apple have pioneered the use of federated learning (FL) in consumer electronics, particularly smartphones. In applications like predictive text input, personalized voice recognition, and language modelling, FL allows these companies to train algorithms directly on users' devices. This ensures that sensitive user data—such as messages or voice inputs—never leave the device. Updates to the global model are based solely on encrypted parameters rather than raw data. This approach not only enhances privacy but also adapts the AI to individual usage patterns. The result is a faster, more personalized user experience. It also showcases how FL can operate efficiently at scale across millions of devices.
- **NVIDIA Clara:** NVIDIA Clara is an advanced federated learning platform designed for healthcare, particularly in the domain of medical imaging. It allows multiple hospitals and research institutions to collaboratively train AI models on diagnostic tasks—such as identifying lung lesions or tumours in radiographs—without ever sharing actual patient data. This preserves data confidentiality while leveraging the diversity of datasets across institutions. Clara supports secure model aggregation and offers real-time monitoring for training performance. By enabling decentralized learning, it accelerates innovation in medical diagnostics. Hospitals benefit from AI tools built on a richer, more diverse foundation of patient cases. Clara is a leading example of secure, scalable FL in clinical practice.
- **Owkin:** Owkin is a biotechnology company utilizing federated learning to accelerate cancer research while upholding strict data privacy standards. Their platform connects hospitals and pharmaceutical companies to build AI models on real-world patient data without transferring it. This is particularly important in oncology, where access to large, diverse datasets enhances predictive modelling for tumour progression, drug response, and biomarker discovery. Owkin's approach allows institutions to retain full control of sensitive data while benefiting from collective intelligence. Through FL, they facilitate breakthroughs in drug development and clinical trial optimization. The model also helps meet stringent European data protection regulations, fostering trust and collaboration across research ecosystems.

6 Chapter

PHARMACOGENOMICS AND DRUG DEVELOPMENT

6.0 INTRODUCTION: AN OVERVIEW

Pharmacogenomics, a cornerstone of personalized medicine, investigates how an individual's genetic makeup influences drug response. Rooted in both pharmacology and genomics, it aims to optimize therapeutic efficacy while minimizing adverse drug reactions by tailoring medications to the genetic profile of each patient. As healthcare shifts away from the traditional one-size-fits-all approach, pharmacogenomics plays an increasingly pivotal role in drug discovery, clinical trials, and prescribing practices. Interindividual variability in drug metabolism, efficacy, and toxicity has long challenged clinicians. While environmental factors and comorbidities contribute to this diversity, genetic differences—particularly single nucleotide polymorphisms (SNPs)—have emerged as key determinants of how patients absorb, transport, metabolize, and eliminate drugs. For instance, polymorphisms in genes encoding cytochrome P450 enzymes (like CYP2D6 and CYP2C19) significantly alter the metabolism of antidepressants, antiplatelet agents, and opioids. By identifying these genetic variants, clinicians can now adjust drug selection or dosing to reduce risks and enhance outcomes. Beyond pharmacokinetics (what the body does to the drug), pharmacogenomics also addresses pharmacodynamics (what the drug does to the body). Variants in drug targets—such as receptors, ion channels, or enzymes—can modulate therapeutic response. For example, mutations in the VKORC1 gene impact warfarin sensitivity, necessitating dosage adjustments. Similarly, HER2 overexpression in breast cancer patients determines the suitability of trastuzumab therapy, illustrating how genomic profiling informs targeted treatments (Fig. 1).

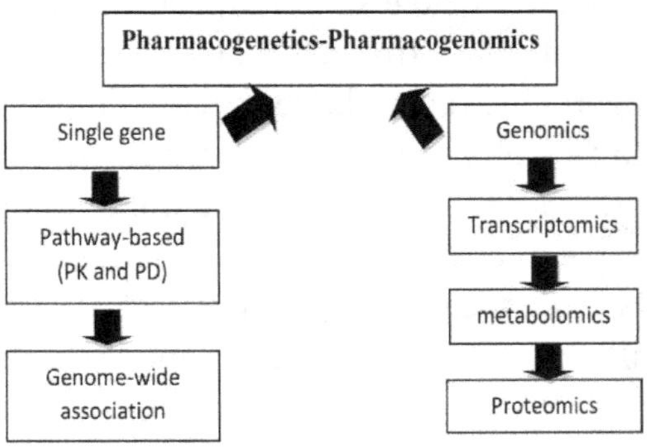

Fig. 1 Applications, and Recent Developments in Pharmacogenomics

The implications of pharmacogenomics extend across the entire drug development pipeline. In preclinical research, genomic insights guide the identification of druggable targets and mechanisms of action. In clinical trials, pharmacogenomic stratification enables more precise inclusion criteria, reducing variability and improving the likelihood of success. Adaptive trial designs can incorporate real-time genetic data to assess differential responses, facilitating faster regulatory approval and safer market entry. Moreover, post-marketing surveillance increasingly relies on pharmacogenomic data to monitor long-term safety in genetically diverse populations. Pharmaceutical companies are embracing this paradigm shift, integrating genomic biomarkers into research and development strategies. Companion diagnostics—tests co-developed with drugs to identify suitable candidates—are now common in oncology and expanding into fields like cardiology and psychiatry. This approach not only enhances therapeutic precision but also offers commercial advantages by reducing development costs, minimizing trial failures, and differentiating products in competitive markets. Governmental and regulatory bodies have also responded proactively. The U.S. FDA has incorporated pharmacogenomic information into drug labelling for dozens of medications, including guidelines on genetic testing. International agencies are developing frameworks to ensure that pharmacogenomic advancements are safely and equitably implemented. Ethical considerations—such as informed consent, data privacy, and access to testing—are central to these efforts, highlighting the need for interdisciplinary collaboration between clinicians, geneticists, policymakers, and patient advocacy groups. Despite its promise, several challenges remain. Limited genetic literacy among healthcare providers, unequal access to genomic testing, and the underrepresentation of diverse populations in genomic databases can hinder equitable implementation. Additionally, the clinical significance of many genetic variants is still uncertain, necessitating further research and real-world evidence. To overcome these barriers, initiatives are underway to expand biobanks, integrate pharmacogenomic data into electronic health records, and develop user-friendly decision support tools. In the era of precision medicine, pharmacogenomics represents a transformative force in how drugs are discovered, developed, and prescribed. It bridges the gap between molecular science and clinical care, enabling treatments that are not only effective but also safer and more personalized. As genomic technologies become more affordable and widely adopted, the integration of pharmacogenomics into routine practice will likely accelerate, shaping the future of therapeutic innovation and individualized healthcare. This chapter explores the scientific principles, clinical applications, technological advances, and societal implications of pharmacogenomics, with a focus on its growing influence on drug development and patient care.

6.1 UNDERSTANDING DRUG-GENE INTERACTIONS

Drug-gene interactions refer to how variations in a person's DNA affect their response to a specific drug. These interactions can alter a drug's pharmacokinetics (absorption, distribution, metabolism, excretion) or pharmacodynamics (mechanism of action, target interaction). The significance of DGIs lies in their potential to optimize therapy, reduce adverse drug reactions, and improve clinical outcomes. Understanding DGIs helps shift medical practice from reactive treatment to proactive prevention and personalization.

6.1.1 Genetic Variants Influencing Drug Response

Genetic variants, particularly single nucleotide polymorphisms (SNPs), play a pivotal role in determining how individuals respond to medications. These subtle changes in a single DNA base can significantly alter the function or expression of genes involved in drug metabolism, transport, or target interaction. Variants in metabolizing enzymes such as CYP2D6, CYP2C19, and CYP3A4 can lead to rapid, slow, or absent drug metabolism, influencing drug efficacy and toxicity. Similarly, mutations in drug transporter genes like ABCB1 or SLCO1B1 affect how drugs are absorbed, distributed, and eliminated. Changes in drug targets—like receptors or enzymes—may render therapies ineffective or hypersensitive. Some variants also modulate gene expression through promoter or regulatory region changes. The clinical implications of these variants are profound, necessitating genotype-guided drug selection and dosing. Their prevalence can vary widely among ethnic groups, influencing population-specific treatment guidelines. Understanding and integrating these genetic differences into prescribing decisions is central to personalized medicine Genetic variants, especially single nucleotide polymorphisms (SNPs), are the most common contributors to DGIs. These variations may:

- Change the activity of drug-metabolizing enzymes (e.g., CYP450 family).
- Alter drug transporter proteins (e.g., ABCB1).
- Affect drug targets such as receptors or enzymes (e.g., VKORC1 for warfarin sensitivity).

Some individuals may metabolize drugs too quickly or too slowly, leading to under-dosing or toxicity, respectively. Others may not respond to drugs at all due to dysfunctional or absent targets.

6.1.2 Pharmacokinetic Interactions

Pharmacokinetic drug-gene interactions (DGIs) refer to genetic influences on the body's absorption, distribution, metabolism, and excretion (ADME) of drugs. These interactions are largely governed by polymorphisms in genes encoding drug-metabolizing enzymes, particularly cytochrome P450 isoenzymes such as CYP2D6,

CYP2C9, CYP2C19, and CYP3A4. For example, individuals carrying non-functional alleles of CYP2D6 may be poor metabolizers of drugs like codeine, leading to reduced therapeutic effect or toxic accumulation. Conversely, ultra-rapid metabolizers may clear the drug too quickly, compromising efficacy. Transporter proteins like SLCO1B1 and ABCB1 also exhibit polymorphisms that influence drug distribution and clearance—impacting statins or chemotherapeutic agents. Variants in conjugation enzymes like UGT1A1 (involved in glucuronidation) further affect drug detoxification. These inherited differences cause inter-individual variability in drug plasma concentrations, half-lives, and bioavailability. Clinically, this variability translates into the need for dose adjustments or alternative therapies to achieve optimal outcomes. Pharmacokinetic DGIs are critical considerations in avoiding underdosing, overdosing, and adverse drug reactions, making pharmacogenetic testing a key component of personalized therapy. For example:

- CYP2D6 polymorphisms affect the metabolism of antidepressants, opioids, and beta-blockers.
- CYP2C19 variants alter the activation of prodrugs like clopidogrel. Individuals can be classified as poor, intermediate, extensive, or ultra-rapid metabolizers, depending on their enzyme activity, which directly influences dosing decisions.

6.1.3 Pharmacodynamic Interactions

Pharmacodynamic drug-gene interactions (DGIs) refer to genetic variations that influence how a drug interacts with its biological targets, such as receptors, enzymes, or signalling molecules, thereby affecting drug efficacy or toxicity. These interactions do not alter drug levels in the body but rather the sensitivity or responsiveness of the target site. For instance, polymorphisms in the VKORC1 gene, which encodes the vitamin K epoxide reductase enzyme targeted by warfarin, can significantly alter anticoagulant response, necessitating dose adjustments. Similarly, mutations in ADRB1 or ADRB2—genes encoding β-adrenergic receptors—affect the therapeutic response to beta-blockers in cardiovascular disease. In oncology, EGFR gene mutations can influence the success of targeted therapies like gefitinib or erlotinib. Additionally, serotonin transporter gene variants (SLC6A4) and serotonin receptor polymorphisms (HTR2A) are associated with variable antidepressant responses. These pharmacodynamic DGIs underscore the importance of understanding a patient's genetic profile to predict drug response more accurately. Integrating such insights into treatment planning allows for optimized therapeutic strategies, minimizing side effects while maximizing clinical benefit. For instance:

- VKORC1 gene variants affect warfarin sensitivity by modifying the target enzyme involved in vitamin K recycling.

- HER2 amplification in breast cancer patients determines response to trastuzumab.Understanding these variations helps clinicians select the most effective drug and predict therapeutic efficacy.

6.1.4 Transporter Gene Variants

Transporter proteins play a crucial role in the pharmacokinetics of drugs by regulating their absorption, distribution, and excretion across cellular membranes. Genetic polymorphisms in transporter genes can significantly alter drug bioavailability and tissue targeting, contributing to variability in drug response. One well-known example is the SLCO1B1 gene, which encodes the hepatic transporter OATP1B1 responsible for the uptake of statins into liver cells. Variants like SLCO1B1 c.521T>C reduce transporter activity, increasing statin plasma levels and the risk of myopathy. Similarly, polymorphisms in the ABCB1 gene, encoding P-glycoprotein, can affect drug efflux from the brain and gut, impacting the efficacy and toxicity of drugs such as digoxin, chemotherapeutics, and antiretrovirals. Mutations in ABCC2 and SLC22A1 are also associated with altered drug handling and adverse effects. These transporter gene variants influence drug exposure at target sites and in systemic circulation, making them important considerations in dose optimization. Pharmacogenomic screening of transporter variants can improve therapeutic precision by guiding drug choice and dosage based on an individual's transport efficiency and risk for side effects Transport proteins influence drug absorption and distribution. Variants in genes encoding these proteins can lead to altered drug bioavailability:

- SLCO1B1 gene polymorphisms affect the hepatic uptake of statins, increasing the risk of statin-induced myopathy.
- ABCB1 polymorphisms can impact blood-brain barrier penetration of drugs like antiepileptics or antidepressants. Such interactions highlight the need for personalized dosing or drug substitution.

6.1.5 Clinical Consequences of DGIs

The clinical outcomes of DGIs include:

- **Adverse Drug Reactions (ADRs):** Adverse drug reactions are one of the most serious consequences of drug–gene interactions (DGIs), often stemming from impaired metabolism or heightened sensitivity due to genetic variants. For example, patients with thiopurine S-methyltransferase (TPMT) deficiency or NUDT15 variants cannot properly metabolize thiopurines such as azathioprine or mercaptopurine, resulting in severe myelosuppression or life-threatening toxicity. Similarly, CYP2C9 or VKORC1 variants can lead to warfarin overdose, increasing the risk of bleeding. These ADRs are often predictable when genetic information is known and can be prevented through pharmacogenomic testing. Thus, pre-emptive screening can drastically reduce hospitalization, morbidity, and healthcare costs due to ADRs, highlighting the clinical significance of integrating pharmacogenomics into routine care.

- **Therapeutic Failure:** Genetic variability may impair drug efficacy by affecting metabolic activation, receptor binding, or downstream signalling, resulting in therapeutic failure. A well-documented case involves CYP2C19 poor metabolizers who are unable to convert clopidogrel into its active form, leading to reduced antiplatelet activity and increased risk of cardiovascular events. Another example includes EGFR mutations conferring resistance to certain tyrosine kinase inhibitors in cancer therapy. In such instances, the standard drug regimen may appear ineffective, prompting unnecessary changes in therapy unless the underlying DGI is identified. Pharmacogenomic insights enable physicians to tailor therapy more accurately, ensuring that patients receive drugs that are likely to work based on their genetic profiles.
- **Need for Alternative Therapies:** When genetic testing reveals a potential risk of ADRs or treatment failure, alternative medications or adjusted dosing become necessary to ensure safety and efficacy. For instance, patients with TPMT deficiency may be prescribed reduced thiopurine doses or non-thiopurine immunosuppressants. In clopidogrel non-responders, alternative antiplatelet agents like prasugrel or ticagrelor may be preferred. Similarly, warfarin dosing can be optimized using CYP2C9 and VKORC1 genotypes to prevent complications. This individualized approach shifts the clinical paradigm from "trial and error" to precision-based prescribing. It reinforces the importance of incorporating pharmacogenetic data into clinical workflows, especially for drugs with narrow therapeutic indices or known pharmacogenetic liabilities.

6.1.6 Examples of Clinically Relevant DGIs

- **lopidogrel & CYP2C19:** Clopidogrel is a prodrug that requires metabolic activation by the enzyme CYP2C19. Individuals with CYP2C19 loss-of-function alleles (such as CYP2C19 *2 or *3) are poor metabolizers and cannot effectively convert clopidogrel into its active form. This leads to reduced platelet inhibition and a higher risk of adverse cardiovascular events, such as stent thrombosis or myocardial infarction. Genotype-guided therapy, where alternative antiplatelet agents like ticagrelor or prasugrel are selected for poor metabolizers, has been shown to significantly improve outcomes in high-risk patients.
- **Warfarin & VKORC1/CYP2C9:** Warfarin, a widely used anticoagulant, exhibits significant inter-individual variability in dosing requirements due

to genetic differences. VKORC1 polymorphisms affect the sensitivity of the vitamin K epoxide reductase complex, the drug's target, while CYP2C9 variants impair metabolic clearance of warfarin. Patients with certain genotypes are at a higher risk of bleeding or inadequate anticoagulation if standard dosing is used. Pharmacogenomic testing enables more accurate dose prediction, allowing safer and more effective initiation of therapy, especially during the critical early phase of anticoagulation.

- **Codeine & CYP2D6:** Codeine is metabolized into morphine by the CYP2D6 enzyme. Ultra-rapid metabolizers with multiple copies of active CYP2D6 alleles convert codeine to morphine more quickly and extensively, which can lead to dangerously high morphine levels in the blood. This increases the risk of respiratory depression and even fatal outcomes, particularly in children and breastfeeding infants. Conversely, poor metabolizers experience little or no analgesic effect. Due to this variability, pharmacogenomic screening is recommended, and many guidelines now advise against using codeine in patients with known CYP2D6 ultra- or poor-metabolizer status.

6.1.7 Tools and Databases

Tools and databases play a pivotal role in translating pharmacogenomic discoveries into clinical practice. Key resources like PharmGKB (Pharmacogenomics Knowledgebase) curate comprehensive information on gene-drug interactions (DGIs), including variant annotations, pathway maps, and clinical summaries. The Clinical Pharmacogenetics Implementation Consortium (CPIC) provides peer-reviewed, evidence-based guidelines that assist clinicians in adjusting drug therapy based on specific genetic variants. These guidelines help determine whether genetic testing is warranted and how results should influence prescribing decisions. The FDA's Table of Pharmacogenomic Biomarkers further supports clinicians by listing approved drugs with known pharmacogenomic information on their labels, encouraging safer and more effective use. Together, these tools bridge the gap between genomic research and clinical implementation, promoting personalized medicine. They also enable consistent, standardized interpretation across healthcare systems, enhancing drug safety, efficacy, and patient outcomes.

6.1.8 Limitations and Considerations

While pharmacogenomics offers transformative potential in personalizing drug therapy, several critical limitations and contextual factors must be acknowledged to ensure accurate interpretation and responsible application:

- **Ethnic Variability:** Genetic variants influencing drug metabolism or response often exhibit significant differences in frequency across ethnic groups. For instance, CYP2D6 ultra-rapid metabolizer alleles are more common in North African and Middle Eastern populations, while CYP2C9 and VKORC1 variants affecting warfarin sensitivity are prevalent in European and Asian groups, respectively. These population-level disparities complicate the generalizability of pharmacogenomic findings and highlight the need for ethnically diverse datasets when developing dosing guidelines or therapeutic recommendations.

Table: 1 Concise Summary of the Limitations and Considerations in Pharmacogenomics

Limitation/ Consideration	Description	Example/Implication
Ethnic Variability	Genetic variants differ across populations, affecting drug metabolism.	CYP2D6 UMs in North Africans; VKORC1 variants more common in Asians.
Gene–Gene Interactions	Multiple genes may interact, influencing drug response unpredictably.	Epistasis may mask or enhance effects of individual variants.
Gene–Environment Interactions	Environmental factors (diet, smoking, etc.) alter gene function.	Enzyme activity affected by lifestyle or concurrent medications.
Incomplete Penetrance	Presence of a variant doesn't always result in a clinical effect.	Not all carriers of risk alleles show altered drug response.
Variable Expressivity	The same genetic variant can cause varying phenotypic effects.	Drug response may differ by age, sex, or organ function.
Population-Specific Data Gaps	Lack of diverse genomic datasets limits guideline applicability.	Dosing algorithms may not suit underrepresented ethnic groups.
Single-Gene Testing Limitations	Single-gene tests may not capture full drug response complexity.	Polygenic models or systems biology may be needed.
Clinical Context Dependency	Genotype interpretation must consider broader clinical factors.	Disease state, organ impairment, or co-morbidities influence decisions.

- **Gene–Gene and Gene–Environment Interactions**: Drug response is rarely governed by a single gene. Interactions among multiple genes (epistasis) or between genes and environmental factors (e.g., diet, smoking, concurrent medications, or microbiome composition) can significantly alter drug efficacy or toxicity. For instance, a polymorphism that reduces enzyme activity might be compensated by upregulation of a parallel metabolic pathway or influenced by environmental inducers or inhibitors. These complex networks require systems biology approaches to model accurately and limit the predictive power of single-gene testing.

- **Incomplete Penetrance and Variable Expressivity:** Even when a pharmacokinetically relevant variant is present, it does not always lead to a predictable clinical phenotype. This phenomenon, known as incomplete penetrance, means some individuals may not manifest altered drug responses despite harbouring a known risk allele. Factors like age, sex, organ function, coexisting diseases, or compensatory mechanisms may influence how strongly a genotype translates into a phenotype. Thus, genotype alone may not be sufficient to guide therapy without considering broader clinical context (Table-1).

6.2 PERSONALIZED DOSING AND METABOLISM

Personalized dosing represents a cornerstone of precision medicine, aiming to tailor drug regimens to an individual's unique genetic makeup, physiological characteristics, and environmental exposures. Unlike traditional dosing, which relies on average population responses, personalized dosing accounts for inter-individual variability that significantly influences drug efficacy and toxicity. A key enabler of this approach is pharmacogenomics—the study of how genetic variations, particularly in genes encoding drug-metabolizing enzymes (e.g., CYP450 family), transporters (e.g., ABCB1), and drug targets (e.g., VKORC1), affect drug behaviour in the body. These genetic factors can classify individuals as poor, intermediate, extensive, or ultra-rapid metabolizers, impacting plasma drug concentrations and therapeutic response. Personalized dosing also considers non-genetic influences such as age, sex, body weight, liver and kidney function, diet, comorbidities, and concurrent medications. Incorporating this multidimensional information into clinical practice allows for more accurate dose selection, reduced adverse drug reactions, and improved treatment outcomes. Clinical tools and guidelines—like CPIC recommendations and dosing algorithms—support healthcare providers in translating complex pharmacogenomic data into actionable decisions. This shift from a "one-size-fits-all" model toward individualized therapy is transforming the safety and effectiveness of pharmacological interventions..

6.2.1 Role of Drug-Metabolizing Enzymes

Drug-metabolizing enzymes, especially those belonging to the cytochrome P450 (CYP450) family, play a pivotal role in determining how quickly or slowly a drug is metabolized and cleared from the body. Variations in the genes encoding these enzymes can lead to significant differences in drug levels, influencing both efficacy and toxicity. For instance, individuals with reduced CYP2C19 activity may accumulate higher levels of drugs like clopidogrel, increasing the risk of adverse effects. Conversely, ultra-rapid CYP2D6 metabolizers may clear certain antidepressants too quickly, rendering them ineffective. Understanding these enzyme activities is essential for guiding personalized dosing strategies and improving therapeutic outcomes (Fig. 2).

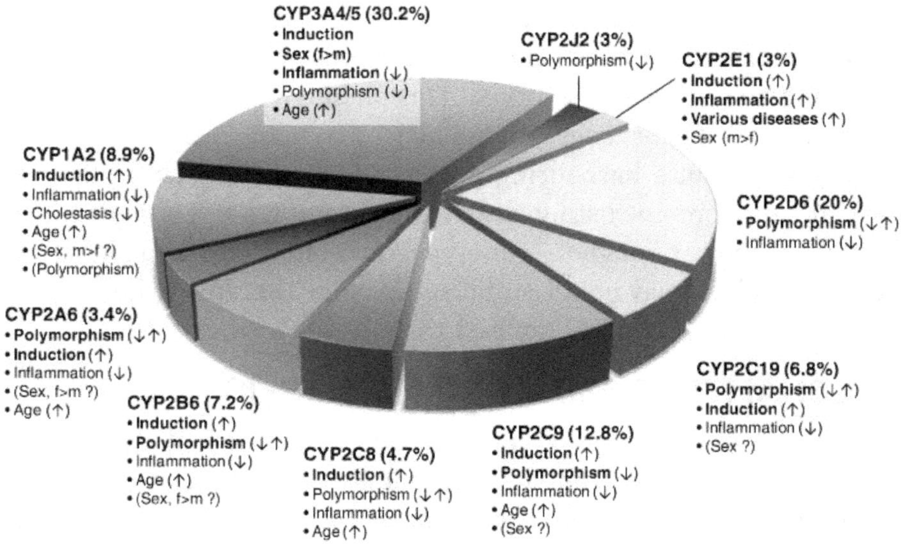

Fig. 2 Cytochrome P450 enzymes in drug metabolism

Genetic polymorphisms in these enzymes can classify individuals into different metabolizer categories:

- **Poor Metabolizers (PM):** Poor metabolizers possess little to no functional activity of a specific drug-metabolizing enzyme, often due to homozygous loss-of-function genetic variants. This leads to a significant reduction in drug clearance from the body, resulting in elevated plasma drug concentrations. As a consequence, poor metabolizers are at increased risk of dose-dependent adverse drug reactions (ADRs) and toxicity. For example, PMs of CYP2D6 may experience exaggerated effects or toxicity from codeine or tricyclic antidepressants. These individuals typically require lower-than-standard doses or alternative therapies. Pre-emptive genotyping can help identify PMs before initiating therapy. Recognizing PM status is critical in narrow therapeutic index drugs. Failure to adjust the dose accordingly may result in life-threatening consequences. Personalized treatment plans improve safety and efficacy in PM patients.

- **Intermediate Metabolizers (IM):** Intermediate metabolizers have reduced enzymatic activity due to heterozygous alleles with one normal and one non-functional variant or two partially functioning alleles. This group exhibits a slower-than-normal metabolism but not as impaired as poor metabolizers. Drug clearance is somewhat reduced, which may cause moderate drug accumulation and increased side effects, though not always reaching toxic levels. IMs often require dose adjustments, especially for drugs with a tight therapeutic window. For example, CYP2C19 IMs may have a suboptimal response to clopidogrel, leading to reduced antiplatelet effects. Pharmacogenetic testing can help guide clinicians in modifying doses or choosing alternative therapies. IMs also represent an important population for dose monitoring. Treatment strategies for IMs may vary depending on the drug involved and clinical context. Recognizing IM status aids in refining therapeutic precision.

- **Extensive/Normal Metabolizers (EM):** Extensive or normal metabolizers carry fully functional alleles, allowing for standard enzymatic activity and predictable drug metabolism. They represent the baseline reference group for whom standard drug dosing guidelines are typically designed. EMs efficiently convert prodrugs to active forms and clear active drugs at expected rates. For most medications, EMs are expected to achieve therapeutic levels with standard doses, minimizing risks of either toxicity or therapeutic failure. However, being an EM does not guarantee uniform response, as other genetic and environmental factors may still influence outcomes. For example, diet, age, renal function, and drug interactions can alter expected pharmacokinetics. Nevertheless, EMs are considered the safest group for conventional dosing unless other clinical variables intervene. Understanding EM status helps determine if deviations from expected outcomes are likely due to non-genetic factors.
- **Ultra-Rapid Metabolizers (UM):** Ultra-rapid metabolizers have increased enzymatic activity due to gene duplications or highly active alleles. This leads to accelerated drug metabolism, often resulting in reduced therapeutic drug levels when standard doses are administered. For prodrugs, however, UMs may convert them too quickly, producing excessive active metabolites and potential toxicity. An example is codeine: UMs convert it rapidly to morphine, risking respiratory depression, especially in children. These individuals often require higher-than-standard doses or alternative medications not affected by the same enzyme. Identifying UM status is crucial to avoid treatment failure or adverse events. UMs may not benefit from medications that require steady-state levels for efficacy. Pharmacogenomic testing enables timely identification and optimal therapy selection. UMs highlight the value of precision dosing in clinical practice. They are key candidates for genotype-guided prescribing to ensure efficacy and safety.

6.2.2 Pharmacokinetic Profiling

Pharmacokinetics (PK) is the study of how a drug moves through the body over time, encompassing the four key processes of absorption, distribution, metabolism, and excretion (ADME). Absorption determines how quickly and efficiently a drug enters the bloodstream, while distribution describes how it is transported to various tissues and organs. Metabolism—primarily occurring in the liver—involves the biochemical transformation of the drug into active or inactive metabolites, influencing both efficacy and toxicity. Excretion, mainly through the kidneys or bile, governs how rapidly the drug and its byproducts are eliminated. In personalized medicine, PK profiling is crucial for tailoring dosing regimens to an individual's genetic makeup, age, organ function, and lifestyle factors. By understanding these parameters, clinicians can optimize therapeutic outcomes, minimize side effects, and avoid under- or overdosing, especially for drugs with narrow therapeutic windws. Personalized dosing uses genetic markers to predict PK parameters, including:

- Clearance rates
- Half-life
- Bioavailability
- Peak plasma concentrations

In individuals with reduced metabolic capacity, the drug remains longer in circulation, increasing toxicity risk. Conversely, ultra-rapid metabolizers may require higher or more frequent dosing.

6.2.3 Genotype-Guided Dosing Algorithms

Genotype-guided dosing algorithms are evidence-based tools designed to integrate a patient's genetic profile into clinical decision-making for drug selection and dosage optimization. These algorithms typically combine pharmacogenomic data—such as single nucleotide polymorphisms (SNPs) in drug-metabolizing enzymes, transporters, or drug targets—with clinical variables like age, body weight, organ function, and co-medications. By incorporating known gene–drug interactions (e.g., CYP2C9 and VKORC1 variants in warfarin therapy, CYP2C19 in clopidogrel metabolism, or TPMT in thiopurine dosing), they help predict an individual's likely pharmacokinetic and pharmacodynamic responses. This approach reduces trial-and-error prescribing, lowers the risk of adverse drug reactions, and improves therapeutic efficacy. Many of these algorithms are embedded in electronic health records (EHRs) with clinical decision support systems, enabling real-time dosing recommendations at the point of care. When implemented systematically, genotype-guided dosing bridges the gap between genomic research and routine clinical practice, paving the way for safer and more precise pharmacotherapy. Examples include:

- **Warfarin Dosing:** Algorithms incorporating CYP2C9 and VKORC1 genotypes.
- **Thiopurines (azathioprine, 6-MP):** Adjusted dosing based on TPMT and NUDT15 status.
- **Tacrolimus:** Dosage adjustments based on CYP3A5 genotype.

These tools improve dosing precision, reduce time to therapeutic effect, and lower adverse event rates.

6.2.4 Population Variability in Metabolic Genes

Allele frequencies of drug-metabolizing enzymes differ significantly among populations, influencing both pharmacokinetic profiles and therapeutic outcomes. Variations in genes encoding enzymes such as CYP2D6, CYP2C19, CYP2C9, NAT2, and UGT1A1 can lead to distinct metabolizer phenotypes—poor, intermediate, extensive, or ultra-rapid—within different ethnic or geographic groups. For example, CYP2D6 ultra-rapid metabolizer alleles are more common in North African and Middle Eastern populations, while CYP2C19 poor metabolizer variants are more prevalent in East Asians. These differences affect drug efficacy and toxicity risks, making population-specific considerations essential in global pharmacotherapy. Understanding these patterns helps refine genotype-guided dosing algorithms, supports equitable access to effective treatments, and informs the design of clinical trials that accurately reflect genetic diversity. In personalized medicine, acknowledging and addressing such variability ensures that therapeutic recommendations are both scientifically robust and culturally relevant.

For example:

- CYP2C19 poor metabolizers are more common in Asians (~15–20%).
- CYP2D6 gene duplications leading to ultra-rapid metabolism are more frequent in North Africans and Middle Easterners.

Understanding this variability is crucial for implementing population-specific dosing strategies and avoiding one-size-fits-all recommendations.

6.2.5 Clinical Implementation Challenges

While personalized dosing strategies are supported by strong scientific evidence and have demonstrated clear benefits in improving drug safety and efficacy, their translation into routine clinical practice remains uneven. The integration of pharmacogenomic insights into day-to-day healthcare is hindered by systemic, logistical, and educational barriers. Limited availability of cost-effective and timely pharmacogenomic testing restricts patient access, while inconsistent insurance coverage and reimbursement policies discourage widespread adoption. Additionally, many healthcare providers lack adequate training to interpret complex genetic data and apply it effectively to dosing decisions. Technical challenges, such as embedding genomic information into electronic health records with functional clinical decision support, further slow implementation. Overcoming these obstacles is essential to fully realize the promise of genotype-guided therapy in personalized medicine.

Despite robust scientific evidence, personalized dosing faces several hurdles:

- Limited access to pharmacogenomic testing in routine settings.
- Variable insurance coverage and reimbursement.
- Need for clinician training in interpreting and applying test results.
- Integration into electronic health records and clinical workflows.

These factors impact the scalability of personalized dosing in standard care.

6.2.6 Benefits of Personalized Dosing

When implemented effectively, personalized dosing offers:

- Improved efficacy through precise therapeutic levels.
- Reduced adverse drug reactions (ADRs) by avoiding toxic exposures.
- Shorter time to therapeutic effect by reducing trial-and-error prescribing.
- Optimized drug costs through fewer hospitalizations and dosage titrations.

6.2.7 Future Directions

The future of personalized dosing is poised to become increasingly adaptive, data-rich, and patient-centric, driven by technological and scientific advancements. Artificial intelligence (AI) will play a central role by developing dynamic dose prediction models that continuously learn from large-scale, multi-source patient data, enabling real-time adjustments based on evolving clinical parameters. Wearable sensor technologies, such as continuous glucose monitors, smart inhalers, or cardiac rhythm trackers, will provide live physiological feedback, allowing dosing regimens—particularly for drugs with narrow therapeutic ranges—to be refined on the fly. The integration of multi-omics data—including genomics, proteomics, metabolomics, and transcriptomics—will create a more holistic understanding of drug-body interactions, capturing influences beyond genetics alone. In combination, these innovations will enable a shift from static, one-time dosing recommendations to continuous, precision-guided therapy. As these tools mature, they will demand robust clinical validation, interoperable data systems, and ethical frameworks to ensure their safe and equitable implementation.

The future of personalized dosing includes:

- Artificial intelligence (AI) integration for dynamic dose prediction models.
- Wearable sensor feedback to refine real-time dosing (e.g., glucose sensors for insulin).
- Multi-omics incorporation, combining genetic, proteomic, and metabolomic data for more nuanced dosing decisions.

6.3 PGX GUIDELINES AND CLINICAL IMPLEMENTATION

6.3.1 Introduction to PGx Guidelines

Pharmacogenomics (PGx) guidelines provide standardized, evidence-based recommendations for integrating genetic information into drug therapy decisions. Developed by expert consortia and regulatory bodies, these guidelines bridge the gap between genomic research and clinical application. They outline how specific genetic variants influence drug selection, dosing, and monitoring, enabling healthcare providers to deliver safer and more effective treatments.

6.3.2 Key Organizations and Resources

- Clinical Pharmacogenetics Implementation Consortium (CPIC) – Focuses on translating genetic test results into actionable prescribing guidance.
- Dutch Pharmacogenetics Working Group (DPWG) – Provides dosing and drug selection recommendations based on genotype.
- U.S. Food and Drug Administration (FDA) – Maintains a list of drugs with pharmacogenomic labeling.
- European Medicines Agency (EMA) – Issues guidance on genetic testing requirements for certain drugs.
- PharmGKB Database – A comprehensive resource for gene–drug associations, guideline summaries, and supporting literature.

6.3.3 Clinical Implementation Workflow

- Patient Identification – Determining candidates for pharmacogenomic testing based on medical history, drug regimen, or disease risk.
- Genetic Testing and Reporting – Conducting validated laboratory tests to identify relevant genetic variants.
- Data Interpretation – Applying PGx guidelines to translate genetic results into clinical recommendations.
- Decision Support Integration – Embedding PGx information into electronic health records (EHR) with clinical decision support (CDS) tools for point-of-care use.
- Therapeutic Action – Adjusting drug type or dosage based on PGx-informed recommendations.

6.3.4 Barriers to Implementation

- Limited availability of cost-effective genetic testing in routine practice.
- Lack of clinician training in pharmacogenomics and guideline use.

- Variable insurance coverage and reimbursement policies.
- Challenges in integrating PGx data into EHRs and CDS systems.
- Need for standardized reporting formats and interoperability.

6.3.5 Strategies to Enhance Adoption

- **Expanding Pre-emptive Genetic Testing Programs in Healthcare Systems:** Pre-emptive pharmacogenomic testing involves screening patients for key genetic variants before medication is prescribed, allowing immediate access to results when needed. By integrating such programs into routine health check-ups or hospital admissions, healthcare systems can avoid delays in treatment decisions. Large-scale initiatives, such as biobank-linked testing, can help identify population-specific allele frequencies and improve dosing guidelines. This proactive approach reduces adverse drug reactions, enhances treatment efficacy, and builds a valuable genomic database for future research.
- **Providing Targeted Education and Training for Clinicians, Pharmacists, and Nurses:** Effective PGx implementation depends on the competency of healthcare professionals to interpret and apply genetic test results. Targeted training programs—offered through workshops, online modules, and continuing medical education—can enhance their understanding of gene–drug interactions and relevant guidelines. Interdisciplinary education fosters collaboration between prescribers, pharmacists, and genetic counsellors. Training should also address the communication of genetic information to patients in a clear, non-technical manner. Ultimately, this empowers clinicians to make confident, evidence-based prescribing decisions.
- **Developing User-Friendly EHR Integration with Automated PGx Alerts:** Embedding pharmacogenomic data into electronic health records (EHRs) with automated alerts ensures that clinicians receive timely, actionable information at the point of care. Such systems can flag potential drug–gene interactions, suggest alternative therapies, or recommend dosage adjustments based on the patient's genotype. The interface should be intuitive, minimizing workflow disruption while maximizing clinical utility. Advanced integration can also link to relevant CPIC or DPWG guidelines for immediate reference. A well-designed EHR PGx module can significantly improve adherence to evidence-based recommendations.
- **Strengthening Policy and Reimbursement Frameworks to Support Routine Use:** Sustainable PGx adoption requires supportive health policy and reimbursement mechanisms. Clear regulations should define testing

standards, reporting formats, and data privacy safeguards. Insurance coverage for pharmacogenomic testing can remove financial barriers for patients and encourage clinicians to use such tools. Governments and health agencies can incentivize adoption by funding pilot programs and including PGx in national health priorities. Strong policy frameworks not only promote equitable access but also ensure consistent quality of testing across institutions.

- **Encouraging Patient Engagement and Understanding of Pharmacogenomics:** Patient awareness and understanding are critical for the acceptance and success of pharmacogenomic testing. Educational campaigns—through clinics, pharmacies, and digital platforms—can inform patients about the benefits, limitations, and privacy safeguards of PGx. Shared decision-making models encourage patients to actively participate in their treatment planning based on their genetic profile. Providing clear explanations of test results and their implications can build trust and adherence to therapy. Engaged patients are more likely to support data-sharing initiatives that drive further PGx research.

6.3.6 Future Outlook

As sequencing costs decline and bioinformatics capabilities grow, PGx guidelines will become more comprehensive, covering a broader range of drugs and genetic variants. AI-driven decision support, real-time monitoring tools, and integration with multi-omics data will make clinical implementation more precise and individualized. Global harmonization of guidelines and collaborative data-sharing initiatives will further enhance their utility and reach.

6.4 INTEGRATION OF PGX IN DRUG DISCOVERY PIPELINES

6.4.1 Role of Pharmacogenomics in Target Identification

Pharmacogenomics (PGx) plays a crucial role in the earliest stage of drug discovery by helping researchers identify genetic variations that influence disease susceptibility and drug response. By analysing large-scale genomic datasets, scientists can pinpoint disease-related genes, protein targets, and signalling pathways that vary among individuals or populations. This information allows for the selection of drug targets that are more likely to produce consistent therapeutic effects across genetically diverse patients. PGx also helps in identifying subpopulations that may benefit most from a particular therapy, thus improving the precision of drug development. Integrating PGx at this stage reduces the likelihood of later-stage failures due to unanticipated variability in efficacy or safety.

6.4.2 Preclinical Studies and Genetic Models

In the preclinical phase, PGx insights guide the development of genetically relevant models—such as transgenic animals, gene-edited cell lines, and organoids—that mimic specific human genetic variations. These models enable researchers to assess how genetic differences affect drug metabolism, target binding, and therapeutic efficacy before entering clinical trials. For example, CYP450 enzyme variants can be modelled to predict metabolism-related drug clearance rates. This approach helps detect genotype-dependent toxicity risks early and refine drug formulations accordingly. By incorporating PGx into preclinical workflows, researchers can enhance the predictive accuracy of safety and efficacy data, making the transition to clinical testing more efficient and targeted.

6.4.3 Clinical Trial Design and Patient Stratification

Pharmacogenomics transforms clinical trial design by enabling the stratification of participants based on genetic markers associated with drug metabolism, efficacy, or risk of adverse reactions. Instead of treating the trial population as homogeneous, PGx-guided studies enrol participants in subgroups—such as poor, intermediate, or ultra-rapid metabolizers—allowing for targeted dosing and tailored endpoints. This strategy increases the likelihood of detecting a drug's true benefit and reduces the noise caused by genetic variability. Regulatory bodies increasingly support adaptive trial designs that incorporate PGx data, as they can shorten timelines, reduce costs, and enhance the probability of success in demonstrating safety and efficacy.

6.4.4 Regulatory Considerations and PGx Labelling

Regulatory agencies such as the U.S. FDA, EMA, and PMDA encourage the inclusion of PGx data in new drug applications (NDAs) and biologics license applications (BLAs). Incorporating PGx findings into drug labelling—such as required genetic testing before prescription or genotype-specific dosing recommendations—ensures safer and more effective use of new therapies. This step often involves close collaboration between pharmaceutical companies and regulators to ensure that the PGx evidence is robust, reproducible, and clinically relevant. Drugs with built-in PGx labelling, such as abacavir (HLA-B*57:01 testing) or trastuzumab (HER2 status), illustrate how regulatory integration can improve patient outcomes and reduce adverse events.

6.4.5 Post-Marketing Surveillance and Real-World Evidence

Even after a drug reaches the market, PGx continues to play a critical role through pharmacovigilance programs and real-world evidence (RWE) studies. Post-marketing surveillance can identify rare genotype-specific adverse events that were not observed during clinical trials due to limited sample sizes. Real-world PGx data, derived from electronic health records, biobank studies, and registries, provide insights into how genetic variability impacts drug performance in broader, more diverse populations. This ongoing feedback loop allows for continuous refinement of dosing recommendations, potential expansion of therapeutic indications, and updates to PGx labelling. In the long term, integrating PGx into surveillance systems strengthens the safety and efficacy profile of marketed drugs.

7 Chapter

PERSONALIZED MEDICINE IN MAJOR DISEASE AREAS

7.0 INTRODUCTION: AN OVERVIEW

In recent decades, the paradigm of healthcare has shifted from a generalized approach toward one that is increasingly patient-specific — a shift that has led to the emergence and expansion of personalized medicine. Also referred to as precision medicine, personalized medicine involves tailoring medical treatment to the individual characteristics of each patient. It incorporates information about a person's genetic makeup, environmental exposures, and lifestyle choices to develop more accurate diagnoses, prognoses, and therapeutic strategies. Rather than applying a one-size-fits-all model, personalized medicine aims to optimize medical care based on variability in genes, biomarkers, phenotypes, and psychosocial factors. This approach is transforming how we understand, detect, and treat a wide spectrum of diseases, particularly in major areas such as oncology, cardiology, neurology, infectious diseases, and rare genetic disorders. In these domains, traditional treatment methods often fall short due to inter-individual differences in disease progression and drug response. Personalized medicine offers an innovative alternative by integrating molecular profiling and advanced diagnostics to predict disease susceptibility, prevent onset, and choose the most effective interventions for each patient. In oncology, for example, targeted therapies now enable clinicians to treat cancers based on specific mutations rather than tumour location. Similarly, in cardiovascular diseases, pharmacogenomics is guiding the prescription of drugs like clopidogrel and warfarin, improving safety and efficacy. In neurology, personalized strategies are emerging for complex conditions like Alzheimer's disease and epilepsy, where conventional treatments often yield variable outcomes. Infectious disease management is also evolving through the use of genomic sequencing and precision diagnostics to combat antibiotic resistance and guide vaccine development (Fig. 1).

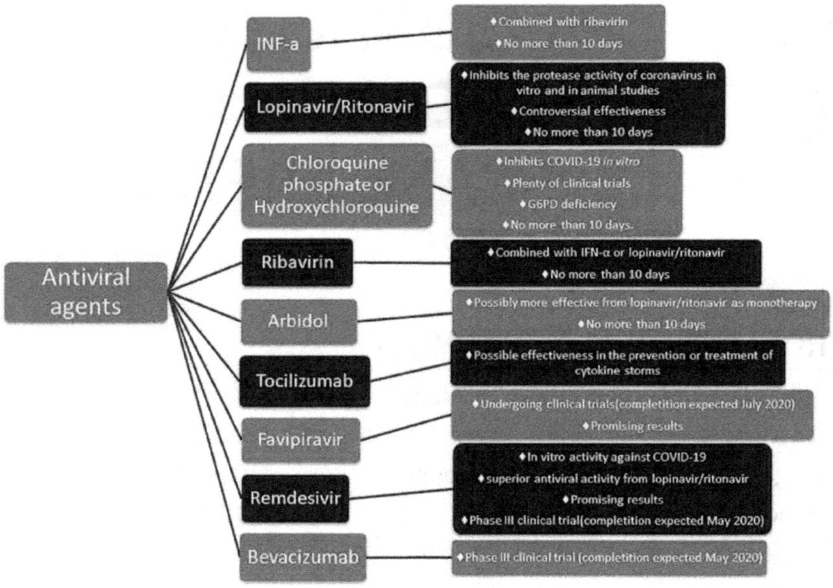

Fig. 1 Milestones in Personalized Medicine

These advances are underpinned by a growing understanding of genomics, proteomics, metabolomics, and systems biology. The integration of large-scale data (big data), artificial intelligence, and digital health platforms further accelerates the development and deployment of personalized interventions. Advances in bioinformatics and computational biology have enabled researchers and clinicians to make sense of complex biological data, identifying patterns and predictive biomarkers that were previously inaccessible. Moreover, patient stratification, companion diagnostics, and predictive modelling are making healthcare more proactive than reactive. Instead of waiting for disease symptoms to manifest, personalized medicine encourages early detection and even pre-emptive treatment. It is reshaping clinical trial designs through adaptive methodologies that focus on smaller, molecularly defined subpopulations, leading to more robust and relevant outcomes. The benefits of personalized medicine extend beyond clinical outcomes. Economically, it promises to reduce the burden of ineffective treatments, hospitalizations, and adverse drug reactions. Ethically, it empowers patients through informed decision-making and shared treatment planning. Despite these advantages, the integration of personalized medicine into clinical practice is not without challenges. These include high costs, data privacy concerns, disparities in access, and the need for healthcare system readiness.

Nonetheless, as healthcare systems across the globe move toward value-based care, personalized medicine is becoming increasingly central to achieving better health outcomes. National and international efforts are underway to implement precision health initiatives, supported by government funding, academic research, and private sector innovation. Initiatives like the U.S. Precision Medicine Initiative and Europe's 1+ Million Genomes Project are testaments to this growing momentum. Personalized medicine is not merely a scientific trend but a fundamental rethinking of how diseases are understood and treated. It holds the potential to redefine standards of care across major disease areas by aligning treatment strategies with individual biological profiles. As we enter an era of more precise, predictive, and preventative medicine, the promise of personalized healthcare continues to grow — offering hope for improved patient outcomes and a more sustainable healthcare future.

7.1 ONCOLOGY

Cancer is a complex and heterogeneous disease, characterized by uncontrolled cell growth and the accumulation of genetic and epigenetic alterations. Traditional treatment strategies in oncology — such as surgery, chemotherapy, and radiation — have historically followed a generalized approach. However, these conventional modalities often yield variable responses among patients, primarily due to the underlying genetic differences in tumour biology. Personalized medicine in oncology has revolutionized this field by introducing tumour profiling and targeted treatments, enabling more precise and effective therapeutic strategies. This section explores the process, significance, and applications of these two components in detail.

7.1.1 Tumour Profiling

Tumour profiling refers to the comprehensive analysis of cancer cells to identify specific genetic mutations, gene expression patterns, protein markers, and other molecular characteristics that drive tumour growth. It provides critical insights into the biological behaviour of individual tumours and serves as the cornerstone of personalized oncology.

- **Genomic Profiling:** Genomic profiling plays a pivotal role in the personalization of cancer treatment by providing detailed insight into the genetic alterations driving tumour development and progression. At the forefront of this innovation is Next-Generation Sequencing (NGS), a high-throughput technology that enables the rapid and simultaneous analysis of hundreds to thousands of cancer-related genes within a single assay. This comprehensive method allows oncologists to identify clinically significant driver mutations that influence tumour behaviour, prognosis, and treatment response. Mutations in genes such as EGFR (epidermal growth factor receptor), KRAS, BRAF, ALK, and PIK3CA have been strongly associated with various cancer types and are now routinely assessed to guide targeted therapies. For example, detecting an EGFR mutation in non-small cell lung cancer (NSCLC) can make a patient eligible for tyrosine kinase inhibitors like erlotinib or osimertinib. Similarly, ALK and ROS1 rearrangements can be targeted with crizotinib, offering improved clinical outcomes over standard chemotherapy. NGS can be applied to both tumour tissue and liquid biopsies, offering flexibility and non-invasive alternatives for monitoring. Moreover, advanced forms of NGS such as whole-exome sequencing (WES) and whole-genome sequencing (WGS) enable the detection of both somatic mutations (acquired in tumour cells) and germline mutations (inherited and present in all cells). This dual capability is crucial not only for therapy selection but also for assessing hereditary cancer risk, as seen in BRCA1/2 mutation carriers. The depth and breadth of information generated through genomic profiling are transforming cancer care, making it possible to classify tumours more precisely and match patients with the most effective, personalized treatments. As technologies evolve and costs decline, genomic profiling is poised to become a standard component of oncologic diagnostics worldwide.

- **Transcriptomic and Epigenetic Profiling:** Transcriptomic and epigenetic profiling are essential tools in understanding the functional dynamics of cancer cells beyond DNA mutations. Transcriptomic profiling involves the comprehensive analysis of messenger RNA (mRNA) expression levels in tumour cells, providing insights into which genes are actively transcribed and to what extent. By examining the transcriptome, researchers and clinicians can determine the activity status of oncogenes and tumour suppressor genes, both of which play critical roles in cancer development, progression, and response to treatment. For example, overexpression of genes like MYC or HER2 may signal aggressive tumour behaviour, while decreased expression of tumour suppressors like TP53 may indicate loss of regulatory control over cell division. This type of profiling is particularly useful in subtyping tumours, identifying prognostic gene signatures, and predicting response to specific therapies. In breast cancer, for instance, transcriptomic assays such as Oncotype DX and MammaPrint help determine the likelihood of recurrence and the potential benefit of chemotherapy, guiding more personalized treatment decisions. Furthermore, transcriptomic data can reveal tumour microenvironment activity, including immune cell infiltration, which has implications for immunotherapy responsiveness. Epigenetic profiling, on the other hand, focuses on heritable but reversible modifications that regulate gene expression without altering the DNA sequence. Key epigenetic mechanisms include DNA methylation, histone modification (such as acetylation and methylation), and chromatin remodelling. In cancer, hypermethylation of tumour suppressor gene promoters often leads to gene silencing, while global hypomethylation can result in genomic instability and activation of oncogenic pathways. Similarly, alterations in histone modification patterns can shift chromatin from a relaxed to a condensed state, affecting gene accessibility and expression. These epigenetic changes are increasingly recognized as critical contributors to tumorigenesis and therapeutic resistance. Importantly, because epigenetic marks are reversible, they present promising targets for novel therapies, such as DNA methyltransferase inhibitors and histone deacetylase inhibitors. Integrating transcriptomic and epigenetic data with genomic information enhances our ability to fully understand cancer biology and develop multidimensional treatment strategies tailored to the individual patient.

- **Proteomic and Metabolomic Profiling:** While genomics and transcriptomics reveal the underlying genetic and transcriptional changes in cancer, proteomic and metabolomic profiling provide critical insights into the functional and biochemical states of tumour cells. Proteomics involves the large-scale study of proteins—the primary effectors of cellular functions—to identify abnormal protein expression patterns, post-translational modifications, and disruptions in cell signalling pathways that contribute to cancer progression. Since proteins ultimately dictate cellular behaviour, analysing their expression and interactions can help pinpoint active oncogenic drivers and resistance mechanisms that might not be evident at the DNA or RNA level. For instance, overexpression or phosphorylation of proteins like HER2, AKT, or mTOR can indicate activated signalling cascades that support cell proliferation, invasion, or survival. Advanced techniques such as mass spectrometry, reverse-phase protein arrays (RPPA), and immunohistochemistry (IHC) are commonly used in proteomic profiling. These tools can identify both diagnostic and prognostic protein biomarkers, and guide treatment decisions—particularly in cases where protein expression is the primary determinant of therapy eligibility, such as HER2-targeted therapies in breast cancer or PD-L1 expression levels for immunotherapy suitability in lung cancer. Metabolomics, on the other hand, examines the dynamic profile of small-molecule metabolites within cancer cells and their microenvironment. Cancer metabolism is notoriously reprogrammed to support rapid growth and survival—seen in phenomena like the Warburg effect, where tumour cells Favor glycolysis even in the presence of oxygen. By profiling metabolites such as lactate, glutamine, lipids, and nucleotides, researchers gain insight into the biochemical pathways active in a particular tumour type. These metabolic fingerprints can reveal new biomarkers for early detection, monitor treatment response, and uncover novel therapeutic vulnerabilities. The integration of proteomic and metabolomic data with genomic information enriches our understanding of tumour biology, offering a systems-level view of cancer. Together, these profiling strategies not only contribute to the identification of actionable targets but also support the development of multi-omics-based precision therapies, ultimately enhancing the personalization of cancer care.

- **Liquid Biopsies:** Liquid biopsies represent a groundbreaking, non-invasive diagnostic technique in personalized oncology, offering a safer and more dynamic alternative to traditional tissue biopsies. This method involves the analysis of tumour-derived components circulating in bodily fluids—primarily blood—including circulating tumour DNA (ctDNA), circulating tumour cells (CTCs), and exosomes. These biomarkers originate from primary tumours, metastases, or even minimal residual disease and carry crucial molecular information about the cancer's genetic makeup and activity. Circulating tumour DNA consists of fragmented DNA released into the bloodstream from cancer cells undergoing apoptosis or necrosis. ctDNA can be analysed using sensitive techniques such as digital PCR and next-generation sequencing, enabling the detection of specific mutations, gene fusions, copy number variations, and methylation patterns. Its presence and concentration can reflect tumour burden, making ctDNA a powerful tool for early cancer detection, identifying actionable mutations, and monitoring treatment response in real time. Circulating tumour cells (CTCs) are intact cancer cells shed into the blood from primary or metastatic sites. They can be isolated and analysed for genetic and phenotypic characteristics, offering insights into tumour heterogeneity, metastatic potential, and resistance mechanisms. CTCs are particularly valuable in cancers like breast, prostate, and lung, where tissue access may be limited or invasive procedures carry high risk. Exosomes, which are small extracellular vesicles secreted by tumour cells, carry DNA, RNA, proteins, and lipids that reflect the molecular status of the tumour. Exosomal content can serve as a rich source of biomarkers for diagnosis and prognosis and may also play a role in cell-to-cell communication and immune modulation. Liquid biopsies are especially useful for detecting minimal residual disease (MRD) after treatment, identifying early relapse, and guiding the adaptation of therapy in a timely manner. Unlike static tissue biopsies, liquid biopsies can be performed serially, providing ongoing insights into tumour evolution, clonal selection, and the emergence of drug resistance. As technology advances and standardization improves, liquid biopsies are poised to become a routine element in the personalized management of cancer, supporting more precise, responsive, and patient-friendly care.

7.1.2 Targeted Treatments

- **Tailoring Therapy to the Tumour's Biology:** Targeted therapy represents a paradigm shift in oncology, offering a more precise and effective alternative to traditional treatments by directly attacking cancer cells based on their unique molecular features. Unlike chemotherapy, which broadly affects both healthy and malignant cells, targeted therapies are designed to interfere with specific molecular pathways that are essential for cancer cell growth, survival, and spread. These treatments rely heavily on the results of tumour profiling, which identifies genetic mutations, protein overexpression, or signalling abnormalities that drive malignancy. Once such targets are identified—such as EGFR, HER2, BRAF, or ALK—clinicians can select drugs specifically engineered to block these drivers. Mechanisms of action vary, including inhibition of tyrosine kinases, blocking of growth factor receptors, induction of apoptosis, and disruption of angiogenesis. Targeted therapies may come in the form of small-molecule inhibitors, which work inside cells, or monoclonal antibodies, which bind to targets on the cell surface. These drugs not only improve treatment efficacy but often result in fewer side effects, as they spare normal tissues. Importantly, targeted treatments are also used in combination with other modalities such as immunotherapy or chemotherapy to overcome resistance and enhance outcomes. As cancer evolves, targeted therapy allows for adaptive treatment strategies, offering real-time response adjustments based on emerging tumour characteristics. This personalized approach is transforming cancer care by increasing survival, improving quality of life, and moving closer to the goal of precision oncology.

- **Tyrosine Kinase Inhibitors (TKIs):** Tyrosine Kinase Inhibitors (TKIs) are a critical class of targeted therapies that work by blocking specific enzymes—tyrosine kinases—that regulate various cellular processes, including growth, proliferation, and survival. In many cancers, these kinases become overactive or mutated, leading to uncontrolled cell division and tumour progression. TKIs are designed to inhibit these faulty signalling pathways, thereby halting cancer development at the molecular level. By occupying the ATP-binding site of the kinase domain, TKIs prevent phosphorylation and downstream signalling required for malignant cell activity. One of the earliest and most notable TKIs is Imatinib, which revolutionized the treatment of chronic myeloid leukaemia (CML) by targeting the BCR-ABL fusion protein, a constitutively active tyrosine kinase formed by a chromosomal translocation. In non-small cell lung cancer (NSCLC), Erlotinib and Gefitinib specifically inhibit EGFR mutations, providing substantial benefits in patients whose tumours harbour these alterations.

Another important TKI, Crizotinib, targets ALK rearrangements in NSCLC, offering improved progression-free survival compared to conventional chemotherapy. TKIs are often taken orally and generally have more favourable side-effect profiles compared to cytotoxic agents. However, resistance can develop through secondary mutations or pathway bypass mechanisms, necessitating the use of second- and third-generation TKIs like Osimertinib for EGFR or Alectinib for ALK. Despite these challenges, TKIs remain a cornerstone of precision oncology, exemplifying how molecular insights can directly inform therapeutic strategies and dramatically improve patient outcomes.

- **Monoclonal Antibodies:** Monoclonal antibodies (mAbs) are lab-engineered immune proteins designed to recognize and bind to specific antigens expressed on the surface of cancer cells. By precisely targeting these tumour-associated proteins, mAbs can block crucial signalling pathways, flag cancer cells for immune destruction, or deliver cytotoxic agents directly to malignant tissues. This level of specificity allows for enhanced anti-tumour activity with reduced damage to healthy cells, making monoclonal antibodies a powerful component of targeted cancer therapy. One of the most widely known mAbs is Trastuzumab, used in HER2-positive breast cancer. By binding to the overexpressed HER2 receptor, Trastuzumab inhibits downstream signalling and promotes immune-mediated cytotoxicity. In colorectal cancer, Cetuximab targets the epidermal growth factor receptor (EGFR), blocking the receptor's activation and interrupting cell proliferation in tumours with wild-type RAS genes. Similarly, Rituximab is used to treat CD20-positive non-Hodgkin lymphoma by binding to the CD20 antigen on B cells, marking them for immune destruction via complement activation and antibody-dependent cellular cytotoxicity. Beyond these mechanisms, monoclonal antibodies can also be conjugated with chemotherapy agents, radioisotopes, or toxins, forming antibody-drug conjugates (ADCs) for enhanced therapeutic effect. Some mAbs are also used in combination with chemotherapy or other targeted therapies to improve response rates. As tumour profiling becomes more advanced, the use of monoclonal antibodies continues to expand across cancer types, solidifying their role in the era of personalized medicine.
- **Immune Checkpoint Inhibitors (a subtype of immunotherapy):** Immune checkpoint inhibitors are a transformative class of immunotherapy drugs that work by unleashing the body's immune system to recognize and destroy cancer cells. Normally, immune checkpoints such as PD-1 (programmed cell death protein 1), PD-L1 (programmed death-ligand 1), and CTLA-4 (cytotoxic T-lymphocyte-associated protein 4) act as regulatory "brakes"

on immune responses to prevent excessive activity that could damage healthy tissue. However, many tumours exploit these pathways to evade immune detection. Immune checkpoint inhibitors block these proteins, thereby restoring T-cell activity and enhancing the immune system's ability to attack the tumour. These agents have shown remarkable success in several cancers, including melanoma, non-small cell lung cancer (NSCLC), bladder cancer, renal cell carcinoma, and head and neck cancers. Drugs like Nivolumab and Pembrolizumab (anti-PD-1), Atezolizumab (anti-PD-L1), and Ipilimumab (anti-CTLA-4) are now standard treatments in various cancer types, often producing durable responses even in advanced disease. Eligibility and likelihood of response are increasingly guided by molecular and immunologic profiling. PD-L1 expression levels in tumour or immune cells can predict benefit from anti-PD-1/PD-L1 therapies. Additionally, microsatellite instability (MSI-high) and high tumour mutational burden (TMB) are biomarkers associated with greater neoantigen load, making tumours more recognizable to immune cells. The success of checkpoint inhibitors marks a significant leap in personalized cancer care, offering patients with specific immunogenic profiles a powerful and often long-lasting therapeutic option.

- **Hormonal Therapies:** Hormonal therapies play a vital role in the management of hormone-driven cancers, particularly breast cancer and prostate cancer, by targeting the endocrine pathways that fuel tumour growth. These therapies are tailored based on the tumour's receptor status, which is determined through testing for hormone receptors such as estrogen receptor (ER), progesterone receptor (PR), and androgen receptor (AR). In breast cancer, tumours that express ER and/or PR are often dependent on these hormones for proliferation, making them susceptible to treatments that either block hormone production or interfere with receptor signalling. Common strategies include the use of selective estrogen receptor modulators (SERMs) like tamoxifen, which block estrogen receptors, or aromatase inhibitors such as anastrozole and letrozole, which reduce estrogen production in postmenopausal women. In prostate cancer, androgen deprivation therapy (ADT) reduces levels of testosterone or blocks androgen receptors to slow disease progression, with agents like leuprolide or enzalutamide frequently used. Hormonal therapies tend to have fewer toxicities compared to chemotherapy and can be administered for long durations, often in adjuvant or metastatic settings. Accurate receptor testing guides treatment decisions, ensuring that only patients with hormone-sensitive tumours receive these therapies, thereby maximizing benefit and minimizing unnecessary exposure. As understanding of hormone receptor biology advances, newer agents continue to emerge, further refining the personalization of endocrine treatment in cancer care.

- **Antibody-Drug Conjugates (ADCs):** Antibody-Drug Conjugates (ADCs) represent an innovative fusion of targeted therapy and chemotherapy, designed to maximize cancer cell killing while minimizing damage to healthy tissue. ADCs combine the specificity of monoclonal antibodies with the potent cytotoxic effects of chemotherapy agents by chemically linking a toxic drug to an antibody that selectively binds to antigens expressed on cancer cells. This targeted delivery system allows the cytotoxic payload to be released directly inside tumour cells, significantly enhancing treatment efficacy and reducing systemic side effects common with traditional chemotherapy. A prominent example is Trastuzumab emtansine (T-DM1), which targets the HER2 receptor on breast cancer cells. The monoclonal antibody component of T-DM1 binds specifically to HER2-positive cells, delivering the conjugated chemotherapeutic agent emtansine directly into the tumour. This targeted approach disrupts microtubule function, leading to cell death, while sparing normal tissues that lack HER2 overexpression. ADCs have expanded treatment options for patients with difficult-to-treat cancers, including HER2-positive breast cancer, certain lymphomas, and other solid tumours. New generations of ADCs continue to be developed, improving drug delivery, minimizing off-target effects, and overcoming resistance mechanisms. By integrating precise tumour targeting with potent cytotoxicity, ADCs exemplify the evolving landscape of personalized medicine, offering tailored, highly effective treatment strategies for cancer patients.

7.1.3 Clinical Applications and Outcomes

Tumour profiling and targeted therapies have revolutionized the management of many cancers, enabling more precise and effective treatment strategies. By identifying specific genetic and molecular alterations within tumours, clinicians can tailor therapies to exploit these vulnerabilities. This personalized approach has led to significant improvements in survival rates, treatment responses, and quality of life for patients. As a result, molecular testing is now an integral part of routine cancer care. The ongoing integration of targeted therapies continues to reshape clinical outcomes across diverse cancer types. Tumour profiling and targeted therapies have already transformed clinical outcomes in several cancers:

- **Lung Cancer:** The advent of targeted therapies against mutations such as EGFR, ALK, and ROS1 has revolutionized the treatment landscape for lung cancer, particularly non-small cell lung cancer (NSCLC). Patients harbouring these genetic alterations experience significantly prolonged progression-free survival and overall survival compared to traditional chemotherapy. These inhibitors not only improve outcomes but also often have better tolerability, allowing patients to maintain quality of life. Routine molecular profiling has become a standard, enabling timely and precise therapeutic decisions. As resistance mechanisms emerge, newer generation inhibitors continue to advance patient care.

- **Melanoma:** Targeted therapies against BRAF mutations in melanoma have dramatically changed prognosis for patients with this aggressive skin cancer subtype. BRAF inhibitors, often combined with MEK inhibitors, deliver rapid tumour regression and durable responses in a majority of treated patients. This approach marks a significant improvement over previous treatments that offered limited survival benefit. Molecular testing for BRAF mutations is now an essential diagnostic step to guide personalized treatment. The integration of targeted therapy with immunotherapy holds promise for even better long-term control.
- **Breast Cancer:** HER2-targeted therapies, such as trastuzumab and newer agents like pertuzumab and T-DM1, have transformed outcomes for HER2-positive breast cancer patients who previously faced poor prognoses. These treatments have substantially increased survival rates and decreased recurrence risk in both early-stage and metastatic disease. HER2 testing is a cornerstone of breast cancer diagnosis, ensuring that patients receive the most effective targeted treatments. The success of HER2-targeted therapy exemplifies how molecular characterization can personalize treatment and improve quality of life. Ongoing research continues to refine these approaches and overcome resistance.
- **Colorectal Cancer:** In colorectal cancer, routine testing for RAS mutations has become standard to determine patient eligibility for anti-EGFR monoclonal antibodies such as cetuximab and panitumumab. Patients with wild-type RAS tumours benefit from these targeted therapies, which improve response rates and survival outcomes, whereas those with RAS mutations do not, preventing ineffective treatments and unnecessary toxicity. This stratification has refined treatment selection and optimized therapeutic efficacy. Molecular profiling guides clinicians in tailoring therapies based on tumour genetics, emphasizing the role of precision medicine in colorectal cancer management. Additional biomarkers like BRAF and MSI status further personalize care.

7.1.4 Companion Diagnostics

Companion diagnostics are specialized tests developed alongside targeted therapies to precisely identify patients who are most likely to benefit from a specific treatment based on their tumour's molecular profile. These diagnostics detect critical biomarkers such as gene mutations, protein overexpression, or chromosomal rearrangements that predict response or resistance to particular drugs. By enabling this precise matching of therapy to tumour biology, companion diagnostics improve treatment effectiveness and minimize unnecessary exposure to ineffective or potentially harmful therapies. Regulatory agencies, including the FDA, have recognized their importance and increasingly mandate biomarker testing before approving certain targeted drugs. For example, HER2 testing is required prior to initiating trastuzumab in breast cancer patients, while EGFR mutation analysis is essential before prescribing erlotinib or osimertinib in non-small cell lung cancer. The integration of companion diagnostics into clinical practice ensures that personalized medicine moves beyond theory to become a practical, life-saving reality. These tests employ advanced molecular techniques, such as immunohistochemistry, fluorescence in situ hybridization, and next-generation sequencing, to provide accurate and timely results that guide therapeutic decisions. As targeted therapies expand, companion diagnostics will continue to play a pivotal role in optimizing cancer treatment and improving patient outcomes.

Example-1: Before initiating trastuzumab therapy in breast cancer patients, HER2 testing is mandatory to confirm overexpression or gene amplification of the HER2 receptor. This testing ensures that only patients whose tumours rely on HER2 signalling receive the treatment, maximizing efficacy and minimizing unnecessary exposure. Accurate HER2 status determination is critical for guiding therapy decisions and improving patient outcomes. It is typically performed using immunohistochemistry (IHC) and fluorescence in situ hybridization (FISH) assays.

Example-2: EGFR mutation testing is a prerequisite before prescribing targeted tyrosine kinase inhibitors such as erlotinib or osimertinib for non-small cell lung cancer patients. This test identifies specific activating mutations in the EGFR gene that predict sensitivity to these drugs. By selecting patients based on mutation status, clinicians can offer therapies with higher response rates and better progression-free survival. Testing is commonly performed using PCR-based methods or next-generation sequencing for precise molecular characterization.

7.1.5 Challenges and Future Directions

While personalized oncology has made substantial progress, it also faces several challenges

- **Tumour Heterogeneity:** Tumour heterogeneity refers to the genetic and molecular variability that exists not only within a single tumour but also between the primary tumour and its metastatic sites. This complexity can cause differential responses to targeted therapies, as some cancer cell populations may lack the specific mutations targeted by treatment.

Such variability challenges effective therapy selection and contributes to treatment resistance. Understanding and addressing tumour heterogeneity is essential for improving personalized treatment strategies. Advanced profiling techniques, including multi-region biopsies and liquid biopsies, help capture this diversity.

- **Acquired Resistance:** While targeted therapies often produce impressive initial responses, many patients eventually develop acquired resistance, wherein the cancer evolves mechanisms to bypass drug effects. Secondary mutations in the target gene, activation of alternative signalling pathways, or phenotypic changes can all contribute to this resistance. Overcoming acquired resistance requires ongoing molecular monitoring and the development of next-generation inhibitors or combination therapies. This dynamic interplay underscores the need for adaptive treatment strategies in precision oncology. Continuous research is focused on predicting and managing resistance mechanisms.
- **Cost and Accessibility:** The advanced molecular diagnostics and targeted therapies integral to personalized medicine often come with high costs, limiting their accessibility, especially in low-resource or rural settings. Expensive reagents, specialized equipment, and trained personnel are required for accurate biomarker testing, while targeted drugs can be prohibitively costly for many healthcare systems. This disparity creates significant barriers to equitable cancer care worldwide. Efforts to reduce costs, expand insurance coverage, and develop affordable technologies are crucial to broadening access. Increasing global collaboration and innovation may help democratize these life-saving advances.
- **Integration into Clinical Workflows:** Successful implementation of personalized medicine requires seamless integration of tumour profiling and targeted therapy into everyday clinical workflows. This process demands close collaboration among multidisciplinary teams, including oncologists, pathologists, molecular biologists, and bioinformaticians. The interpretation of complex genomic data and translating it into actionable treatment decisions pose significant challenges. Additionally, healthcare systems must adopt advanced data management tools and develop standardized protocols. Investing in training and infrastructure is key to optimizing the clinical utility of precision oncology.

Future strategies include:

- Combination therapies to overcome resistance.
- Artificial intelligence and machine learning for better biomarker discovery.

- Pan-cancer molecular profiling and basket trials that match treatments to molecular features regardless of cancer type.
- Expansion of liquid biopsy applications for early diagnosis and surveillance.

Tumour profiling and targeted treatments lie at the heart of personalized medicine in oncology. By identifying the molecular drivers of cancer and intervening with highly specific therapies, clinicians can improve survival rates, reduce toxicity, and personalize patient care like never before. The integration of precision diagnostics with individualized treatment strategies is not only changing the clinical landscape but also offering renewed hope for millions of cancer patients worldwide.

7.2 CARDIOLOGY

Genetic Testing for Risk and Response: Genetic testing has emerged as a powerful tool in cardiology, enabling the identification of inherited genetic variants that influence an individual's risk of developing cardiovascular diseases. These tests help detect mutations associated with conditions such as hypertrophic cardiomyopathy, long QT syndrome, and familial hypercholesterolemia, often before clinical symptoms appear. Early identification allows for timely interventions and personalized monitoring strategies, improving patient outcomes. Beyond risk assessment, pharmacogenomic testing plays a crucial role in guiding cardiovascular drug therapy by predicting how patients metabolize medications like clopidogrel, reducing the risk of adverse effects and optimizing treatment efficacy. Genetic screening is also vital in familial cardiac disorders, facilitating cascade testing among relatives to prevent sudden cardiac events. Additionally, genetic insights can predict susceptibility to drug-induced cardiotoxicity, enabling safer medication choices. The integration of genetic testing into cardiology practice exemplifies the move toward precision medicine, offering tailored prevention, diagnosis, and treatment strategies. Multidisciplinary collaboration and advanced molecular technologies continue to enhance the clinical utility of these tests. As research advances, genetic testing is expected to become increasingly central to cardiovascular care. Overall, genetic testing provides a comprehensive approach to managing cardiac health on an individualized basis.

7.2.1 Genetic Risk Assessment

Genetic testing in cardiology helps identify inherited variants that increase susceptibility to cardiovascular diseases such as hypertrophic cardiomyopathy, long QT syndrome, familial hypercholesterolemia, and arrhythmogenic right ventricular cardiomyopathy. By analysing mutations in genes related to cardiac structure, ion channels, or lipid metabolism, clinicians can stratify patients' risk profiles early—sometimes before symptoms develop—enabling timely preventive measures and surveillance.

7.2.2 Pharmacogenomics in Cardiology

Pharmacogenomic testing evaluates how genetic variations influence an individual's response to cardiovascular drugs. For example, variants in the CYP2C19 gene affect metabolism of clopidogrel, an antiplatelet agent, impacting its efficacy and safety. Identifying such polymorphisms allows clinicians to personalize drug choice and dosage, reducing adverse events and optimizing therapeutic outcomes in conditions like atrial fibrillation or coronary artery disease.

7.2.3 Genetic Testing for Familial Disorders

In families with a history of inherited cardiac conditions, genetic testing provides critical information for cascade screening and early diagnosis of at-risk relatives. Testing for mutations in genes such as MYH7, TNNT2, or LDLR informs clinical management, including lifestyle modifications, medical therapy, or implantable devices to prevent sudden cardiac death or heart failure progression.

7.2.4 Predicting Drug-Induced Cardiotoxicity

Certain cardiovascular drugs, including some chemotherapeutic agents or antiarrhythmics, carry risks of cardiotoxicity that may be influenced by genetic factors. Genetic screening can identify patients predisposed to adverse cardiac effects, guiding safer drug selection and monitoring strategies.

7.2.5 Integration into Clinical Practice

Incorporating genetic testing into cardiology requires coordinated efforts among cardiologists, genetic counsellors, and laboratory specialists. Developing guidelines for test utilization, interpretation, and patient education ensures the clinical utility of genetic information, facilitating precision cardiology that improves prevention, diagnosis, and treatment. Overview of genetic testing applications in cardiology for risk stratification and personalized drug response is given in Table-1.

Table: 1 Overview of Genetic Testing Applications in Cardiology for Risk Stratification and Personalized Drug Response

S. No.	Description	Examples / Key Genes	Clinical Impact
1.Genetic Risk Assessment	Identifies inherited variants increasing susceptibility to cardiovascular diseases. Early risk stratification enables preventive care.	Hypertrophic cardiomyopathy, Long QT syndrome, Familial hypercholesterolemia, Arrhythmogenic right ventricular cardiomyopathy	Early detection and surveillance before symptoms appear.

S. No.	Description	Examples / Key Genes	Clinical Impact
2. Pharmacogenomics in Cardiology	Tests genetic variants influencing drug metabolism and response to tailor cardiovascular drug therapy.	CYP2C19 (clopidogrel metabolism)	Optimizes drug choice/dose; reduces adverse drug reactions.
3. Genetic Testing for Familial Disorders	Provides information for cascade screening in families with inherited cardiac diseases, aiding early diagnosis.	MYH7, TNNT2, LDLR	Guides clinical management and preventive interventions.
4. Predicting Drug-Induced Cardiotoxicity	Identifies genetic predisposition to cardiotoxicity from certain drugs, enabling safer treatment plans.	Various genetic markers (dependent on drug)	Prevents adverse cardiac effects; guides monitoring.

7.3 NEUROLOGY AND PSYCHIATRY

Pharmacogenetics in mental health is an emerging field that studies how genetic differences influence an individual's response to psychiatric medications. Mental health disorders such as depression, schizophrenia, bipolar disorder, and anxiety affect millions worldwide, and treatment responses can vary widely between patients. Genetic variations, particularly in drug-metabolizing enzymes and receptor genes, play a crucial role in determining drug efficacy and risk of side effects. By understanding these genetic factors, clinicians can personalize medication choices, dosages, and treatment plans. This approach aims to reduce the traditional trial-and-error method in psychiatry, minimizing adverse effects and improving treatment outcomes. Pharmacogenetic testing is increasingly being integrated into clinical practice to guide antidepressant and antipsychotic therapies. Although challenges remain in implementation, such as cost and clinical guidelines, the potential benefits for patient care are substantial. As research advances, pharmacogenetics promises to enhance precision medicine in neurology and psychiatry, leading to more effective and safer mental health treatments. This personalized strategy ultimately aims to improve quality of life for patients by tailoring therapies to their unique genetic makeup.

7.3.1 Role of Pharmacogenetics in Psychiatry

Pharmacogenetics explores how genetic differences among individuals influence their response to psychiatric medications, with the goal of optimizing treatment efficacy and minimizing adverse effects. Psychiatric disorders such as depression, bipolar disorder, schizophrenia, and anxiety often require long-term medication, but responses vary widely due to genetic variability. By identifying genetic markers associated with drug metabolism, receptor sensitivity, and neurotransmitter pathways, clinicians can personalize medication regimens. This tailored approach helps avoid the traditional trial-and-error prescribing, which can delay symptom relief and increase the risk of side effects. Pharmacogenetics also aids in predicting which patients may experience toxicity or poor therapeutic response, thereby improving adherence and overall outcomes. As mental health conditions carry significant personal and societal burdens, pharmacogenetics represents a promising strategy to advance precision psychiatry and transform care.

7.3.2 Genetic Variants Affecting Drug Metabolism

Genetic polymorphisms in cytochrome P450 enzymes, particularly CYP2D6 and CYP2C19, significantly impact the metabolism of many psychotropic drugs. Individuals classified as poor metabolizers may have slower drug clearance, leading to increased drug levels and heightened risk of side effects or toxicity. Conversely, ultra-rapid metabolizers process drugs too quickly, potentially resulting in subtherapeutic drug concentrations and treatment failure. These variations affect not only antidepressants but also antipsychotics, mood stabilizers, and anxiolytics. Understanding a patient's metabolizer status allows clinicians to adjust drug choice and dosing appropriately, improving both safety and efficacy. Genetic testing for these variants is becoming more accessible and is increasingly integrated into clinical decision-making, providing a critical tool in personalized mental health care.

7.3.3 Impact on Antidepressant Therapy

Pharmacogenetic testing can guide the selection and dosing of antidepressants, such as selective serotonin reuptake inhibitors (SSRIs) and tricyclic antidepressants, by revealing individual genetic factors that influence drug metabolism and receptor interactions. For instance, CYP2C19 and CYP2D6 variants determine how quickly these drugs are metabolized, affecting their plasma concentrations and clinical effects. Additionally, variations in serotonin transporter genes or receptor genes may alter drug response or susceptibility to side effects like weight gain or sexual dysfunction. By incorporating pharmacogenetic insights, clinicians can choose antidepressants with a higher likelihood of effectiveness and tolerability for each patient. This personalized approach reduces the time needed to find an effective treatment, decreases adverse effects, and improves patient adherence and quality of life in managing depression and other mood disorders.

7.3.4 Antipsychotic Drug Response and Safety

Genetic testing also plays a vital role in optimizing antipsychotic therapy by identifying variants that affect drug metabolism and receptor binding, thereby influencing both efficacy and risk of side effects. For example, polymorphisms in CYP2D6 can affect plasma levels of drugs like risperidone and aripiprazole, necessitating dose adjustments. Genetic differences in dopamine and serotonin receptor genes may also modulate therapeutic response and susceptibility to extrapyramidal symptoms or metabolic side effects such as weight gain and diabetes. Tailoring antipsychotic treatment based on genetic information can improve symptom control while minimizing harmful effects, which are major causes of treatment discontinuation. This precision approach enhances overall treatment success and patient quality of life in disorders like schizophrenia and bipolar disorder.

7.3.5 Implementation Challenges and Clinical Utility

Despite the promise of pharmacogenetic testing in mental health, several challenges hinder widespread adoption. Standardized guidelines for test utilization and result interpretation remain limited, causing variability in clinical application. Additionally, insurance coverage and reimbursement for these tests are inconsistent, limiting patient access. Many clinicians lack formal training in genetics, creating barriers to integrating pharmacogenetic data into treatment planning. Ethical and privacy concerns around genetic information also require careful management. However, accumulating evidence supports pharmacogenetics' potential to improve treatment outcomes, reduce adverse events, and decrease the trial-and-error approach common in psychiatry. Ongoing research, education, and policy efforts aim to overcome these challenges and embed pharmacogenetics as a routine part of personalized mental healthcare.

7.4 INFECTIOUS DISEASES

Personalized medicine has significantly advanced the management of infectious diseases, particularly HIV, hepatitis, and COVID-19, by integrating genetic insights from both the pathogen and the host. In HIV care, viral genotyping identifies drug resistance mutations, enabling clinicians to tailor antiretroviral therapy for maximum efficacy. Additionally, host genetic factors such as the HLA-B*57:01 allele can predict hypersensitivity reactions to specific drugs like abacavir, improving treatment safety. Similarly, in hepatitis B and C infections, viral genotyping and host genetic polymorphisms, including IL28B variants, guide the selection and duration of antiviral therapies, enhancing response rates. Pharmacogenomics also plays a critical role in identifying patients at risk of drug-induced toxicities, helping to optimize drug regimens and reduce adverse effects. The COVID-19 pandemic has further highlighted the importance of genetic factors in infectious diseases; variations in genes related to immune response and viral entry, such as ACE2 receptor polymorphisms, influence susceptibility and disease severity. By understanding these genetic differences, healthcare providers can develop personalized preventive and therapeutic strategies, improving patient outcomes. Overall, the integration of pathogen genomics, host genetics, and pharmacogenomics forms the cornerstone of precision medicine in infectious diseases, enabling tailored treatment approaches that are more effective and safer. This personalized approach not only enhances individual care but also supports public health efforts by addressing the genetic diversity of both hosts and pathogens. As genomic technologies continue to evolve, their application in infectious diseases promises to further revolutionize diagnosis, treatment, and prevention strategies worldwide.

7.4.1 Genetic Profiling in HIV Management

Genetic profiling in HIV management focuses primarily on analysing the viral genome to identify mutations that confer resistance to antiretroviral drugs. HIV's high mutation rate leads to the emergence of drug-resistant strains, which can compromise therapy effectiveness. By performing viral genotyping, clinicians can detect these resistance-associated mutations before or during treatment, allowing for the selection of an optimal antiretroviral therapy (ART) regimen tailored to the patient's viral profile. This precision reduces the risk of treatment failure and the spread of resistant strains. Beyond viral genetics, host genetic factors also play a critical role in therapy personalization. For example, the presence of the HLA-B*57:01 allele predicts hypersensitivity to the drug abacavir, which can cause severe immune reactions. Testing for this allele prior to initiating abacavir treatment is now standard clinical practice, significantly enhancing patient safety. Furthermore, other host genetic markers influence drug metabolism and immune responses, offering additional avenues to customize treatment. Together, viral and host genetic profiling form the foundation for precision HIV medicine, aiming to maximize treatment efficacy, reduce adverse effects, and improve long-term outcomes for patients living with HIV.

7.4.2 Personalized Therapy in Hepatitis B and C

In hepatitis B and C infections, personalized therapy hinges on the detailed genetic analysis of both the virus and the host. Hepatitis viruses exhibit multiple genotypes and subtypes, each responding differently to antiviral treatments. Viral genotyping is crucial for choosing the most effective antiviral agents, determining treatment duration, and predicting the likelihood of achieving sustained virologic response (SVR). For hepatitis C, certain genotypes respond better to direct-acting antivirals, while others may require longer or combination therapies. Host genetics also critically influence treatment success. Polymorphisms in the IL28B gene, for example, are strongly associated with response to interferon-based therapies in hepatitis C patients. Patients with favourable IL28B variants tend to clear the virus more effectively when treated with interferon and ribavirin. Although direct-acting antivirals have largely replaced interferon, IL28B genotyping remains relevant in some clinical settings and for predicting spontaneous viral clearance. Similarly, host genetic factors impact immune responses and liver disease progression in hepatitis B infection, helping guide monitoring and therapy decisions. By integrating viral and host genetic data, clinicians can design personalized treatment strategies that maximize cure rates, minimize side effects, and improve patient prognosis.

7.4.3 Pharmacogenomics and Drug Toxicity

Pharmacogenomics plays a pivotal role in managing drug-induced toxicities in infectious disease treatment, particularly for antiviral therapies. Certain genetic variants in patients can predispose them to adverse reactions such as mitochondrial toxicity, hepatotoxicity, or hypersensitivity, which can significantly impact treatment adherence and outcomes. For example, some nucleoside reverse transcriptase inhibitors (NRTIs) used in HIV therapy may cause mitochondrial dysfunction in genetically susceptible individuals. Pharmacogenetic testing helps identify these patients before initiating therapy, enabling clinicians to avoid or adjust the offending drugs accordingly. Similarly, genetic variations affecting liver enzyme function can increase the risk of hepatotoxicity during hepatitis treatment. Recognizing these risks through genetic screening allows for closer monitoring, dose adjustments, or alternative therapies to reduce harm. Additionally, pharmacogenomics aids in understanding drug–drug interactions and variable drug metabolism, supporting safer and more effective medication regimens. By tailoring antiviral therapy based on individual genetic susceptibility to toxicity, healthcare providers can improve patient safety, reduce treatment discontinuations, and enhance overall therapeutic success in infectious diseases.

7.4.4 COVID-19

Genetic Factors Influencing Susceptibility and Severity: The COVID-19 pandemic has underscored the critical influence of host genetics on susceptibility to SARS-CoV-2 infection and disease severity. Genetic variations in key immune response genes, such as those encoding the ACE2 receptor—which SARS-CoV-2 uses to enter cells—and components of the innate immune system, modulate individual responses to the virus. For example, certain ACE2 polymorphisms may affect viral binding efficiency, influencing infection risk and viral load. Other genetic variants involved in inflammatory pathways can determine the severity of the immune response, contributing to the development of severe symptoms or complications like cytokine storms. Understanding these genetic factors enables better risk stratification, allowing high-risk individuals to receive prioritized preventive measures such as vaccination or early therapeutic interventions. Additionally, genetic insights have facilitated the identification of novel therapeutic targets and informed the development of precision medicine approaches, including personalized antiviral therapies and immunomodulatory treatments. As research evolves, integrating host genetic profiling with clinical data holds promise for improving COVID-19 patient management and outcomes on an individualized basis.

7.4.5 Precision Medicine Approaches in Infectious Diseases

Precision medicine in infectious diseases integrates pathogen genomics, host genetic information, and pharmacogenomics to deliver highly tailored healthcare. This comprehensive approach improves diagnosis, guides therapeutic choices, and predicts treatment responses with greater accuracy than traditional methods. Viral genomic sequencing enables the identification of resistance mutations, emerging variants, and epidemiologic tracking, informing public health strategies and individualized treatments. Concurrently, host genetic profiling identifies susceptibilities to infections, drug metabolism capabilities, and risks for adverse drug reactions. Pharmacogenomic data allow for drug regimen optimization, minimizing toxicity and maximizing efficacy. Together, these tools enable personalized prevention, diagnosis, and treatment plans that reflect the genetic diversity of both patients and pathogens. Such strategies are particularly vital in managing complex infections like HIV, hepatitis, and COVID-19, where genetic variability significantly influences clinical outcomes. Moreover, precision medicine supports antimicrobial stewardship by reducing inappropriate drug use and combating resistance development. As genomic technologies become more accessible and cost-effective, their integration into infectious disease management promises to transform patient care and public health worldwide.

7.5 RARE AND GENETIC DISORDERS

Rare and genetic disorders, though individually uncommon, collectively affect millions of people worldwide. These conditions often arise from single-gene mutations and present with complex, varied symptoms that challenge traditional diagnostic methods. Personalized medicine offers a transformative approach by leveraging genomic technologies such as whole-exome and whole-genome sequencing to accurately identify disease-causing mutations. Early diagnosis not only ends the diagnostic odyssey but also allows timely intervention that can prevent or slow disease progression. Moreover, treatments can now be tailored to a patient's specific genetic mutation, enhancing effectiveness and reducing side effects. Innovations like gene therapy and CRISPR-based editing are pushing the boundaries of what is possible in terms of cures. Carrier screening and genetic counselling further support informed reproductive decisions and family planning. Despite these advances, challenges such as high costs, limited access, and ethical concerns remain significant barriers. Nonetheless, with growing global collaboration and data sharing, personalized medicine continues to reshape the landscape of care for rare and genetic disorders.

7.5.1 Importance of Genomic Sequencing in Rare Diseases

Rare diseases are often monogenic and highly heterogeneous, making diagnosis through clinical presentation alone extremely challenging. Traditional diagnostic approaches can take years and involve numerous tests, leading to what is commonly referred to as a "diagnostic odyssey." The advent of whole-exome sequencing (WES) and whole-genome sequencing (WGS) has revolutionized the diagnostic process by enabling comprehensive analysis of a patient's DNA in a single test. These technologies allow for the identification of previously undetectable or misdiagnosed mutations, especially in genes with complex or variable expression. In many cases, WES or WGS not only leads to an accurate diagnosis but also reveals potential therapeutic targets. For paediatric patients with developmental delay, unexplained metabolic crises, or progressive neurological conditions, genomic sequencing can provide answers that influence medical decisions, family planning, and eligibility for emerging therapies or clinical trials. Furthermore, these techniques are now more accessible and cost-effective than ever, making them a first-line diagnostic tool in many genetic centres. Ultimately, genomic sequencing transforms rare disease management by turning years of uncertainty into actionable insight within weeks.

7.5.2 Early Diagnosis and Intervention

Timely identification of rare genetic disorders is critical for initiating interventions that may prevent irreversible damage or disease progression. Many genetic diseases, especially inborn errors of metabolism or neuromuscular disorders, manifest symptoms only after a critical threshold is crossed. By identifying at-risk individuals early—sometimes even during the newborn period—clinicians can implement dietary modifications, enzyme replacement therapies, or surveillance strategies that significantly improve quality of life. For example, early diagnosis of phenylketonuria (PKU) allows dietary management that prevents intellectual disability. In conditions like spinal muscular atrophy (SMA), where treatment efficacy is highest before symptom onset, genetic newborn screening can be life-saving. Precision diagnostics also help stratify patients based on disease severity, enabling tailored therapeutic approaches. Moreover, early detection supports families in planning care, connecting with support networks, and understanding the prognosis. Genetic counselling can accompany early testing to prepare families for decisions ahead. In sum, early diagnosis not only improves clinical outcomes but also reduces healthcare costs and emotional distress for families.

7.5.3 Tailored Treatment Based on Mutational Profile

One of the most powerful applications of personalized medicine in rare diseases is the ability to align treatment strategies with the specific genetic mutation a patient carries. Rather than using a one-size-fits-all approach, therapy can be tailored to correct or compensate for the defective gene product. For instance, in cystic fibrosis, the development of ivacaftor and other CFTR modulators targets the functional defect caused by specific CFTR gene mutations, resulting in improved lung function and quality of life. Similarly, enzyme replacement therapy (ERT) is used in lysosomal storage disorders such as Gaucher disease or Pompe disease, where recombinant enzymes replace deficient ones. Some therapies even vary based on the exact mutation subtype, ensuring optimal efficacy. Precision treatment approaches are now being explored for conditions like Duchenne muscular dystrophy, where exon-skipping therapies target specific deletions. By matching the therapy to the molecular profile, clinicians can achieve better outcomes, reduce unnecessary side effects, and offer patients more hope. This mutation-guided approach marks a significant evolution from generalized symptom management to targeted care.

7.5.4 Gene Therapy and Emerging Modalities

Gene therapy represents a transformative advancement in treating rare and genetic disorders. Unlike conventional treatments that manage symptoms, gene therapy aims to address the root cause by delivering a correct copy of the faulty gene into the patient's cells. One of the landmark therapies is Zolgensma, approved for spinal muscular atrophy (SMA), which delivers the SMN1 gene through an adeno-associated virus vector, restoring motor function in infants and reducing mortality. Other gene therapies are being developed for conditions such as haemophilia, Leber congenital amaurosis, and beta-thalassemia, offering the potential for long-term or even permanent cures. Alongside viral-based therapies, gene-editing technologies such as CRISPR-Cas9 allow for precise correction of genetic mutations at the DNA level, showing promise for monogenic conditions like sickle cell disease and Tay-Sachs disease. However, these technologies are still in early clinical stages and pose challenges related to delivery, safety, and off-target effects. As these modalities mature, they are expected to become more accessible and cost-effective, redefining therapeutic landscapes for many previously untreatable rare diseases.

7.5.5 Carrier Screening and Genetic Counselling

Carrier screening identifies individuals who harbour mutations for recessive genetic disorders, even if they are asymptomatic. This information is crucial for reproductive decision-making, particularly in couples with a family history of genetic disease or in populations with high prevalence of specific conditions. Expanded carrier screening panels now test for dozens or hundreds of genetic conditions, including Tay-Sachs, cystic fibrosis, spinal muscular atrophy, and fragile X syndrome. When both partners are found to be carriers of the same condition, they can explore reproductive options such as preimplantation genetic diagnosis (PGD), use of donor gametes, or in vitro fertilization (IVF). Genetic counselling plays a vital role in this process by helping individuals and families understand inheritance patterns, test results, emotional impacts, and medical options. Counselling is also essential in supporting patients' post-diagnosis, guiding them through treatment planning, support resources, and anticipatory care. In the era of personalized medicine, genetic counselling ensures that medical decisions are informed, ethically sound, and aligned with the patient's values and goals.

7.5.6 Challenges in Implementation

Despite remarkable advancements, the implementation of personalized medicine for rare diseases faces several barriers. High costs of genomic testing, specialized therapies, and gene therapies limit widespread access, particularly in low- and middle-income countries. Even when testing is available, there may be a lack of infrastructure, trained professionals, and awareness among clinicians to interpret and apply the data effectively. Ethical concerns also arise regarding the storage, sharing, and use of sensitive genetic information, including potential discrimination and privacy breaches. In some regions, insurance coverage for genetic testing and counselling remains inconsistent. Furthermore, while diagnosis is improving, therapeutic options are still unavailable for many ultra-rare conditions due to the high cost and complexity of drug development. This creates disparities in care and limits the potential impact of early diagnosis. Addressing these challenges requires coordinated efforts between governments, healthcare systems, researchers, and industry stakeholders to ensure equitable and sustainable access to personalized medicine.

7.5.7 Role of Registries and Data Sharing

Due to the low prevalence of individual rare diseases, accumulating sufficient clinical and genetic data for research and treatment development is difficult. Rare disease registries and international data-sharing platforms help overcome this challenge by pooling anonymized patient data across institutions and borders. These databases support natural history studies, inform clinical trial design, and enable the identification of patient subgroups most likely to benefit from emerging therapies. Platforms like Orphanet, Global Genes, and initiatives from organizations like EURORDIS foster collaboration among researchers, clinicians, and patient communities. Sharing genomic and phenotypic data in a standardized and secure manner accelerates biomarker discovery, treatment development, and regulatory approval processes. Moreover, registries empower patients by offering them a voice in research prioritization and access to trials. As data-sharing technology and privacy protections evolve, such initiatives are essential for advancing personalized medicine in rare diseases and ensuring that no patient is left behind due to rarity. Personalized medicine approaches in rare and genetic disorders is summarised in Table-2.

Table-2: Personalized Medicine Approaches in Rare and Genetic Disorders

S. No.	Area	Key Insights
1.	Genomic Sequencing in Diagnosis	WES and WGS help identify disease-causing mutations, reducing diagnostic delays in rare conditions.
2.	Early Diagnosis and Intervention	Early genetic detection enables timely, sometimes life-saving, treatment before symptom onset.
3.	Tailored Treatment Based on Mutation	Therapies like ERT and mutation-specific drugs (e.g., ivacaftor) are selected based on genetic profile.
4.	Gene Therapy and Emerging Modalities	Therapies like Zolgensma and CRISPR offer potential cures for monogenic disorders.
5.	Carrier Screening & Genetic Counselling	Identifies at-risk individuals; informs reproductive decisions and supports affected families.
6.	Challenges in Implementation	High cost, access issues, ethical concerns, and limited treatment options hinder widespread use.
7.	Registries & Data Sharing	Global databases support research, clinical trial recruitment, and knowledge sharing in rare diseases.

8 Chapter

DIGITAL HEALTH AND PERSONALIZED CARE

8.0 INTRODUCTION: AN OVERVIEW

The fusion of digital health and personalized care represents a paradigm shift in how healthcare is delivered and experienced. It moves the focus from reactive, episodic treatment to proactive, preventive, and precision-based management. By leveraging real-time data, intelligent systems, and individualized insights, digital personalized healthcare holds the potential to improve outcomes, enhance quality of life, and make healthcare more efficient and equitable. As this field continues to evolve, its success will depend on our collective ability to harness technology responsibly, inclusively, and innovatively in the service of better health for all.

The landscape of modern healthcare is undergoing a profound transformation, driven by the convergence of digital technologies and personalized medicine. Digital health refers to the use of information and communication technologies—including mobile health (mHealth), wearable devices, telemedicine, health information systems, artificial intelligence (AI), and big data analytics—to improve health outcomes, efficiency, and patient engagement. Personalized care, on the other hand, emphasizes tailored treatment approaches based on an individual's unique genetic makeup, lifestyle, environment, and health history. When integrated, digital health and personalized care form a synergistic model that empowers both patients and providers, ushering in a new era of precision healthcare. Traditionally, medicine has operated on a "one-size-fits-all" model, where patients with similar conditions received similar treatments, often without consideration of biological differences. However, advances in genomics, biomarkers, and clinical data analytics have revealed the need for more individualized approaches. Personalized care leverages this insight, delivering therapies that are optimized for the individual rather than the average. Digital health tools are key enablers in this process, offering real-time data collection, continuous monitoring, and decision-support systems that translate complex information into actionable insights at the point of care. Wearable technologies and mobile applications have made health monitoring more accessible than ever before. Devices that track heart rate, sleep, glucose levels, and physical activity allow patients to participate actively in their care, promoting preventive behaviours and early detection of health issues. These data streams, when integrated with electronic health records (EHRs), create a comprehensive digital profile that supports dynamic and responsive healthcare delivery. Telemedicine has further expanded access to personalized care, especially for patients in rural or underserved areas, by connecting them to specialists and services without the need for travel.

Artificial intelligence plays a pivotal role in transforming vast amounts of health data into personalized care pathways. Machine learning algorithms can predict disease risk, optimize treatment regimens, and support early diagnosis with unprecedented accuracy. AI-driven tools are already being used in radiology, dermatology, mental health, and oncology to guide clinical decisions based on patterns recognized across millions of data points. This enhances the precision of diagnosis and treatment while reducing variability in care delivery. Furthermore, digital health platforms enable the seamless integration of multi-omics data—genomics, proteomics, metabolomics—with lifestyle and behavioural data to create truly individualized care models. Such platforms support the delivery of "N-of-1" medicine, where treatments are developed, tested, and optimized for a single patient. This level of personalization has major implications for managing chronic diseases such as diabetes, cardiovascular conditions, and mental health disorders, which require ongoing, adaptive care strategies. Personalized digital health is also revolutionizing population health management. By identifying at-risk groups through predictive analytics, public health officials can implement targeted interventions, reducing disease burden and healthcare costs. For healthcare providers, digital tools support clinical workflows, improve documentation accuracy, and enable data-driven decision-making. For patients, digital platforms offer greater transparency, education, and empowerment in managing their health journey. Despite its immense promise, the integration of digital health and personalized care is not without challenges. Issues such as data privacy, interoperability, cybersecurity, algorithmic bias, and the digital divide must be addressed to ensure equity, safety, and trust. Additionally, regulatory frameworks must evolve to keep pace with rapidly developing technologies while safeguarding ethical standards. Clinical validation of digital tools and their integration into routine care pathways require strong collaboration between healthcare systems, tech developers, and policymakers (Fig. 1).

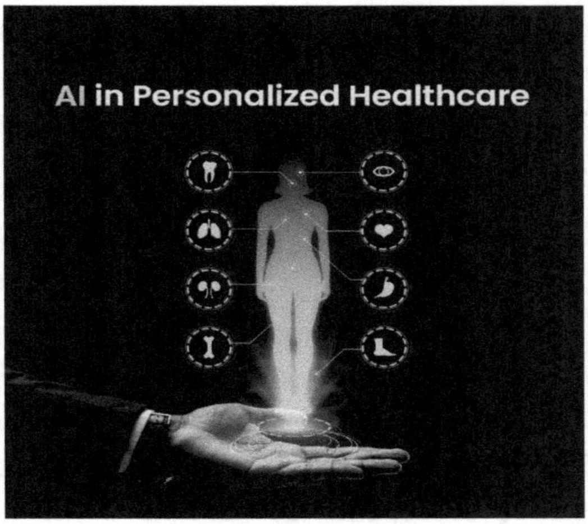

Fig. 1 The Role of AI in Personalized Healthcare

8.1 MOBILE HEALTH (MHEALTH) AND REMOTE MONITORING

Mobile Health (mHealth) and remote monitoring represent transformative components of digital healthcare, enabling real-time, patient-centred care beyond traditional clinical settings. Through smartphones, wearable devices, and mobile applications, individuals can now track their health metrics, manage chronic conditions, and engage in virtual consultations from virtually anywhere. Remote monitoring tools, such as continuous glucose monitors and smartwatches, provide clinicians with timely data for proactive interventions and personalized treatment adjustments. These technologies enhance patient engagement, improve adherence to care plans, and reduce hospital visits. Especially valuable in chronic disease management and post-discharge care, mHealth tools are also expanding access to healthcare in underserved regions. As connectivity improves globally, mHealth is becoming a cornerstone of preventive and precision medicine. However, issues like data privacy, device accuracy, and digital literacy remain challenges. Despite this, the potential of mHealth and remote monitoring to reshape healthcare delivery is immense and rapidly growing.

8.1.1 Definition and Scope of mHealth

Mobile Health (mHealth) is a rapidly evolving subset of digital health that harnesses the power of mobile technologies—such as smartphones, tablets, smartwatches, and wireless biosensors—to deliver healthcare services and information. It encompasses a broad range of applications including health monitoring, disease prevention, patient education, treatment adherence, teleconsultation, and lifestyle management. By enabling health data collection and communication in real time, mHealth bridges the gap between patients and healthcare providers, facilitating a more dynamic and proactive model of care. The scope of mHealth spans multiple dimensions of healthcare. It supports chronic disease management by allowing patients to monitor blood glucose, blood pressure, or respiratory function through mobile apps or connected devices. Medication adherence apps remind users to take prescriptions on time, reducing complications and hospitalizations. mHealth tools also promote preventive health by tracking steps, sleep, nutrition, and mental well-being, encouraging users to adopt healthier lifestyles. Women's health apps monitor menstrual cycles, pregnancy progress, and fertility windows, while mental health platforms offer mindfulness exercises, mood tracking, and access to virtual therapy. In clinical settings, mHealth enhances workflow efficiency and patient communication. Providers can remotely review patient data, offer virtual follow-ups, and intervene early when adverse trends are detected. For populations in remote or underserved areas, mHealth breaks down barriers to access by offering mobile-based consultations and health education. Public health programs increasingly rely on mHealth for disease surveillance, vaccination tracking, and emergency health alerts, especially during outbreaks or natural disasters. Overall, mHealth represents a paradigm shift toward personalized, connected, and decentralized care. As mobile technology becomes more affordable and widespread, its role in promoting health equity, patient empowerment, and system-wide efficiency continues to grow. However, to realize its full potential, challenges such as data privacy, user literacy, device interoperability, and regulatory oversight must be carefully addressed.

8.1.2 Types of mHealth Applications

Mobile health (mHealth) applications have become integral tools in modern healthcare, offering a wide range of functions that support both patients and healthcare providers. These apps are designed to enhance accessibility, promote self-care, and enable real-time health monitoring across various domains. From chronic disease management and mental health support to fitness tracking and teleconsultation, mHealth solutions are transforming how individuals engage with their health. Their versatility makes them suitable for both preventive and therapeutic purposes. Many apps integrate with wearable devices, allowing continuous data collection and feedback. As these technologies evolve, they are playing a critical role in advancing personalized and patient-centred care. mHealth apps cover a wide range of functions including:

- **Chronic Disease Management:** mHealth applications are highly effective in managing chronic conditions such as diabetes, hypertension, asthma, and cardiovascular diseases. These apps allow patients to track vital signs, medication schedules, and symptoms daily. Some integrate with wearable devices or glucose monitors to send real-time data to healthcare providers. This continuous feedback loop enables early intervention, better disease control, and reduced hospital admissions. Personalized alerts and educational content further empower patients to understand and manage their condition proactively.

- **Mental Health Support:** A growing number of mHealth apps focus on mental health by offering tools for cognitive behavioural therapy (CBT), stress management, and mood tracking. These applications often include guided meditation, breathing exercises, journaling, and AI-powered chatbots for emotional support. Users can monitor their emotional patterns and access mental wellness resources discreetly. Some platforms also offer virtual therapy sessions with licensed professionals. Such tools are especially valuable for people in remote areas or those hesitant to seek in-person care.
- **Medication Adherence Reminders:** Medication non-compliance is a major issue in chronic illness management, and mHealth apps address this by sending personalized medication reminders. These apps can alert users to take their pills on time, track missed doses, and even notify caregivers if doses are skipped. Some platforms include barcode scanning to ensure the correct drug is taken. By improving adherence, mHealth helps reduce complications, improve outcomes, and decrease healthcare costs. Integration with pharmacies can also streamline prescription refills.
- **Lifestyle and Fitness Tracking:** mHealth tools play a vital role in promoting healthy lifestyle habits through apps that track physical activity, sleep patterns, nutrition, and heart rate. These apps motivate users with daily goals, visual progress charts, and gamified experiences. Integration with wearable fitness devices enhances accuracy and consistency in data collection. Over time, the gathered data can reveal behavioural trends, aiding in the prevention of obesity, metabolic disorders, and stress-related illnesses. Many apps also offer personalized fitness coaching and diet recommendations.
- **Reproductive and Maternal Health Monitoring:** Women's health apps support users throughout various stages of life, from fertility tracking and pregnancy monitoring to postpartum care. These apps provide menstrual cycle tracking, ovulation prediction, foetal development updates, and appointment reminders. Some also allow symptom logging and connect users with OB/GYNs for virtual consultations. For expectant mothers, mHealth tools help monitor vital signs and manage prenatal health risks. This digital support enhances maternal outcomes and empowers women with information and control over their reproductive health.

- **Teleconsultation and Virtual Triage Services:** Teleconsultation apps enable users to connect with healthcare professionals via video calls, chat, or voice—reducing the need for in-person visits. Virtual triage services assess symptoms through interactive questionnaires or AI-driven tools and guide patients to the appropriate level of care. These apps are particularly valuable in rural or underserved regions where access to clinics is limited. They offer convenience, reduce wait times, and help in early diagnosis. During pandemics or emergencies, they serve as critical tools for continuity of care.

8.1.3 Wearable Devices in Remote Monitoring

Wearable devices have emerged as powerful tools in remote patient monitoring, offering continuous, real-time data collection that supports proactive and personalized healthcare. These devices—ranging from smartwatches and fitness bands to biosensors and smart patches—track a wide array of physiological parameters including heart rate, respiratory rate, oxygen saturation (SpO_2), body temperature, electrocardiogram (ECG), sleep patterns, blood glucose levels, and physical activity. Their non-invasive nature and ease of use make them particularly suitable for long-term monitoring without disrupting the patient's daily routine. One of the most significant advantages of wearables is their ability to detect subtle physiological changes that may indicate early signs of deterioration, even before symptoms appear. For patients with chronic illnesses such as diabetes, heart failure, hypertension, or COPD, wearables can alert both the patient and healthcare providers to abnormalities, enabling timely interventions that can prevent hospitalizations or complications. Continuous glucose monitors (CGMs), for instance, help diabetic patients maintain tighter glycaemic control, while smartwatches with ECG functions can detect atrial fibrillation or arrhythmias. Wearables also promote patient engagement and self-awareness. By offering real-time feedback and personalized health insights, they encourage users to stay active, monitor trends, and adhere to treatment plans. Many devices sync with mobile apps or cloud-based dashboards, allowing clinicians to remotely access and analyse patient data. This connectivity enhances telemedicine workflows and supports data-driven decision-making without requiring in-person visits. Moreover, wearable technology is proving valuable in post-operative care, rehabilitation, geriatric monitoring, and even early detection of infectious disease symptoms. As artificial intelligence and machine learning are integrated into these platforms, wearables are evolving from passive trackers to intelligent health companions capable of predicting risks and guiding behaviour change. Despite their benefits, challenges remain, including concerns about data privacy, accuracy, interoperability with health systems, and patient adherence. Nonetheless, as technology advances and clinical validation improves, wearable devices are set to play a central role in remote, personalized, and preventive healthcare delivery.

8.1.4 Integration with Electronic Health Records (EHRs)

The integration of data from mobile health (mHealth) applications and wearable devices into Electronic Health Records (EHRs) marks a transformative step toward fully connected, data-driven healthcare systems. Traditionally, EHRs captured static, episodic data from clinic visits or hospital stays. Now, with the rise of health-tracking technologies, clinicians can access continuous streams of real-world data that reflect a patient's health status beyond the clinical setting. Wearables and apps generate rich datasets—tracking heart rate, glucose levels, physical activity, sleep patterns, and more—which, when fed directly into EHRs, create a dynamic and longitudinal health profile. This ongoing flow of information helps healthcare providers monitor disease progression, assess treatment response, and make more informed decisions in real time. For instance, blood pressure trends captured at home can supplement in-clinic readings, offering a more comprehensive understanding of cardiovascular risk. Integration also supports early intervention by enabling alerts for abnormal readings, reducing reliance on patient self-reporting, and facilitating timely outreach. Over time, it allows care teams to identify patterns that would otherwise go unnoticed, especially in chronic disease management. Furthermore, embedding patient-generated data into the EHR fosters collaborative care by giving multiple providers access to consistent, up-to-date information. From the patient's perspective, this integration increases engagement and trust, as they can see their daily efforts directly influencing their care plans. It also enables personalized health coaching, automated reminders, and feedback loops that encourage adherence and lifestyle modifications. However, challenges persist, including the need for standardized data formats, secure data sharing, and the avoidance of clinician data fatigue. Still, as interoperability improves, and data analytics tools become more sophisticated, the seamless flow between mHealth tools and EHRs is poised to redefine clinical workflows, enhance preventive care, and improve patient outcomes at scale.

- **Connecting mHealth to Clinical Workflows:** Integration of mHealth applications and wearable data with Electronic Health Records (EHRs) bridges the gap between patient-generated data and clinical decision-making. It allows real-time health information collected outside the clinic—such as blood pressure, glucose levels, heart rate, and physical activity—to become part of the official patient record. This streamlines communication between patients and providers and enriches the clinical context during consultations.

- **Enabling Continuous, Real-World Data Collection:** By incorporating continuous data from mHealth tools, EHRs are no longer limited to sporadic, in-clinic measurements. Instead, they can reflect dynamic health patterns across days or weeks, offering a more accurate picture of a patient's health status. This helps clinicians identify early warning signs of deterioration or improvement trends that may not be visible in isolated appointments.
- **Enhancing Data-Driven Decision-Making:** Access to real-time and longitudinal data supports evidence-based clinical decisions. For example, a cardiologist can review weeks of heart rate variability data from a smartwatch to evaluate medication effectiveness or arrhythmia patterns. This data-rich environment promotes tailored treatment planning, risk stratification, and timely interventions.
- **Improving Chronic Disease Management:** In chronic disease care—such as diabetes, hypertension, and COPD—integrated mHealth-EHR systems support proactive management. Alerts can be set for out-of-range metrics, enabling care teams to contact patients before a condition worsens. Automated dashboards can highlight trends and support collaborative decision-making among multidisciplinary teams.
- **Enhancing Patient Engagement and Shared Decision-Making:** Patients benefit from seeing their health data reflected in their official medical records. This transparency fosters a sense of ownership and involvement in their care. Shared access to charts and progress over time strengthens patient-provider communication and encourages adherence to treatment goals.
- **Challenges and Considerations:** While integration offers clear benefits, challenges persist. These include interoperability between diverse mHealth platforms and EHR systems, standardization of data formats, privacy and consent management, and the risk of data overload for clinicians. Ensuring cybersecurity and regulatory compliance is also critical to maintaining patient trust.
- **The Path Forward:** Future advancements in health IT standards (like HL7 FHIR) and APIs are making integration more seamless. As machine learning and analytics tools become embedded in EHR platforms, the value of mHealth data will only grow. Integrated systems will support predictive modelling, personalized care pathways, and population health management initiatives.

8.1.5 Benefits of mHealth and Remote Monitoring

Mobile health (mHealth) and remote monitoring technologies are reshaping the landscape of modern healthcare by enabling continuous, real-time interaction between patients and providers. These digital tools extend care beyond traditional clinical settings, empowering individuals to actively participate in their own health management. With the help of smartphones, wearable devices, and connected health platforms, patients can monitor vital signs, track symptoms, receive reminders, and access personalized health information—anytime, anywhere. For clinicians, remote monitoring offers a valuable stream of real-world data that enhances clinical decision-making and supports early intervention. By capturing ongoing trends and deviations from baseline, healthcare teams can intervene proactively rather than reactively. This not only improves health outcomes but also reduces hospital visits, admissions, and associated healthcare costs. Furthermore, mHealth encourages patient engagement, improves treatment adherence, and fosters health literacy through interactive, user-friendly interfaces. In underserved or rural areas, these tools help close access gaps, bringing care to populations that may otherwise face barriers. Overall, mHealth and remote monitoring represent a major leap forward in delivering more responsive, equitable, and personalized healthcare solutions.

- **Improved Access to Care, Especially in Rural or Underserved Regions:** One of the most significant benefits of mHealth and remote monitoring is the improvement in healthcare access, particularly for populations in rural, remote, or underserved areas. Traditional healthcare services often require patients to travel long distances, which can lead to delayed diagnoses and treatment. Mobile health technologies overcome geographical barriers by providing virtual consultations, remote monitoring, and access to health information via mobile devices. This allows patients to connect with healthcare providers without leaving their homes, reducing travel time and associated costs. Moreover, these digital tools enable continuous monitoring for chronic disease management, ensuring timely interventions without the need for frequent in-person visits. For healthcare systems, expanding digital access can alleviate the burden on overtaxed facilities, while improving health equity. By bridging gaps in healthcare infrastructure, mHealth empowers communities that might otherwise face systemic disadvantages, contributing to better population health outcomes.
- **Enhanced Patient Engagement Through Self-Monitoring and Education:** mHealth platforms significantly boost patient engagement by encouraging active participation in health management. Self-monitoring tools such as mobile apps and wearable devices enable patients to track vital signs, symptoms, medication schedules, and lifestyle factors in real time. This constant involvement fosters greater awareness and responsibility for one's health, which can lead to improved adherence to treatment plans. Additionally, many mHealth apps incorporate educational content tailored

to individual needs, helping users understand their conditions and the importance of lifestyle changes. Interactive features such as reminders, goal-setting, and feedback loops motivate patients to maintain healthy behaviours and recognize early warning signs. Enhanced engagement not only improves clinical outcomes but also strengthens the patient-provider relationship by facilitating informed discussions and shared decision-making. Overall, empowered patients are more likely to achieve sustained health improvements through these personalized, technology-driven interventions.

- **Early Detection of Health Issues via Real-Time Alerts and Data Trends:** Remote monitoring technologies continuously collect and analyse physiological and behavioural data, enabling the early detection of potential health problems before they escalate. Real-time alerts triggered by abnormal readings—such as irregular heart rhythms, blood glucose fluctuations, or blood pressure spikes—can prompt timely medical review or emergency intervention. By identifying subtle trends over days or weeks, healthcare providers gain insights into disease progression or treatment effectiveness, allowing for proactive adjustments. This continuous surveillance is particularly valuable for chronic conditions like diabetes, hypertension, or heart failure, where early intervention can prevent severe complications and hospitalizations. Additionally, remote monitoring can identify adherence lapses or lifestyle changes that might adversely affect health. Such early warnings improve patient safety, reduce acute episodes, and enhance overall disease management by shifting care from reactive to preventive, thus minimizing the risk of adverse outcomes.
- **Reduced Hospital Visits and Readmissions:** The integration of mHealth and remote monitoring into healthcare delivery has proven effective in decreasing hospital visits and readmission rates. By enabling continuous outpatient monitoring and early detection of clinical deterioration, these technologies allow healthcare providers to intervene earlier, often avoiding emergency department visits or inpatient admissions. Patients can receive timely adjustments to medications or lifestyle recommendations without the need for hospital stays. Additionally, remote monitoring supports better post-discharge care by tracking recovery progress and alerting clinicians to potential complications, reducing the likelihood of readmission. This approach not only improves patient comfort by minimizing disruptive hospital stays but also alleviates financial strain on healthcare systems by lowering costs associated with acute care. Enhanced communication and data sharing between patients and providers further streamline care

coordination, ensuring a smooth transition from hospital to home and supporting long-term health stability.

- **Personalized Care Based on Real-Time Health Data and Feedback:** Personalized care is a cornerstone of mHealth and remote monitoring, with real-time data enabling highly individualized treatment plans. Continuous collection of health metrics provides a comprehensive picture of each patient's unique physiological patterns, lifestyle, and treatment response. This data allows clinicians to tailor interventions precisely, adjusting medications, therapies, or recommendations based on up-to-date information. Patients receive customized feedback through apps or wearable devices, empowering them to make informed decisions and maintain adherence. Personalized insights also help identify triggers or behaviours impacting health, fostering targeted lifestyle modifications. Moreover, the integration of artificial intelligence and predictive analytics enhances the ability to forecast disease exacerbations and optimize care pathways. This dynamic, patient-centred approach improves outcomes by addressing the specific needs and circumstances of each individual, moving beyond the one-size-fits-all model of traditional healthcare.

8.1.6 Applications in Chronic Disease Management

Remote monitoring has become a transformative tool in the management of chronic diseases, offering unprecedented opportunities to enhance patient care beyond traditional clinical settings. Chronic conditions such as hypertension, diabetes, cardiovascular diseases, chronic obstructive pulmonary disease (COPD), and asthma require ongoing monitoring to prevent complications and maintain optimal health. By leveraging wearable devices, mobile health applications, and connected sensors, healthcare providers can continuously track vital health parameters remotely in real time. This approach allows for timely detection of abnormalities, enabling early intervention before conditions worsen or emergencies arise. Remote monitoring empowers patients to actively participate in their own care by providing immediate feedback and educational resources, which fosters better adherence to treatment regimens and healthier lifestyle choices. Moreover, it reduces the need for frequent in-person visits, lowering healthcare costs and minimizing the burden on healthcare systems. In rural and underserved areas where access to specialized care is limited, remote monitoring bridges the gap by ensuring continuous clinical oversight without geographical constraints. The ability to collect and analyse longitudinal health data helps clinicians tailor treatment plans according to individual patient trends and responses, advancing personalized medicine. Ultimately, integrating remote monitoring into chronic disease management not only improves health outcomes but also enhances quality of life by promoting proactive, patient-centred care that is timely, efficient, and accessible.

- **Hypertension:** Remote blood pressure (BP) monitoring has revolutionized the management of hypertension by providing continuous and real-time data outside the clinical setting. Patients use automated BP monitors at home, which record readings throughout the day and transmit the information to healthcare providers. This constant surveillance helps detect abnormal blood pressure fluctuations or sustained hypertension episodes that may go unnoticed during occasional clinic visits. Early identification of such changes allows physicians to adjust medications promptly and provide timely lifestyle recommendations. Moreover, patients become more engaged in their health management, as immediate feedback motivates adherence to treatment and lifestyle modifications such as diet, exercise, and stress reduction. Remote monitoring also aids in distinguishing white-coat hypertension from true hypertension, reducing unnecessary medication changes. It supports risk stratification by identifying patients at higher risk for cardiovascular events, enabling targeted interventions. Ultimately, BP remote monitoring reduces complications like stroke, heart attack, and kidney disease by ensuring optimal blood pressure control through proactive management.
- **Diabetes:** Continuous glucose monitoring (CGM) systems have transformed diabetes care by providing patients and clinicians with a comprehensive, real-time picture of blood glucose fluctuations. Unlike traditional finger-prick tests, CGM devices measure glucose levels continuously via a small sensor inserted under the skin, sending data wirelessly to smartphones or dedicated monitors. This allows for early detection of hyperglycaemia and hypoglycaemia, both of which can be dangerous if left unmanaged. CGM helps patients understand the impact of diet, exercise, and medications on their glucose levels, empowering them to make informed decisions and improve glycaemic control. Clinicians use the data to tailor treatment plans more precisely, adjusting insulin doses or oral medications to maintain glucose within target ranges. Remote monitoring through CGM reduces the risk of long-term complications such as neuropathy, retinopathy, and cardiovascular disease. It also decreases emergency hospital visits by enabling timely interventions for glucose abnormalities. As a result, CGM systems enhance quality of life and support more effective, personalized diabetes management.
- **Cardiovascular Diseases:** Remote monitoring devices play a critical role in managing cardiovascular diseases by enabling early detection of arrhythmias, heart failure exacerbations, and other cardiac abnormalities.

Wearable ECG monitors and implantable devices such as pacemakers and defibrillators continuously track heart rhythm, sending alerts when irregularities occur. This timely information allows cardiologists to intervene promptly, adjusting medications or recommending procedures to prevent severe complications like stroke or sudden cardiac arrest. For patients with heart failure, remote monitoring tracks parameters such as heart rate, blood pressure, and fluid status, helping to identify early signs of decompensation before symptoms become severe. This proactive approach reduces hospital admissions and improves survival rates by maintaining better clinical stability. Additionally, patients feel more secure knowing their condition is closely observed, which can reduce anxiety and encourage adherence to treatment plans. Integration of remote monitoring data with clinical care facilitates personalized therapy adjustments, optimizing outcomes in this high-risk population.

- **COPD and Asthma:** Remote monitoring technology has significantly improved the management of respiratory diseases like chronic obstructive pulmonary disease (COPD) and asthma by tracking respiratory metrics and medication usage. Devices such as portable spirometers and wearable sensors measure lung function parameters, oxygen saturation, respiratory rate, and physical activity levels continuously. This data helps detect early signs of exacerbations, enabling healthcare providers to intervene before hospitalizations become necessary. Additionally, smart inhalers record medication usage patterns, ensuring patients follow prescribed regimens and alerting clinicians to non-adherence or incorrect inhaler technique. By providing real-time feedback, remote monitoring empowers patients to manage symptoms proactively, recognize triggers, and adjust lifestyle factors such as smoking cessation and environmental exposure. It also facilitates personalized care by tailoring therapy based on individual respiratory patterns and response to treatment. Overall, remote monitoring improves disease control, reduces emergency visits, and enhances the quality of life for patients living with COPD and asthma (Table-1).

Table-1: Utilization of Remote Monitoring for Effective Chronic Disease Management

Chronic Disease	Remote Monitoring Application	Key Benefits
Hypertension	Blood pressure (BP) monitors alert patients and doctors of abnormal readings	Enables timely adjustments to treatment; prevents complications
Diabetes	Continuous glucose monitoring (CGM) systems	Improves glycaemic control; reduces hypoglycaemia and hyperglycaemia episodes

Cardiovascular Diseases	Devices that detect arrhythmias or early signs of heart failure	Early detection allows prompt intervention; reduces hospitalizations
COPD and Asthma	Track respiratory metrics and medication usage	Enhances symptom management; reduces exacerbations and emergency visits

8.1.7 Role in Mental Health Support

Mobile health (mHealth) technologies are increasingly playing a pivotal role in mental health support by providing accessible, scalable, and personalized solutions. These digital tools include mood tracking apps, guided meditation and mindfulness programs, cognitive behavioural therapy (CBT) platforms, and virtual counselling services that empower users to actively engage with their mental well-being. By allowing individuals to monitor their symptoms daily, mHealth apps help detect early signs of anxiety, depression, or mood fluctuations, facilitating timely intervention. These tools also offer psychoeducation, coping strategies, and self-help exercises, promoting resilience and emotional regulation. For many, especially those in underserved or remote areas with limited access to mental health professionals, mHealth bridges critical gaps by providing confidential and immediate support. Virtual therapy sessions and chat-based counselling increase convenience and reduce stigma by allowing users to seek help from the privacy of their homes. Moreover, these platforms often include personalized feedback based on real-time data, enabling tailored care that adapts to an individual's evolving needs. Integration with wearable devices further enhances monitoring of physiological indicators linked to mental health, such as heart rate variability or sleep patterns. Collectively, mHealth tools expand mental health service reach, reduce barriers to care, and complement traditional treatment models, ultimately improving overall patient outcomes and quality of life.

- **Increasing Importance of mHealth in Mental Health:** Mobile health (mHealth) technologies are rapidly becoming essential tools in mental health care, offering accessible and scalable solutions that transcend traditional healthcare boundaries. These technologies help reach diverse populations, including those who may face barriers such as geographic isolation, stigma, or lack of specialist availability. By delivering personalized interventions through mobile platforms, mHealth empowers individuals to take a more active role in managing their mental health. This democratization of care supports earlier detection and ongoing management, fostering better outcomes. The flexibility and convenience offered by mHealth tools also align well with modern lifestyles, encouraging consistent engagement with mental health resources.

- **Types of Digital Mental Health Tools:** The landscape of digital mental health tools is diverse and continually expanding, offering options tailored to various needs and preferences. Mood tracking applications allow users to log their emotional states regularly, providing valuable data to identify patterns or triggers. Guided meditation and mindfulness programs promote stress reduction and emotional balance through structured exercises. Cognitive Behavioural Therapy (CBT) platforms provide evidence-based techniques in a self-guided or therapist-supported format, enhancing accessibility. Virtual counselling services, including chat or video therapy, offer direct connection to mental health professionals. Together, these tools provide comprehensive support from self-care to professional intervention, making mental health care more approachable and user-friendly.
- **Symptom Monitoring and Early Detection:** A key advantage of mHealth apps is their ability to facilitate daily symptom tracking, which enables early identification of changes in mental health status. Regular monitoring helps users recognize subtle shifts in mood, anxiety, or other psychological symptoms that might otherwise go unnoticed. This real-time data empowers both patients and clinicians to intervene promptly, potentially preventing full relapse or crisis. Early detection is crucial in mental health, where delays in treatment can worsen prognosis. Furthermore, symptom monitoring enhances self-awareness, encouraging users to engage in proactive coping strategies and adhere more closely to treatment plans.
- **Psychoeducation and Coping Strategies:** mHealth platforms often incorporate psychoeducational content designed to increase users' understanding of mental health conditions, symptoms, and treatments. By equipping individuals with knowledge, these tools foster empowerment and reduce feelings of helplessness. Additionally, many apps provide practical coping strategies such as relaxation techniques, breathing exercises, and cognitive restructuring activities. These resources support emotional regulation and resilience-building in daily life. Self-help exercises embedded within mHealth apps enable users to practice skills independently, complementing formal therapy and promoting sustained mental wellness. This continuous learning and skill-building can significantly improve long-term management of mental health.
- **Bridging Gaps in Underserved Areas:** In many regions, access to mental health professionals remains limited due to shortages, geographical barriers, or socioeconomic challenges. mHealth technologies help bridge this gap by delivering mental health support directly to users' smartphones or tablets, regardless of location. This accessibility is particularly valuable

for rural populations, low-income groups, and those facing mobility issues. Moreover, mHealth offers an anonymous and confidential environment, reducing stigma associated with seeking mental health care. The immediacy and flexibility of digital access ensure that help is available when needed, which is critical for crisis prevention and ongoing support. By overcoming traditional barriers, mHealth advances equity in mental health services.

- **Virtual Therapy and Stigma Reduction:** Virtual therapy platforms, including video calls and chat-based counselling, have transformed the way mental health services are delivered. These modes of care reduce common barriers such as travel time, scheduling conflicts, and social stigma. Users can access therapy discreetly from their homes, which encourages more people to seek help without fear of judgment. The convenience of virtual sessions often results in higher adherence to treatment plans and more consistent engagement. Furthermore, chat-based counselling provides immediate support during moments of distress, acting as an important supplement to scheduled therapy. This shift towards digital care models fosters a more inclusive and patient-centered mental health landscape.
- **Personalized Feedback and Tailored Care:** Many mHealth applications utilize data analytics and artificial intelligence to provide personalized feedback based on the user's input and behavioural patterns. This approach allows for adaptive care that evolves alongside the individual's mental health status. Personalized insights can highlight triggers, suggest coping mechanisms, or recommend when to seek professional help. Tailored interventions increase the relevance and effectiveness of care, improving motivation and adherence. This dynamic customization ensures that mental health support is not one-size-fits-all but responsive to unique needs and preferences. Ultimately, personalized care facilitated by mHealth enhances therapeutic outcomes and patient satisfaction.
- **Integration with Wearable Devices:** Wearable technologies, such as smartwatches and fitness trackers, complement mHealth applications by providing continuous physiological data linked to mental health. Metrics like heart rate variability, sleep quality, and activity levels offer objective indicators of stress, mood, and overall well-being. Integration of this data with mental health apps enables a holistic view of the user's condition, supporting early warning signs of deterioration or relapse. Wearables facilitate passive monitoring, reducing the burden of self-reporting while enhancing accuracy. This seamless connectivity empowers users and clinicians with comprehensive, real-time insights, fostering timely adjustments to treatment and lifestyle interventions.

- **Overall Impact on Mental Health Services:** The integration of mHealth into mental health care is reshaping the delivery and accessibility of services worldwide. By expanding reach, reducing barriers, and offering personalized, scalable interventions, these technologies complement traditional therapeutic models effectively. mHealth enhances patient empowerment and engagement, driving better self-management and adherence. The data generated also informs clinical decision-making, allowing for more precise and timely care. Collectively, these advances contribute to improved mental health outcomes, reduced healthcare costs, and enhanced quality of life. As technology continues to evolve, mHealth's role in mental health is poised to grow, promising a future of more inclusive, responsive, and patient-centred care.

8.1.8 COVID-19 and the Rise of Remote Monitoring

The COVID-19 pandemic fundamentally transformed healthcare delivery, accelerating the adoption and reliance on mobile health (mHealth) technologies and remote monitoring solutions. As healthcare systems worldwide faced unprecedented challenges, minimizing physical contact became crucial to reduce virus transmission risks. Remote monitoring tools emerged as indispensable resources for tracking symptoms, managing patients in isolation, and providing timely interventions without exposing healthcare workers or other patients to infection. Devices such as pulse oximeters and temperature sensors gained widespread use, allowing continuous, real-time measurement of vital signs like oxygen saturation and body temperature—key indicators for COVID-19 severity. In parallel, symptom-reporting apps enabled individuals to self-monitor and report their health status from home, facilitating early detection of deterioration and guiding decisions on when to seek medical care.

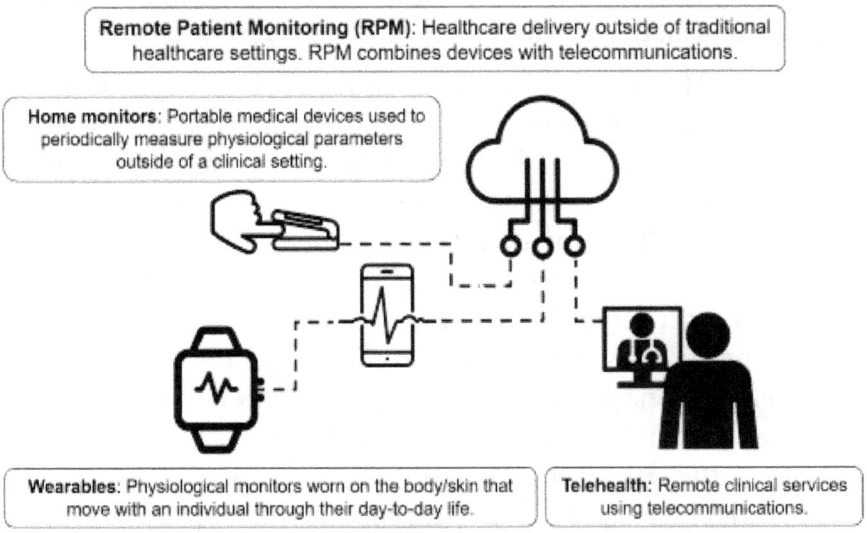

Fig. 2 Remote patient monitoring in the COVID-19 era

These digital tools also supported remote triage, helping prioritize hospital admissions and reduce healthcare burdens. Furthermore, remote monitoring enhanced follow-up care for recovering patients, ensuring ongoing assessment while maintaining quarantine protocols. Beyond individual patient management, aggregated data from these devices provided public health authorities with valuable insights into outbreak trends and resource allocation. The pandemic underscored the critical role of digital health in maintaining continuity of care during crises and highlighted the potential for these technologies to revolutionize future healthcare models. By enabling safe, efficient, and patient-centred management, remote monitoring has become a cornerstone of pandemic response and a lasting legacy for healthcare innovation. Remote patient monitoring in the COVID-19 era is given in Fig. 2.

- **Pandemic-Driven Shift in Healthcare Delivery:** The onset of the COVID-19 pandemic posed unprecedented challenges to traditional healthcare delivery, necessitating rapid adaptation to minimize virus transmission risks. Healthcare providers had to rethink patient interactions, moving away from routine in-person visits to virtual consultations and remote care. This shift was crucial to protect both patients and healthcare workers from potential exposure to the virus, especially given its high contagion and severity. Physical distancing measures and lockdowns further limited access to healthcare facilities, pushing the adoption of telehealth and remote monitoring technologies. These innovations enabled continuity of care for both COVID-19 patients and those with chronic conditions, reducing the burden on overwhelmed hospitals. The pandemic highlighted the vulnerabilities in existing healthcare infrastructures and emphasized the need for scalable, flexible solutions that prioritize patient safety while maintaining high-quality care. This shift laid the groundwork for a long-term transformation in how healthcare is delivered globally.
- **Emergence of Remote Monitoring Tools:** During the pandemic, the rapid deployment of remote monitoring devices became a cornerstone of patient care outside hospitals. Tools such as pulse oximeters, which measure blood oxygen saturation, and digital thermometers allowed continuous tracking of vital signs critical for detecting COVID-19 complications early. These devices provided real-time data, enabling healthcare providers to monitor patients' health remotely and intervene promptly when necessary. The convenience of these tools empowered patients to participate actively in their health management, fostering greater awareness and compliance. Importantly, remote monitoring reduced the need for hospital visits, thereby decreasing the risk of viral exposure in healthcare settings. Additionally, these technologies proved essential for monitoring at-risk populations,

including elderly patients and those with pre-existing conditions. Their widespread use during the pandemic accelerated advancements in wearable health tech and expanded acceptance among patients and clinicians alike.

- **Symptom-Reporting Apps and Self-Monitoring:** Mobile applications designed for symptom tracking played a vital role in managing COVID-19 by enabling individuals to self-report symptoms daily from the safety of their homes. These apps facilitated early identification of warning signs such as fever, cough, or shortness of breath, triggering alerts for medical consultation or testing when necessary. By crowdsourcing symptom data, health authorities gained valuable insights into community spread and emerging hotspots. Users benefited from personalized health recommendations and reminders, promoting adherence to quarantine and isolation guidelines. Moreover, the accessibility and ease of use of these apps bridged gaps for populations with limited access to in-person care. Self-monitoring tools also supported mental health by providing resources for stress management during periods of isolation. The integration of symptom-reporting with other remote monitoring technologies created a comprehensive digital ecosystem for pandemic response.
- **Remote Triage and Care Prioritization:** With healthcare systems overwhelmed by surges in COVID-19 cases, remote triage emerged as a critical strategy to prioritize patient care effectively. Digital platforms and telehealth services allowed clinicians to assess patients' symptoms and severity remotely, determining who required urgent hospital care versus those who could safely isolate at home. This approach helped optimize the allocation of limited resources such as ICU beds, ventilators, and medical staff. Remote triage also reduced unnecessary hospital visits, lowering the risk of healthcare-associated infections. It empowered patients to receive timely guidance and reassurance without leaving their homes. Automated algorithms and decision-support tools enhanced the accuracy and consistency of triage assessments. The ability to prioritize care based on real-time data helped flatten infection curves and improve clinical outcomes by ensuring critically ill patients received prompt attention.
- **Follow-up and Quarantine Management:** Effective follow-up and management of patients recovering from COVID-19, as well as those in quarantine, were crucial to controlling virus spread and ensuring recovery. Remote monitoring enabled healthcare providers to track patients' vital signs, symptoms, and overall well-being continuously during isolation periods. This approach allowed for early detection of deterioration, facilitating timely interventions and hospital admissions when necessary. Regular virtual check-ins via telemedicine platforms provided emotional

support and addressed post-acute COVID-19 complications, often referred to as "long COVID." Remote monitoring also helped enforce quarantine compliance by providing alerts and reminders. For healthcare systems, it reduced the burden on physical facilities and minimized exposure risks for both patients and staff. This comprehensive approach ensured safer, more effective care continuity throughout the pandemic.

- **Public Health Surveillance and Data Insights:** The aggregation of data from remote monitoring devices and symptom-reporting apps provided public health authorities with unprecedented real-time insights into pandemic trends. This wealth of data enabled the tracking of infection rates, identification of emerging clusters, and assessment of intervention effectiveness across different regions. Predictive analytics and machine learning models applied to these datasets helped forecast healthcare demand, guiding resource allocation and policy decisions. Additionally, anonymized data contributed to epidemiological research, improving understanding of virus transmission dynamics. The integration of digital health data with traditional surveillance methods enhanced the responsiveness and precision of public health strategies. This data-driven approach supported contact tracing efforts, vaccine rollout planning, and public communication campaigns, ultimately strengthening pandemic control measures.
- **Lasting Impact on Healthcare Models:** The COVID-19 pandemic catalysed a paradigm shift in healthcare delivery, firmly establishing mHealth and remote monitoring as essential components of modern medicine. These technologies demonstrated their value in enhancing access, safety, and efficiency of care during a global crisis, accelerating their adoption across healthcare systems worldwide. As a result, hybrid care models combining in-person and virtual services are becoming the norm. The experience highlighted the need for robust digital infrastructure, interoperability, and patient data security. Furthermore, the pandemic exposed health disparities, prompting efforts to ensure equitable access to digital health tools. Moving forward, remote monitoring and mHealth are poised to expand beyond infectious diseases to chronic disease management, preventive care, and personalized medicine. This transformation promises to improve patient outcomes, reduce healthcare costs, and create more resilient health systems prepared for future challenges.

8.1.9 Limitations and Challenges

- **Data Privacy and Security Concerns:** One of the foremost challenges in mHealth and remote monitoring is ensuring data privacy and security.

Health data collected through mobile apps and wearable devices are highly sensitive and vulnerable to breaches, unauthorized access, or misuse. Cybersecurity threats such as hacking, phishing, and ransomware attacks pose significant risks, potentially compromising patient confidentiality and trust. Compliance with regulations like HIPAA and GDPR requires robust encryption, secure data storage, and stringent access controls, which can be complex and costly to implement. Additionally, patients often lack full awareness of how their data is used, shared, or stored, raising ethical concerns. Healthcare providers must establish transparent privacy policies and invest in continuous monitoring to safeguard information. Without strong protections, data breaches could deter user adoption and undermine the benefits of digital health technologies.

- **Device Accuracy and Reliability:** The clinical utility of mHealth and remote monitoring depends heavily on the accuracy and reliability of devices such as wearable sensors, glucose monitors, and pulse oximeters. Inaccurate or inconsistent readings can lead to misdiagnosis, delayed treatment, or unnecessary interventions. Variability in device quality, calibration issues, and environmental factors can affect performance. Moreover, consumer-grade devices may lack the rigorous validation required for clinical decision-making. This creates challenges in standardizing device use across diverse patient populations and health conditions. Manufacturers must adhere to strict regulatory standards and conduct thorough clinical trials to ensure reliability. Healthcare providers should also educate patients on proper device use and limitations. Ultimately, ensuring high-quality, validated devices is crucial to maintaining clinical confidence and improving patient outcomes.
- **Digital Literacy Barriers Among Certain Populations:** Despite the widespread availability of mHealth technologies, disparities in digital literacy create significant barriers for many users, particularly older adults, socioeconomically disadvantaged groups, and those with limited education. Navigating apps, understanding health data, or troubleshooting devices can be challenging, reducing engagement and adherence. Language differences and cultural factors may also impede effective use. These barriers can exacerbate health inequities, limiting the benefits of remote monitoring for vulnerable populations. To address this, healthcare systems and developers must design intuitive, user-friendly interfaces and provide comprehensive education and technical support. Community outreach and training programs can empower users to confidently manage their digital health tools. Bridging the digital divide is essential to ensuring equitable access and maximizing the positive impact of mHealth.

- **Integration Difficulties with Legacy Health Systems:** Integrating data from mHealth apps and wearable devices into existing electronic health records (EHRs) and hospital information systems remains a complex challenge. Many legacy systems are not designed to handle large volumes of real-time data or lack standardized interoperability protocols. This fragmentation leads to data silos, limiting comprehensive patient insights and hindering coordinated care. Additionally, healthcare providers face workflow disruptions when incorporating new data streams without adequate infrastructure or training. Vendors and institutions must collaborate to develop universal standards, such as HL7 FHIR, to facilitate seamless integration. Investment in scalable IT infrastructure and staff education is also critical. Overcoming these integration challenges is vital for leveraging the full potential of remote monitoring in personalized medicine and improving clinical decision-making.
- **Overdependence on Technology Without Sufficient Clinical Validation:** While mHealth and remote monitoring technologies offer tremendous promise, there is a risk of overreliance on these tools without adequate clinical validation. Many apps and devices enter the market without rigorous testing, leading to concerns about their safety, efficacy, and appropriate clinical use. Overdependence on unproven technologies may result in missed diagnoses, inappropriate treatment changes, or delayed medical attention. It is essential that digital health solutions undergo thorough validation through clinical trials and regulatory review before widespread adoption. Healthcare professionals must balance technology use with clinical judgment, ensuring patient care remains evidence-based. Ongoing research, monitoring, and feedback loops will help refine these tools, ensuring they complement rather than replace traditional medical assessments. Responsible integration of technology is key to optimizing patient outcomes and maintaining trust in digital health.

8.1.10 Future Prospects

The future of mHealth and remote monitoring is poised to become even more transformative with the integration of advanced technologies like artificial intelligence (AI), machine learning (ML), and real-time data analytics. These tools will enable predictive models that anticipate health deteriorations before they occur, allowing for proactive interventions rather than reactive treatments. AI-driven algorithms can continuously learn from patient data, tailoring recommendations to individual behaviours, environmental factors, and clinical histories. This will shift healthcare from episodic care to continuous, dynamic monitoring. Future innovations may include smart textiles embedded with biosensors that track biometric data through everyday clothing, and implantable devices capable of monitoring internal physiological changes in real time. These tools could provide early warnings for conditions such as heart failure, seizures, or infections. Additionally, therapeutic feedback loops—where interventions are automatically adjusted based on real-time readings—may enable automated drug delivery systems or digital therapeutics that adapt on the fly. Improved interoperability will also support seamless integration of mHealth data into clinical workflows and population health strategies. With regulatory advances, privacy protections, and greater patient empowerment, the next generation of mHealth promises not only more personalized care, but also more equitable, accessible, and preventive healthcare systems across the globe.

8.2 WEARABLES AND SMART SENSORS FOR CONTINUOUS DATA

8.2.1 Scope of Wearables & Smart Sensors

Wearables and smart sensors represent a rapidly evolving class of health technologies, spanning from everyday smartwatches and fitness bands to advanced adhesive patches, sensor-embedded clothing, and even implantable gadgets. These devices continuously and unobtrusively capture an array of physiological and environmental data—ranging from standard metrics like heart rate, body temperature, activity levels, ECG signals, and stress indicators, to emerging biochemical markers such as glucose, sweat metabolites, and respiratory gases. Smart textiles like Hexoskin shirts integrate sensors within fabric to monitor breathing, heart rate variability, and movement in real time . In parallel, energy-autonomous sensors—powered by body heat or movement—are pioneering battery-free monitoring solutions, enhancing wearability and convenience. Cutting-edge prototypes, such as sweat-powered electronic fingertip wraps, track biomarkers like glucose and vitamins without external power sources. Further innovations include contactless wearables that hover above the skin to detect gases associated with hydration, infection, and wound healing—ideal for sensitive populations like newborns or the elderly. These technologies blur the line between clinical-grade monitoring and everyday comfort, enabling long-term, low-effort data collection integrated into daily life. As sensor technology evolves—driven by flexible materials, miniaturized electronics, and novel power solutions—wearables are poised to deliver increasingly precise, yet unobtrusive, health insights. Collectively, they reshape how we capture human health data—on our skin, in our clothes, and even beneath our epidermis—with precision, ease, and continuity.

8.2.2 Types of Sensors and Measured Parameters

Sensors used in modern wearable and biomedical devices serve a diverse range of purposes, enabling real-time monitoring of physiological and biochemical parameters. Photoplethysmography (PPG) sensors are commonly used to track heart rate by measuring blood volume changes in the microvascular bed of tissue using light. Accelerometers detect motion, orientation, and activity levels, helping to assess physical activity, sleep patterns, and fall detection. Temperature sensors monitor skin or core body temperature, which can be vital for early illness detection or tracking menstrual cycles. Electrocardiogram (ECG) electrodes capture the heart's electrical signals, providing more detailed cardiac insights, while electrodermal activity (EDA) sensors measure skin conductivity to gauge stress and emotional responses. More advanced sensors can monitor oxygen saturation (SpO_2) through pulse oximetry, often integrated into wristbands or smart rings. Continuous glucose monitoring (CGM) systems, typically implantable or transdermal, allow non-invasive or minimally invasive tracking of blood sugar levels in diabetic patients. Some emerging technologies can detect lactate, hydration levels, or other biochemical markers via microfluidic patches or skin-contact biosensors. Sweat analysis, for instance, is being explored for tracking electrolytes, hormones, and even drug levels. Implantable biosensors offer continuous internal monitoring, enabling proactive healthcare with minimal patient intervention. Together, these sensors are shaping the future of personalized, preventive, and precision medicine by providing seamless, round-the-clock health data.

8.2.3 Data Collection Techniques and Frequency

Wearable and biomedical devices utilize both passive and active data collection techniques to monitor various physiological parameters over time. Passive data collection occurs automatically in the background, requiring no user intervention—for example, continuous heart rate or movement tracking throughout the day. Active data collection, on the other hand, may require user input or initiation, such as performing a guided ECG reading or logging symptoms manually. The frequency of data acquisition can vary significantly based on the sensor type, use case, and device capabilities. Some sensors operate on a per-minute or per-second basis, enabling near-continuous streaming (e.g., PPG or accelerometers), while others may collect data in intervals or upon specific triggers. Most devices are equipped with local memory and wireless connectivity, allowing them to synchronize data with companion smartphone applications or cloud-based platforms. This synchronization may occur in real time or batch-uploaded at scheduled intervals, depending on connectivity and power constraints. Once transmitted, the data is stored securely, processed using algorithms for trend analysis or anomaly detection, and visualized through user-friendly dashboards. This enables users and healthcare providers to gain actionable insights and support data-driven decision-making. High-frequency and long-duration data capture allows for comprehensive health monitoring and the early detection of deviations from baseline physiological norms.

8.2.4 Clinical and Lifestyle Applications

Wearables support both clinical care and wellness. They are instrumental in disease monitoring (e.g., arrhythmia, sleep disorders), fitness tracking, stress detection, and behavioural monitoring. Continuous data allows for nuanced insights into physiological trends.

- **Clinical Care and Disease Monitoring:** Wearable devices have revolutionized the way chronic and acute conditions are monitored in real time. In cardiology, sensors like ECG and PPG allow for continuous detection of irregular heart rhythms such as arrhythmias and atrial fibrillation, helping in early diagnosis and timely intervention. These devices can also alert patients and physicians in case of abnormal cardiac activity. Sleep tracking wearables are used to monitor sleep duration, stages, and interruptions, playing a role in diagnosing sleep disorders like insomnia and sleep apnea. In diabetes management, continuous glucose monitors (CGMs) enable non-stop tracking of blood glucose levels, minimizing the need for frequent finger pricks and enhancing glycaemic control. Respiratory monitoring devices with pulse oximeters and respiratory rate sensors assist in managing chronic conditions like asthma and COPD, especially during sleep or exercise. These wearables offer crucial data trends that support medication adjustments and lifestyle changes. Their ability to track and send alerts improves clinical outcomes and patient compliance. They also serve as valuable tools in rehabilitation, were continuous monitoring guides recovery. As medical-grade wearables continue to evolve, their role in clinical decision-making will become even more integrated and essential. Their contribution extends to diagnostics, ongoing care, and even emergency detection. Ultimately, they help bridge the gap between home-based care and clinical oversight, improving both convenience and clinical outcomes.
- **Remote Patient Monitoring (RPM):** Remote Patient Monitoring (RPM) allows healthcare professionals to observe patients' health conditions from outside the hospital, especially for chronic disease management. Wearables make RPM feasible by collecting continuous physiological data such as heart rate, respiration, glucose levels, and sleep cycles. These devices transmit data to healthcare platforms, enabling doctors to monitor changes and intervene early if necessary. This reduces hospital visits and readmissions, particularly for post-surgery patients or those with heart failure. For elderly or high-risk individuals, RPM ensures they are constantly monitored without needing to leave their homes. It supports long-term care models, allowing for better resource management within healthcare systems. RPM also plays a vital role in rural or underserved

areas where access to hospitals may be limited. With integration into telemedicine, wearable data enhances virtual consultations, allowing physicians to make informed decisions remotely. The seamless data flow also enables early detection of health deterioration, often before symptoms are noticeable. These systems are also beneficial for medication adherence, alerting patients or caregivers about missed doses. By empowering patients with real-time insights, RPM encourages active engagement in self-care. From cost reduction to improved patient satisfaction, RPM represents a transformative shift in modern healthcare. As technology advances, RPM platforms are becoming more robust, integrating AI for predictive insights. Its continued growth signals a future where proactive, home-based care is the norm rather than the exception.

- **Fitness and Activity Tracking:** Fitness and activity tracking is one of the most widespread applications of wearable technology, used extensively by athletes, fitness enthusiasts, and the general population. These devices track daily step counts, distance travelled, calories burned, and active minutes to provide a comprehensive picture of physical activity. They also monitor heart rate during exercise to ensure workouts remain within optimal zones for fat burning, endurance, or cardiovascular benefit. Activity trackers often feature built-in GPS to map outdoor runs or cycling routes, giving real-time feedback on pace and performance. Sleep monitoring helps users understand their recovery and optimize rest for better athletic output. Some wearables include coaching functions, offering workout suggestions and personalized training plans based on fitness goals and historical data. Advanced devices can distinguish between different activities—like walking, running, swimming, or weightlifting—and automatically log them. The gamification aspect of fitness tracking, including achievements, daily goals, and social challenges, helps maintain motivation. For beginners, these tools are valuable for setting achievable goals and gradually increasing activity levels. They also play a significant role in promoting general wellness by encouraging a more active lifestyle. Through consistent use, users can develop healthier habits and increase awareness of their physical routines. Integration with nutrition and health apps allows for holistic health tracking. Fitness trackers have become essential in preventive health, motivating people to take control of their physical well-being and stay active.
- **Stress and Mental Health Monitoring:** Wearable technology has expanded beyond physical health to address emotional well-being and mental health. Devices equipped with Electrodermal Activity (EDA) sensors and Heart Rate Variability (HRV) analysis can detect physiological signs of stress,

anxiety, and emotional arousal. These metrics help users identify moments of high stress, even if they are not consciously aware of it. Some wearables offer guided breathing exercises and mindfulness sessions in response to elevated stress indicators, encouraging self-regulation. Sleep tracking also contributes to mental health insights, as sleep disturbances are often linked to anxiety and depression. Wearables can help users understand the impact of daily activities, caffeine intake, or screen time on their stress levels and emotional state. By visualizing trends over time, users gain awareness of how lifestyle choices influence their mental health. In clinical settings, wearables can complement therapy by providing data that informs treatment plans. This is especially useful for people with anxiety, PTSD, or mood disorders. Alerts and gentle nudges can prompt users to take breaks, meditate, or seek social interaction during high-stress periods. The discreet nature of these devices makes them ideal for continuous mental health monitoring without stigma. Moreover, by empowering individuals to track and manage their mental well-being proactively, these technologies help reduce burnout and improve overall quality of life. As research continues, wearables are likely to play an increasing role in preventive mental healthcare and emotional resilience.

- **Behavioural and Lifestyle Monitoring:** Behavioural and lifestyle monitoring through wearables provides continuous insights into an individual's daily habits, helping build healthier routines. These devices track a range of parameters including sleep quality, physical activity, sedentary behaviour, hydration, and even nutritional intake. By analysing patterns over days or weeks, wearables can highlight unhealthy behaviours, such as prolonged inactivity or insufficient sleep. Many devices issue reminders to move, drink water, or take medications, promoting adherence to healthier habits. This real-time feedback loop encourages users to make small, consistent changes that lead to long-term wellness. For example, wearables can alert users when they've been inactive too long, helping reduce risks associated with a sedentary lifestyle. They also help monitor adherence to sleep schedules by showing sleep consistency and duration. Over time, users can recognize trends and triggers that impact their well-being, such as late-night screen use or irregular meal times. Behavioural data collected through wearables can be shared with healthcare providers, therapists, or coaches to tailor interventions more effectively. In corporate wellness programs, aggregated data helps companies promote healthier workplaces. In weight management, wearables encourage users to monitor their calorie balance and eating habits. For individuals aiming to change or improve their behaviour—such as quitting smoking or reducing alcohol—

wearables offer support and tracking tools. With personalized nudges and gamified feedback, these devices foster accountability and sustained motivation. Ultimately, they transform passive observation into active health engagement.

- **Preventive and Personalized Healthcare:** Preventive and personalized healthcare are at the forefront of wearable technology's contribution to medicine. By collecting real-time physiological data, wearables can detect subtle changes in health long before symptoms appear, enabling early intervention. This data-driven approach supports preventive healthcare by identifying risk factors for conditions like hypertension, diabetes, or cardiovascular disease. For example, a gradual increase in resting heart rate or reduced HRV may signal stress, overtraining, or illness, prompting timely action. Personalization comes from tailoring health recommendations based on each individual's unique biometrics, activity levels, and lifestyle. Wearables can adjust goals and alerts according to age, fitness level, and medical history, enhancing engagement and relevance. They also support medication adherence by providing timely reminders and tracking intake. In chronic disease management, personalized alerts help users maintain control and avoid complications. Data analytics and AI integration further enhance personalization by predicting health events or suggesting lifestyle changes. Preventive applications extend to detecting infections (like early signs of fever or respiratory changes) and even predicting menstrual cycles. For clinicians, wearable data offers a comprehensive patient profile that complements diagnostic tools. In insurance and wellness programs, data can help assess health risk and guide incentive plans. As wearables evolve, they increasingly function as personalized health assistants, reducing reliance on reactive healthcare models. They empower users to stay ahead of illness and manage health proactively, leading to better outcomes and reduced healthcare costs.
- **Clinical Trials and Research:** Wearable devices are playing a transformative role in clinical research by enabling continuous, real-world data collection. Traditional clinical trials often rely on infrequent, clinic-based assessments, which may not reflect a patient's day-to-day condition. Wearables solve this gap by tracking health parameters continuously in natural environments, offering a more accurate and holistic view of patient outcomes. They improve participant compliance by reducing the burden of travel and manual reporting. Data collected through wearables—such as heart rate, sleep, movement, glucose, or temperature—can be timestamped and stored securely for analysis. This streamlines data collection and enhances reliability. Wearables are especially valuable in long-term studies

where consistent monitoring is critical, such as trials involving chronic diseases or behavioural interventions. They also enable decentralized trials, where patients participate from remote locations, improving accessibility and diversity in research populations. Researchers can monitor adverse effects or therapeutic responses in real time, improving patient safety. Moreover, automated data capture reduces human error and subjectivity in reporting. AI algorithms can analyse large datasets from wearables to uncover patterns, predict outcomes, and optimize study design. By integrating wearable data with other digital health records, researchers gain comprehensive insights into intervention efficacy. In post-market surveillance, wearables help track real-world device performance and side effects. As a result, clinical trials become faster, more efficient, and more patient-centric. Wearables are redefining the research landscape, aligning with the goals of precision medicine and evidence-based practice.

8.2.5 Integration with Digital Health Platforms

Collected data can integrate with electronic health records (EHRs) or digital health dashboards, enriching clinical decision-making and enabling personalized intervention strategies. APIs and interoperability standards (e.g., FHIR) facilitate seamless data flow.

- **Integration with Electronic Health Records (EHRs):** Wearable devices collect vital health information such as heart rate, blood pressure, glucose levels, sleep quality, and physical activity. This data can be integrated into Electronic Health Records (EHRs), allowing healthcare providers to access a more comprehensive and real-time view of a patient's health history. Unlike traditional EHR data, which is often limited to snapshots from clinical visits, wearable data offers continuous monitoring, enhancing diagnostic accuracy. Integration ensures that wearable insights are not siloed but directly available within the existing clinical workflow, making it easier for doctors to correlate symptoms with lifestyle factors or physiological changes over time. This helps in proactive care planning, medication adjustments, and timely interventions.
- **Use of Digital Health Dashboards:** Digital health dashboards provide intuitive and visual representations of complex health data gathered from wearables. These platforms are used by both healthcare providers and patients to track trends over time, identify anomalies, and set personalized health goals. For clinicians, dashboards simplify the interpretation of large datasets, providing alerts, summaries, and AI-generated recommendations. For patients, dashboards offer feedback on health behaviours and progress, encouraging engagement and self-care. Integration with dashboards

transforms raw data into actionable insights, supporting informed decision-making and enhanced communication between patients and providers.

- **Role of APIs (Application Programming Interfaces):** APIs serve as the communication bridge between wearable devices and digital health systems. They allow the secure and structured transfer of data from one system to another, regardless of device manufacturer or software. APIs ensure that data from various wearable brands can be integrated into a common platform, fostering flexibility and scalability. For example, a fitness tracker, glucose monitor, and ECG patch can all feed into a unified health monitoring application using their respective APIs. APIs also support real-time data synchronization, enabling clinicians to respond quickly to health changes without manual data entry or delays.
- **Interoperability Standards – FHIR and Others:** Interoperability is essential for ensuring that health data from wearables is understood and usable across different systems. Standards like FHIR (Fast Healthcare Interoperability Resources), developed by HL7, provide a consistent format for sharing health data. FHIR enables wearable data to be structured and coded in a way that EHR systems, apps, and clinical software can interpret correctly. Other standards like HL7 V2, CDA, and IEEE 11073 may also be used, depending on the system architecture. Adoption of these standards reduces fragmentation and promotes seamless data exchange, especially important in multi-provider or cross-platform environments.
- **Personalized Intervention and Decision Support:** With integrated wearable data, healthcare providers can move toward truly personalized medicine. Data-driven decision support systems can analyse patterns in real-time, flag abnormalities, and suggest tailored interventions. For instance, a rise in resting heart rate combined with poor sleep and reduced activity might trigger a recommendation for stress management or clinical evaluation. These insights can be delivered directly to both the clinician's dashboard and the patient's app. Personalized notifications, coaching tips, and alerts for critical values enhance preventive care and improve outcomes, especially for chronic disease management.
- **Remote Monitoring and Telehealth Integration:** Wearable integration supports remote patient monitoring (RPM) and telehealth services by providing real-time access to patient data during virtual consultations. Clinicians can assess trends, evaluate responses to treatment, and make clinical decisions without in-person visits. This is especially valuable for managing elderly or chronically ill patients who may not be able to attend frequent checkups. The data can also be used for early detection

of deterioration, enabling prompt remote intervention. Integration with telehealth platforms ensures that wearable data becomes an active tool during virtual care delivery.

- **Enhanced Data Security and Compliance:** As wearable data flows into digital health platforms, ensuring data privacy and security becomes paramount. Integrated systems must comply with healthcare regulations like HIPAA (USA), GDPR (Europe), or equivalent local standards to protect patient data. APIs and platforms use encryption, secure authentication protocols, and access controls to safeguard data transmission and storage. Role-based access ensures that only authorized personnel can view sensitive health information. Secure integration builds trust among users and providers and is essential for widespread adoption.
- **Scalability and Future-Proofing:** As wearable technologies continue to evolve, integration frameworks must be scalable and adaptable to new sensors and devices. A well-designed digital health platform can accommodate updates through flexible APIs and modular architecture. Interoperability standards like FHIR ensure that newly developed devices can plug into existing systems without needing complete infrastructure overhauls. This future-proofing is crucial as healthcare increasingly depends on digital and remote monitoring tools.
- **Cross-Platform and Multimodal Integration:** Digital health platforms often integrate not just wearables, but also mobile apps, smart home devices, and diagnostic tools. For example, a patient's smartwatch, smart scale, and blood pressure monitor can all sync into one platform. Cross-platform integration enables multimodal data correlation, offering a holistic view of health and lifestyle. When combined with clinical data from lab tests or imaging, this leads to more comprehensive and precise healthcare delivery.
- **Real-Time Alerts and Clinical Workflow Integration:** Integrated systems can be configured to generate real-time alerts for critical health events such as hypoglycaemia, atrial fibrillation, or oxygen desaturation. These alerts can be sent to clinicians, caregivers, or emergency services depending on severity. Additionally, the data can be embedded into clinical workflow tools like patient management systems, EMR task queues, and decision support modules. This allows for prompt actions, timely documentation, and better coordination among healthcare teams.

8.2.6 Benefits of Continuous Monitoring

Continuous data supports early detection of health deviations, timely alerts to patients and providers, enhanced self-awareness, and improved treatment adherence. Longitudinal insights contribute to more personalized, preventive care.

- **Early Detection of Health Deviations:** Continuous monitoring allows for the real-time tracking of vital signs and physiological parameters, enabling the early identification of abnormal patterns or deviations from an individual's baseline. This proactive approach helps detect the onset of health issues—such as arrhythmias, glucose fluctuations, or respiratory distress—before symptoms become severe. Early warnings can prompt timely medical interventions, reduce complications and improve outcomes.
- **Timely Alerts to Patients and Providers:** Wearables and monitoring systems can generate instant alerts when critical thresholds are crossed or unusual trends emerge. These notifications can be sent directly to patients, caregivers, or healthcare providers, facilitating rapid responses. Timely alerts are crucial for managing chronic conditions, preventing emergencies, and supporting remote patient care. They ensure that health issues are addressed promptly, often before clinical visits.
- **Enhanced Self-Awareness and Patient Engagement:** Continuous data empowers individuals with detailed insights into their own health, increasing awareness of lifestyle factors and behaviours that influence well-being. By tracking trends such as activity levels, sleep quality, or stress responses, users become more motivated to adopt healthier habits. Enhanced self-awareness fosters active participation in health management, encouraging better adherence to treatment plans and lifestyle modifications.
- **Improved Treatment Adherence:** Continuous monitoring supports healthcare providers in evaluating patient adherence to prescribed therapies or lifestyle recommendations. Real-time data can highlight when medication schedules are missed or activity targets are not met, allowing for targeted interventions. Patients receiving feedback and reminders based on their data tend to show higher compliance, leading to better disease control and fewer complications.
- **Longitudinal Insights for Personalized Care:** Collecting data over extended periods enables the development of personalized health profiles that capture individual variability and trends. These longitudinal insights help clinicians tailor treatments and preventive strategies to the patient's unique physiological patterns. Personalized care plans informed by continuous monitoring can optimize medication dosing, lifestyle recommendations, and follow-up schedules, resulting in more effective and efficient healthcare delivery.
- **Support for Preventive Healthcare:** Continuous health monitoring shifts the focus from reactive to preventive care by identifying risk factors and early warning signs before disease progression. This approach reduces

hospitalizations, lowers healthcare costs, and improves quality of life. Wearables facilitate routine health assessments outside clinical settings, making preventive healthcare more accessible and scalable.

- **Facilitating Remote Patient Management:** Continuous data streams enable healthcare providers to monitor patients remotely, reducing the need for frequent in-person visits. This is particularly beneficial for elderly or chronically ill patients who face mobility challenges. Remote monitoring promotes timely interventions and ongoing support while increasing convenience for patients.
- **Enabling Data-Driven Clinical Research:** The vast amounts of continuous health data collected from wearables can also be leveraged for clinical research and population health studies. Longitudinal and real-world data enhance the understanding of disease progression, treatment responses, and health behaviours, driving innovation in medical science and public health strategies.

8.2.7 Challenges and Limitations

Key challenges include maintaining data accuracy, managing large volumes of streaming data, ensuring user compliance, protecting data privacy, and securing interoperability. Technical issues and user acceptance can hinder effectiveness.

- **Data Accuracy and Reliability:** One of the primary concerns with wearable devices is the accuracy and reliability of the data they collect. Consumer-grade wearables may not always match the precision of clinical instruments, particularly for parameters like ECG, SpO_2, or glucose levels. External factors such as skin tone, motion artifacts, sweat, improper placement, or environmental conditions can affect sensor readings. Inaccurate data may lead to false alarms, missed detections, or misleading trends, which can compromise clinical decisions and patient trust. Ensuring device calibration, validation against clinical standards, and improving sensor technology remain ongoing challenges in the field.
- **Data Overload and Management:** Wearables continuously generate massive amounts of real-time data, which can be overwhelming for both users and healthcare providers. Managing, storing, and analysing high-frequency streaming data requires robust backend systems, scalable cloud storage, and efficient data processing frameworks. Without proper filtering or prioritization, important signals can get lost in the noise. For clinicians, reviewing such extensive datasets can be time-consuming and impractical unless intelligent summarization, alerting, and AI-driven insights are in place. Ensuring meaningful use of data while avoiding "information fatigue" is a growing concern.

- **User Compliance and Engagement:** For wearables to be effective, consistent usage and proper handling by users are essential. However, user compliance can vary due to multiple factors such as discomfort, battery life issues, lack of motivation, or loss of interest over time. Devices may be removed, forgotten, or improperly worn, leading to gaps in data or misleading trends. Additionally, not all users are tech-savvy, which may limit adoption, especially among older adults or individuals with disabilities. Designing wearables that are comfortable, user-friendly, and seamlessly integrated into daily life is crucial for long-term adherence.
- **Data Privacy and Security Risks:** As wearables collect sensitive health data, ensuring privacy and security is a top concern. These devices transmit personal information wirelessly to apps or cloud platforms, which can be vulnerable to hacking, data breaches, or unauthorized access. Weak encryption, poor authentication protocols, or insecure APIs can compromise data integrity. Inadequate compliance with healthcare regulations such as HIPAA, GDPR, or local data protection laws can lead to legal and ethical violations. Protecting patient confidentiality requires rigorous security frameworks, informed consent, and transparent data handling policies.
- **Interoperability and Integration Challenges:** Despite advances in interoperability standards like FHIR, many wearable devices still operate within proprietary ecosystems, making it difficult to integrate data across different platforms, devices, and healthcare systems. Lack of standardization can lead to data silos, inconsistencies, and duplication. Healthcare providers often face difficulty in combining wearable data with Electronic Health Records (EHRs) or using it effectively in clinical workflows. Seamless integration requires standard data formats, open APIs, and cooperative industry frameworks, which are still evolving.
- **Technical and Hardware Limitations:** Many wearables face technical limitations related to hardware design, such as short battery life, limited processing power, or low memory capacity. Continuous monitoring consumes significant energy, and frequent charging can reduce usability and compliance. Sensor miniaturization and cost-effective design also introduce trade-offs in data quality or durability. Device malfunctions, software bugs, or firmware incompatibility can disrupt data collection or introduce errors. In rugged environments or extreme climates, performance may degrade further, impacting real-world reliability.
- **Regulatory and Clinical Validation Gaps:** A significant number of wearables in the market are not medically certified, which limits their use in clinical settings. Regulatory approval from bodies like the FDA or CE is

essential for medical-grade wearables but is often a lengthy and expensive process. Devices lacking clinical validation may provide health-related insights that are not scientifically reliable, leading to skepticism among clinicians. The gap between consumer wearables and clinically approved medical devices remains a major barrier to full integration into healthcare systems.

- **User Interpretation and Health Anxiety:** While wearables empower users with health data, misinterpretation of that data can cause unnecessary worry or self-diagnosis. For example, fluctuations in heart rate or sleep scores may be seen as alarming, even if they're within normal physiological ranges. This can lead to health anxiety, increased healthcare visits, or misuse of medical services. Without appropriate guidance or context, users may also ignore important signs. Education, in-app explanations, and clinician involvement are necessary to ensure users interpret data appropriately

8.3 TELEMEDICINE AND TAILORED PATIENT ENGAGEMENT

Telemedicine leverages digital technology to provide healthcare services remotely, breaking down geographical and logistical barriers between patients and providers. It enables real-time consultations, remote monitoring, and timely medical interventions from the comfort of a patient's home. Tailored patient engagement within telemedicine focuses on customizing communication and care strategies to meet individual needs, enhancing adherence and health outcomes. Together, they transform healthcare delivery into a more accessible, personalized, and efficient experience. This approach is especially valuable for managing chronic conditions and improving preventive care.

8.3.1 Definition and Scope of Telemedicine

Telemedicine refers to the delivery of healthcare services remotely using telecommunications technology. It encompasses virtual consultations, remote monitoring, tele-radiology, and tele-psychiatry, among others. This approach enables patients and healthcare providers to interact without the need for physical presence, breaking geographical barriers and increasing access to care, especially in underserved or rural areas. Telemedicine has expanded significantly with advancements in internet connectivity and digital health tools. Telemedicine revolutionizes healthcare delivery by offering remote access to medical services and continuous patient monitoring. When combined with tailored patient engagement strategies, it enhances communication, adherence, and empowerment, leading to better health outcomes. Despite challenges, advancements in digital health technologies and AI are shaping a future where personalized, accessible, and efficient telemedicine becomes a standard part of care.

8.3.2 Benefits of Telemedicine for Patients

Telemedicine offers convenience, reducing the need for travel and minimizing time spent in waiting rooms. Patients can access specialists regardless of location, improving healthcare equity. It is particularly advantageous for managing chronic diseases, mental health support, and routine follow-ups. Additionally, telemedicine can lead to faster diagnosis and treatment initiation, reduce healthcare costs, and enhance patient satisfaction by offering more flexible appointment scheduling.

8.3.3 Role of Wearables and Remote Monitoring in Telemedicine

Integration of wearable devices with telemedicine platforms enhances remote patient monitoring by providing continuous, real-time physiological data. This enables healthcare providers to track vital signs, medication adherence, and symptom progression remotely. Such data-driven insights support informed clinical decisions during virtual visits and can trigger alerts for early intervention, improving patient outcomes and reducing hospital admissions.

8.3.4 Tailored Patient Engagement: Definition and Importance

Tailored patient engagement involves customizing communication, education, and intervention strategies to meet individual patient needs, preferences, and health conditions. This personalized approach improves patient motivation, adherence to treatment, and overall health outcomes. In telemedicine, tailored engagement is critical as it compensates for the lack of face-to-face interaction by fostering meaningful and relevant patient-provider relationships.

8.3.5 Strategies for Tailored Patient Engagement in Telemedicine

Effective tailored engagement strategies include personalized health education materials, customized care plans, and interactive tools like mobile apps and chatbots. Behavioural nudges, reminders for medication or appointments, and feedback based on patient data help maintain adherence. Additionally, culturally sensitive communication and language options enhance inclusivity. Utilizing patient preferences to determine communication channels (e.g., text, video, email) further supports engagement.

8.3.6 Enhancing Patient Empowerment through Telemedicine

Telemedicine empowers patients by giving them greater control over their health management. Access to personal health data, educational resources, and virtual support tools helps patients make informed decisions. Empowered patients are more likely to engage actively in their care, adhere to treatment regimens, and adopt healthier behaviours, leading to improved health outcomes.

8.3.7 Challenges in Telemedicine and Patient Engagement

Challenges include technological barriers such as limited internet access, low digital literacy, and privacy concerns. Patients may feel less connected or less trusting in virtual environments compared to in-person visits. Additionally, ensuring equity in access and avoiding disparities in care delivery are ongoing issues. Effective engagement requires addressing these barriers through user-friendly platforms, patient education, and robust security measures.

8.3.8 Future Trends: AI and Data Analytics in Tailored Engagement

Emerging technologies like artificial intelligence (AI) and advanced data analytics are enhancing tailored patient engagement by providing predictive insights and personalized recommendations. AI-driven chatbots can offer 24/7 support, answer questions, and triage symptoms. Data analytics can identify adherence patterns and risk factors, enabling proactive outreach. These innovations promise to make telemedicine more responsive, efficient, and patient-centred.

8.4 PREDICTIVE HEALTH AND PREVENTIVE STRATEGIES

Predictive health utilizes data analytics, machine learning, and advanced algorithms to anticipate the onset or progression of diseases before symptoms appear. By analysing genetic, behavioural, environmental, and physiological data, predictive models identify individuals at risk, enabling early interventions.

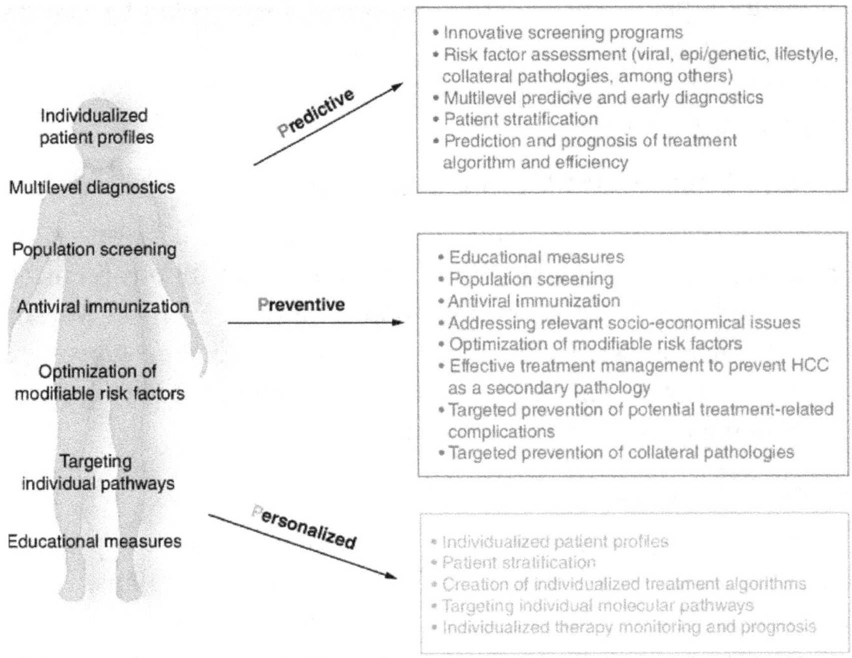

Fig. 2 Principles of Predictive, preventive and personalised medicine

This proactive approach shifts healthcare from reactive treatment to foresight-driven management, aiming to reduce disease burden and improve quality of life. Predictive health and preventive strategies represent a transformative approach to medicine, focusing on forecasting health risks and implementing early interventions. Leveraging big data, AI, genomics, and continuous monitoring, this paradigm shift enables personalized care that emphasizes prevention, improves outcomes, and reduces healthcare costs. While challenges remain, ongoing innovations promise a future where health risks are anticipated and managed proactively for better population health (Fig. 2).

8.4.1 Role of Big Data and Artificial Intelligence (AI)

Big data aggregates vast amounts of health-related information from electronic health records (EHRs), wearables, genomics, and lifestyle apps. AI processes and learns from these complex datasets to recognize patterns and predict health outcomes with increasing accuracy. AI-driven tools can forecast disease risks, recommend personalized preventive measures, and optimize resource allocation, revolutionizing how healthcare anticipates and manages patient needs.

8.4.2 Genetic and Genomic Profiling

Advances in genomics allow the identification of genetic predispositions to various diseases. Genetic profiling helps stratify individuals by risk levels, informing personalized prevention plans. For example, individuals with a family history of certain cancers or cardiovascular diseases can receive tailored screening schedules or lifestyle advice. Integrating genetic data with other health information enhances the precision of predictive models.

8.4.3 Lifestyle and Environmental Risk Assessment

Predictive health also considers behavioural and environmental factors such as diet, physical activity, exposure to pollutants, and stress. Continuous monitoring through wearables and health apps provides real-time data on these variables. Combining this information with clinical data allows for comprehensive risk assessments and supports customized interventions aimed at modifying harmful behaviours and reducing environmental exposures.

8.4.4 Preventive Strategies and Intervention Models

Based on predictive insights, healthcare providers can design targeted preventive strategies such as vaccination programs, lifestyle modification plans, or early therapeutic measures. These interventions focus on risk reduction, health promotion, and delaying or preventing disease onset. Preventive care models may include regular screenings, nutritional counselling, exercise programs, and stress management tailored to individual risk profiles.

8.4.5 Benefits of Predictive and Preventive Healthcare

By identifying risks early and acting proactively, predictive health can reduce hospital admissions, lower healthcare costs, and improve patient outcomes. It fosters a shift from treating illnesses to maintaining wellness, enhancing lifespan and quality of life. Preventive strategies reduce the incidence and severity of chronic diseases, alleviate strain on healthcare systems, and empower patients to take an active role in their health.

8.4.6 Challenges and Ethical Considerations

Despite its promise, predictive health faces challenges such as data privacy concerns, potential biases in AI algorithms, and ensuring equitable access to predictive tools. Ethical dilemmas arise around genetic data use, informed consent, and the psychological impact of risk information on patients. Addressing these issues requires transparent policies, robust data security, and inclusive healthcare frameworks.

8.4.7 Future Directions and Innovations

The future of predictive health lies in integrating multi-omics data, real-time sensor inputs, and sophisticated AI to create dynamic, continuously updated health profiles. Emerging technologies like digital twins—virtual models of patients—could simulate disease progression and treatment responses. Advances in telehealth, personalized medicine, and population health analytics will further enable precision prevention and timely interventions.

9 Chapter

ETHICAL, LEGAL AND SOCIAL IMPLICATIONS (ELSI)

9.0 INTRODUCTION: AN OVERVIEW

The rapid advancement of technology in healthcare—from artificial intelligence (AI) and big data analytics to genetic engineering and wearable health monitoring—has revolutionized how we understand, diagnose, and manage disease. These innovations hold immense promise for improving public health, enabling early interventions, and personalizing treatments. However, alongside these transformative benefits arise complex Ethical, Legal, and Social Implications (ELSI) that demand urgent and ongoing attention. ELSI is a multidisciplinary field of study that explores how new biomedical and technological developments impact individuals, communities, institutions, and broader society. As predictive health tools gain momentum, they collect, process, and interpret vast amounts of personal health data—ranging from genetic sequences and biometric indicators to lifestyle patterns and environmental exposures. While this enables more accurate risk predictions and personalized care, it also raises critical questions about data privacy, consent, and ownership. Who controls the data? How is it stored, shared, or used? Can it be misused for discrimination or surveillance? These concerns are not just technical—they are deeply ethical and legal. Moreover, AI-driven decision-making in healthcare introduces additional dilemmas. Algorithms, if not carefully designed, can perpetuate or exacerbate biases, leading to unfair treatment outcomes for marginalized groups. Ensuring transparency, accountability, and explainability in AI systems is essential to uphold trust and equity in medical practice. Similarly, genomics and genetic testing, while powerful for disease prevention, raise moral issues around genetic determinism, family dynamics, and psychological burden. The knowledge of one's genetic risks can be empowering for some, but overwhelming or stigmatizing for others. Legally, healthcare systems must navigate a maze of regulations to ensure compliance with data protection laws, intellectual property rights, and anti-discrimination statutes. Differences in legal frameworks across regions can hinder global data sharing and collaboration, creating barriers to research and innovation (Fig. 1).

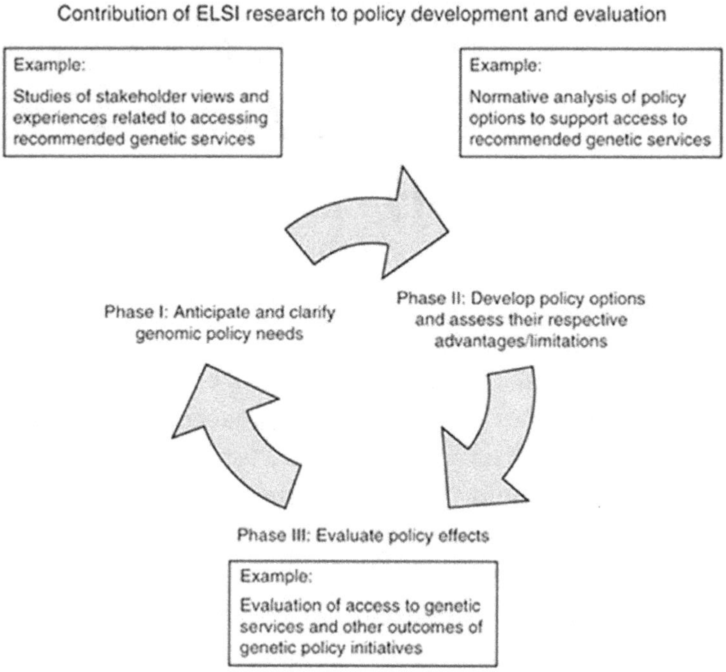

Fig. 1 Ethical, Legal, and Social Implications (ELSI)

Socially, the deployment of predictive health tools may shift the burden of disease prevention onto individuals, risking a culture of blame, over-medicalization, or health anxiety. Additionally, equitable access to predictive and personalized health technologies remains a pressing concern. Without inclusive design and distribution, there is a risk that such advancements will widen existing health disparities, benefitting only affluent or well-connected populations. The concept of health justice—ensuring fair access, participation, and outcomes—must therefore guide the implementation of these technologies. Public engagement, transparency, and interdisciplinary collaboration are vital to address ELSI challenges responsibly. Ethical frameworks must evolve alongside technology, guided by principles such as autonomy, beneficence, non-maleficence, and justice. Legal systems must be robust yet flexible, accommodating innovation while safeguarding rights. Social scientists, ethicists, policymakers, technologists, and the public must work together to shape a future where technological progress aligns with societal values. This chapter explores the multifaceted ELSI landscape in predictive health and related technologies. It examines the dilemmas and debates at the intersection of technology, ethics, law, and society, and offers insights into how these challenges can be addressed through thoughtful design, governance, and education. As healthcare becomes increasingly data-driven and personalized, understanding and integrating ELSI considerations is not optional—it is essential for building a future that is not only innovative, but also ethical, equitable, and just.

9.1 GENETIC PRIVACY AND INFORMED CONSENT

9.1.1 Introduction to Genetic Privacy

Genetic privacy refers to the right of individuals to control access to and use of their genetic information. As genetic data is uniquely identifiable and can reveal deeply personal information—not just about the individual but also their biological relatives and ancestry—it raises significant ethical, legal, and social concerns. With advancements in genomic research and technologies like whole genome sequencing, vast amounts of genetic data are being collected for medical, research, and commercial purposes. This has increased the risk of unauthorized access, data breaches, and potential misuse of genetic information. Misuse could lead to genetic discrimination in employment or insurance, social stigma, or psychological distress. For instance, learning about a predisposition to a serious hereditary illness could cause anxiety or impact life decisions. Because of its far-reaching implications, genetic data must be handled with the highest level of confidentiality and respect. Informed consent becomes crucial in this context, ensuring that individuals fully understand what genetic tests involve, how their data will be used, stored, and who may access it. Consent should be ongoing, allowing individuals to withdraw at any time. Moreover, as genetic findings can affect family members, questions arise about shared privacy and the ethics of disclosure. Thus, protecting genetic privacy requires robust policies, transparent practices, and respect for individual autonomy in both research and clinical settings.

9.1.2 Sensitivity of Genetic Information

Genetic information is among the most sensitive types of personal data because it can reveal intimate details about an individual's health, identity, and lineage. For instance, genetic testing can indicate a predisposition to various hereditary diseases such as cancer, Alzheimer's, or heart conditions, even before symptoms appear. This predictive power, while valuable for preventive care, also makes individuals vulnerable to potential misuse. Beyond medical concerns, genetic data can disclose non-medical traits, such as ancestry, ethnic background, or biological relationships, including paternity. These revelations may have profound personal and social consequences, especially if they conflict with an individual's beliefs or family narratives. If such sensitive data falls into the wrong hands—through data breaches, unauthorized sharing, or inadequate consent—it can lead to stigmatization, discrimination, or even social exclusion. For example, a person identified as genetically predisposed to a mental illness might face prejudice in the workplace or insurance denial. The sensitivity of this data demands stringent privacy protections, ethical safeguards, and legal frameworks to prevent its misuse and ensure individuals retain control over how their genetic information is collected, used, and shared.

9.1.3 Data Ownership and Control

The question of who truly owns genetic data is a contentious and evolving issue in the fields of bioethics, law, and medicine. Unlike general health records, genetic data is permanent, uniquely identifiable, and carries implications not just for individuals but also for their biological relatives. Debates over ownership centre around various stakeholders—individuals, laboratories, biotechnology companies, research institutions, and even governments—all of whom may claim rights to access, use, or store this data. In many current systems, once individuals submit their DNA for testing—whether for medical diagnosis, ancestry exploration, or research—they often relinquish control over how that data is used in the future. This loss of agency can lead to genetic information being stored indefinitely, shared with third parties, or used in studies without the subject's ongoing knowledge or consent. Such practices have sparked increasing concern and criticism, especially as the value of genetic data in both medical research and commercial markets grows. In response, there is a growing call for patient-centric data ownership models. These models prioritize individual autonomy and advocate for full transparency, requiring that data subjects give informed consent not just once, but continuously—especially when new uses arise. They also support mechanisms for individuals to access, monitor, and even delete their genetic data. Emerging technologies, like blockchain and decentralized data storage, are being explored to facilitate secure, individual-led data control. Ultimately, resolving the issue of genetic data ownership is crucial for maintaining trust in genomic science, ensuring ethical research practices, and protecting personal rights in the digital age of medicine.

9.1.4 Risks of Data Breach and Misuse

Genetic data, due to its deeply personal and unchangeable nature, presents a high-value target for cyberattacks and unauthorized access. As more health organizations, biotech companies, and research institutions build vast genetic databases, the risk of data breaches increases significantly. Hackers may target these databases to access sensitive genetic profiles, which can be misused in various harmful ways. One of the most pressing concerns is the potential for genetic discrimination—particularly in employment or insurance settings. For instance, individuals found to have a genetic predisposition to certain diseases like cancer or neurological disorders could be unfairly denied job opportunities or health coverage, even if they are currently healthy. This potential misuse creates fear and mistrust around genetic testing and participation in research. To counteract such threats, legal frameworks like the Genetic Information Non-discrimination Act (GINA) in the United States have been established. GINA prohibits the use of genetic information in employment decisions and health insurance eligibility. However, it has limitations—it does not extend to areas like life insurance or long-term care insurance, nor does it fully regulate all types of genetic data collection and sharing. As technology advances and genetic testing becomes more widespread, existing legal protections must be updated and expanded. In addition, institutions handling genetic data must implement robust cybersecurity measures, ethical oversight, and clear consent processes to ensure privacy is respected and data is not exploited. Without such safeguards, the promise of genetic research could be overshadowed by the risks of misuse and loss of individual autonomy.

9.1.5 Informed Consent in Genetic Testing

Informed consent in genetic testing is a critical ethical requirement that ensures individuals are fully aware of the implications of undergoing such tests. Unlike routine medical procedures, genetic testing can uncover deeply personal information that affects not only the individual but also their biological relatives. Therefore, informed consent must be more than a signed form—it should be a comprehensive process of education, understanding, and voluntary agreement. Patients must clearly understand what the test involves, including the type of genetic information being analysed and the purpose behind it. They should also be informed about what kind of results the test may reveal, such as predispositions to genetic disorders, carrier status, or unexpected findings like non-paternity or unknown family relationships. Equally important is transparency regarding who will have access to the test results—whether healthcare providers, researchers, insurance companies, or third-party labs—and how this data will be stored, shared, or possibly reused in future studies. Patients must also be made aware of the potential consequences of testing, including psychological impacts, insurance or employment risks, and the ethical dilemma of whether or not to share findings with family members who may also be affected. Since genetic data can never be "unknown" once revealed, individuals must be given the opportunity to ask questions, consider the implications, and even withdraw consent if they choose. A meaningful informed consent process empowers individuals, respects their autonomy, and builds trust in medical and research institutions that handle sensitive genetic information.

9.1.6 Challenges in Ensuring Informed Consent

Ensuring truly informed consent in genetic testing poses several significant challenges, largely due to the complexity of the subject matter and the long-term implications of sharing genetic information. Many genetic concepts—such as gene mutations, inheritance patterns, or probabilistic risk—are scientifically dense and often difficult for individuals without a medical or scientific background to fully understand. As a result, patients may agree to testing or data sharing without grasping the full scope of what they are consenting to. This gap in understanding can be further complicated by the emotional stress or urgency often associated with medical decisions, making it harder for individuals to process nuanced information. Another major challenge is that patients may not fully comprehend the potential future uses of their genetic data. Data shared today for clinical diagnosis or research could be stored indefinitely and possibly used in unrelated future studies, sold to third parties, or become vulnerable to data breaches. The long-term implications for the individual and their relatives—such as psychological impacts, disclosure of unexpected familial relationships, or risk of discrimination—may not be immediately evident at the time of testing. Therefore, consent should not be treated as a one-time signature on a form, but rather as an ongoing, dynamic process. Patients should be regularly updated on how their data is used and given opportunities to reaffirm or withdraw their consent as new situations arise. This approach respects individual autonomy, enhances trust in medical and research institutions, and helps ensure that consent is truly informed and ethically sound.

9.1.7 Family and Third-Party Implications

Genetic testing doesn't only affect the individual being tested—it often has far-reaching implications for their biological relatives. Because genes are shared within families, a result indicating a hereditary condition or genetic mutation in one person can suggest that close family members may also be at risk. This can unintentionally reveal highly sensitive information, such as unknown biological relationships (e.g., misattributed paternity or undisclosed adoption) or the presence of inherited health conditions that others in the family were unaware of. These revelations can disrupt family dynamics, create emotional distress, and raise difficult questions about disclosure and responsibility. One of the most pressing ethical challenges is deciding whether, and how, to inform family members who may be affected. While the tested individual has a right to privacy and control over their medical information, withholding potentially life-saving information from relatives can pose serious moral dilemmas. Healthcare professionals often find themselves caught between respecting individual confidentiality and acting in the broader interest of familial well-being. In some cases, there may be a strong ethical argument to encourage or even facilitate disclosure—especially when early intervention or preventive measures could benefit relatives. However, the line between autonomy and obligation is not always clear. This tension highlights the need for clear guidelines, sensitive communication strategies, and possibly legal frameworks to balance individual rights with the collective nature of genetic information.

9.1.8 Genetic Testing in Minors

Genetic testing in minors, especially for adult-onset conditions, brings forth a range of ethical dilemmas that must be approached with caution and sensitivity. One of the main concerns is that children are not yet fully capable of providing informed consent due to their ongoing cognitive and emotional development. This means that decisions about genetic testing are usually made by parents or guardians, whose intentions may be well-meaning but may not always align with the best long-term interests of the child. When testing is done for conditions that will not affect the child until adulthood—and for which no preventive action is necessary during childhood—it can interfere with the child's right to make an informed choice about their own health information later in life. Such testing can also have psychological impacts, potentially causing anxiety or shaping how a child is treated or viewed within the family. On the other hand, some parents argue that knowing their child's genetic risks early allows them to prepare emotionally, financially, or medically. In rare cases where early interventions or lifestyle changes can reduce long-term risks, testing might be justified on the grounds of medical benefit. However, in the absence of immediate medical need, many ethicists and professional organizations recommend delaying testing until the child reaches an age where they can actively participate in the decision. Ultimately, genetic testing in minors demands a careful balance between respecting parental rights, protecting the child's developing autonomy, and considering whether any meaningful health benefits can be gained from early testing.

9.1.9 Commercial Genetic Testing Services

- Commercial genetic testing services, especially direct-to-consumer (DTC) platforms like 23andMe, have rapidly gained popularity by offering individuals easy and affordable access to insights about their ancestry, health risks, and genetic traits. While these services promise convenience and personal empowerment, they also raise significant concerns surrounding data privacy, informed consent, and the ethical use of sensitive genetic information. One of the most pressing issues is that consumers often lack a clear understanding of how their genetic data will be stored, processed, and potentially shared with third parties. Terms of service and privacy policies are frequently lengthy, complex, and written in legal jargon, making it difficult for the average user to grasp the full implications of their participation.

- Many companies reserve broad rights to use genetic data not only for internal research but also for external partnerships, including pharmaceutical companies and marketing firms. While some users may appreciate contributing to scientific advancements, others may be unaware that their DNA is being monetized without explicit, ongoing consent. Unlike traditional medical contexts where genetic testing is tightly regulated and guided by healthcare professionals, DTC tests often bypass those safeguards, leaving users without proper counselling or follow-up. Moreover, once genetic data is shared, it becomes nearly impossible to retract or anonymize completely, especially if it has already been integrated into broader research databases.

- There is also the issue of data security. As genetic data is uniquely identifiable and contains deeply personal information, breaches or misuse could have long-lasting consequences—not just for the individual, but potentially for their biological relatives. Some services allow users to upload their raw genetic data to third-party platforms for further analysis, which further increases exposure to potential data exploitation. Additionally, law enforcement agencies have occasionally accessed DTC databases to identify suspects through familial DNA, raising ethical questions about consent and surveillance. Ultimately, while commercial genetic testing holds exciting potential, it also calls for increased transparency, stronger data protections, and better consumer education to ensure users can make truly informed decisions about their genetic privacy.

9.1.10 Regulatory and Legal Frameworks

- The regulation of genetic data and testing is an evolving and complex challenge that varies significantly across countries and jurisdictions. This fragmented landscape creates inconsistencies in how genetic information is collected, stored, used, and shared, ultimately impacting the protection of individuals' privacy and the integrity of genomic research. In some countries, robust legislation such as the General Data Protection Regulation (GDPR) in the European Union offers strong safeguards for individuals, requiring clear informed consent, data minimization, and strict protocols for data sharing. However, in many other regions, legal frameworks are either outdated, ambiguous, or entirely absent, leaving individuals vulnerable to misuse or exploitation of their sensitive genetic data.
- An effective regulatory framework must address several core elements. First, data security is paramount, as genetic information is not only deeply personal but also permanently identifiable. Laws must mandate rigorous encryption, secure storage practices, and breach notification requirements. Second, informed consent must be clear, specific, and ongoing, ensuring that individuals fully understand what they are agreeing to when they submit their genetic material—particularly regarding secondary uses of their data. Third, regulations must carefully define and control secondary use of data, including research, commercial applications, and third-party access. Participants should have the right to opt in or out of such uses at any point, with transparency about how their data might be monetized or transferred.

- A major regulatory challenge lies in cross-border data sharing, especially as genomic research becomes increasingly international. Data collected in one country may be stored or analysed in another, often without the participant's full awareness or consent. Without aligned regulations, this can lead to legal loopholes and ethical grey areas. Therefore, harmonized legal frameworks at the global level are urgently needed. Such harmonization would support collaborative international research while ensuring that all participants, regardless of nationality or location, enjoy the same high standards of protection.
- Efforts such as the Global Alliance for Genomics and Health (GA4GH) aim to foster standardized policies and technical solutions for responsible data sharing. Still, their success depends on the willingness of nations and corporations to adopt and enforce shared ethical principles. In conclusion, robust and harmonized regulatory and legal frameworks are essential to protect individual rights, maintain public trust, and enable ethical global advancement in genomic science.

9.1.11 Ethical Principles Involved

- **Autonomy- Respecting the Individual's Right to Control Personal Information:** Autonomy is a cornerstone of bioethics and refers to an individual's right to make informed decisions about their own body and personal data. In the context of genetic testing and data collection, this means individuals must be fully informed about how their genetic information will be used, stored, and shared, and must give consent freely—without coercion or manipulation. Informed consent is not a one-time checkbox but a continuous process that allows participants to withdraw or modify their consent as circumstances change. Respecting autonomy also includes ensuring individuals have access to understandable information, especially when dealing with complex scientific and technical terms. This is particularly important in direct-to-consumer genetic testing, where users may not fully realize that their DNA could be used for secondary purposes, such as pharmaceutical research or law enforcement investigations. Without transparent policies and communication, true autonomy is compromised. In addition, autonomy respects cultural and personal values; what may be acceptable for one person may be intrusive for another. Systems must therefore be designed with flexibility and inclusivity to support diverse perspectives and empower users with control over their genetic identity.
- **Beneficence- Using Genetic Data to Improve Health Outcomes:** Beneficence refers to the ethical obligation to promote good and contribute positively to the well-being of individuals and society. In genetics, this

principle supports the responsible use of data to advance medical research, improve diagnostics, develop personalized treatments, and prevent disease. For example, large-scale genomic studies have helped identify genetic markers associated with diseases like cancer, diabetes, and rare disorders, enabling earlier interventions and tailored care. However, beneficence must be carefully balanced with respect for autonomy and privacy. While using genetic data can lead to significant medical breakthroughs, the benefits must be shared equitably, and not just serve the interests of pharmaceutical companies or wealthy nations. Additionally, individuals who contribute data should ideally receive feedback or benefit from any health-related discoveries made through their participation. There's also a duty to ensure that genetic data is interpreted accurately, as incorrect results could lead to unnecessary anxiety, misdiagnosis, or ineffective treatment. In this sense, beneficence also implies a commitment to scientific rigor, transparency, and public education, ensuring that genetic science is used for the collective good while minimizing misinformation.

- **Non-Maleficence- Preventing Harm Through Misuse of Data:** Non-maleficence, meaning "do no harm," is a fundamental ethical principle that is especially critical in the handling of genetic information. Genetic data is highly sensitive, and if misused, it can lead to significant harm—ranging from privacy violations and discrimination to psychological distress or even social stigma. For instance, if a person's genetic predisposition to mental illness or certain diseases is exposed without consent, they may face discrimination in employment or insurance. Inadequate data security, unclear privacy policies, or unauthorized third-party access can further increase risks of harm. Moreover, genetic testing without proper counseling may cause emotional harm when individuals learn of predispositions to untreatable or misunderstood conditions. This is particularly concerning in DTC genetic testing, where medical guidance is often lacking. Ethical frameworks must prioritize robust data protection, transparency about secondary data usage, and systems that prevent misuse by both private and public entities. Policies should also address long-term harms, such as the use of genetic data by future regimes or companies in ways the original user never anticipated. Ultimately, non-maleficence requires a proactive approach to risk management and a deep commitment to safeguarding the dignity and well-being of all data subjects.
- **Justice- Ensuring Fair Access and Protection for All, Especially Vulnerable Populations:** Justice in genetics revolves around fairness, equity, and equal protection, particularly in how genetic data is collected, interpreted, and used. It calls for the equitable distribution of the benefits

and burdens of genetic research and healthcare, ensuring that no group is disproportionately exploited or excluded. Vulnerable populations—such as Indigenous communities, racial minorities, or individuals in low-income regions—have historically been underrepresented or misrepresented in genomic databases, leading to biased medical results and limited access to advances in genetic medicine. Ethical justice requires proactive inclusion of diverse populations in research, ensuring their specific genetic traits and health risks are understood and addressed. It also involves protecting those groups from being exploited for data without adequate benefit-sharing or consent. Justice extends to accessibility as well—genetic testing and the resulting medical benefits should not be limited to the wealthy or privileged. Legal protections against genetic discrimination, such as those provided by the Genetic Information Non-discrimination Act (GINA) in the U.S., are also essential components of justice. In global research contexts, justice demands that low- and middle-income countries not be relegated to mere data sources but be treated as equal partners, receiving fair benefits from the research outcomes.

9.1.12 The Future of Genetic Privacy and Consent

As genetic technologies evolve and the volume of personal genomic data grows, the future of genetic privacy and consent is poised for significant transformation. Traditional, static models of consent—where individuals agree once and permanently relinquish control over their data—are increasingly viewed as inadequate in the face of complex, long-term data usage. In response, there is a growing shift toward dynamic consent models, which empower individuals to manage their data permissions over time. This flexible, user-centric approach allows participants to grant or withdraw consent for specific uses of their data, such as research, commercial use, or cross-border sharing. Dynamic consent not only enhances autonomy but also builds trust between users and data handlers by promoting transparency and ongoing engagement. Technological innovations are also playing a critical role in strengthening genetic privacy. Emerging blockchain and decentralized data systems offer promising alternatives to centralized databases, which are more vulnerable to breaches and unauthorized access. Blockchain's immutable ledger and decentralized architecture allow for secure, traceable, and user-controlled access to genetic information. For example, individuals could choose to share specific parts of their genetic profile with researchers while keeping the rest private, all with the ability to revoke access at any time. These systems can also automate consent management through smart contracts, ensuring that data is used exactly as agreed. However, these advancements cannot be fully effective without significant improvements in public education and awareness. Genetic data is complex, and individuals must be empowered with not only control over their information but also the knowledge to make informed decisions. This includes understanding what their data reveals, how it can be used, and the implications of sharing it with commercial entities or research institutions. Educational initiatives must be inclusive, accessible, and culturally sensitive, addressing diverse populations with varying levels of literacy and technological access. Governments, healthcare providers, and private companies all share responsibility in ensuring the public is equipped to navigate the genetic data landscape safely. Looking ahead, a future that balances innovation with ethical responsibility will depend on coordinated efforts to create user-centric systems, enforce robust regulations, and foster a well-informed society. By integrating dynamic consent, decentralized technology, and public engagement, we can move toward a model of genetic data governance that respects individual rights while enabling scientific progress.

9.2 DATA OWNERSHIP AND SHARING

9.2.1 Introduction to Data Ownership in Healthcare:

- In the age of digital health and precision medicine, health and genetic data have emerged as some of the most valuable and powerful resources in the healthcare ecosystem. These data—ranging from electronic health records (EHRs) and biometric readings to DNA sequences and personal health behaviours—are central to clinical decision-making, disease research, and the development of personalized treatments. As a result, the question of who owns this data has become one of the most critical and hotly debated ethical and legal issues in modern healthcare. Unlike physical property, data ownership is not universally defined, leading to varying interpretations among stakeholders. For many patients, the assumption is that because the data comes from their bodies, they naturally "own" it. This view is supported by ethical principles like autonomy and the right to control one's personal information. Patients may expect to decide who can access their data, how it is used, and whether it can be sold or shared. However, in practice, the ownership and control of health data often rest in the hands of healthcare institutions, laboratories, or technology companies that collect, store, and analyse the information. Electronic health record systems, for example, are typically managed by hospitals or third-party vendors, limiting patients' direct access or control over their own health histories. Understanding data ownership and data rights is given in Fig. 2.

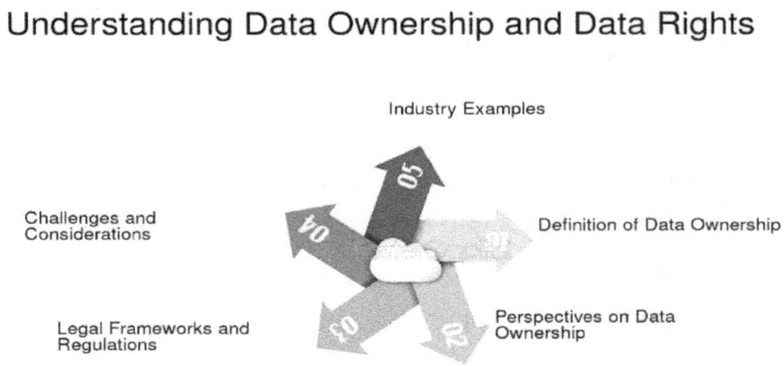

Fig. 2 Understanding data ownership and data rights

- Researchers and biotech firms add another layer to this debate. They rely heavily on aggregated health and genetic datasets to identify disease patterns, develop new therapies, and drive innovation. While such research can yield public health benefits, it also raises concerns when conducted without patients' explicit knowledge or consent, especially if the findings are monetized. Tech companies further complicate matters. Many digital health apps and wearables collect vast amounts of user data—often under opaque terms of service—and then use it for analytics, targeted advertising, or partnerships with pharmaceutical firms, blurring the lines between health service and data commercialization. The lack of clear, legally binding definitions of data ownership leads to uncertainty and ethical dilemmas, particularly around consent, privacy, and profit-sharing. Who decides whether a patient's data can be sold to third parties? Should patients receive a share of the revenue generated from their information? What rights do individuals have to delete or transfer their data? These unresolved questions highlight the urgent need for frameworks that clearly define ownership while balancing individual rights with public health goals.
- Ultimately, defining ownership is not only a legal issue but also a moral one. It shapes how data is collected, who benefits from it, and how trust is built—or broken—within the healthcare system. Clear, equitable policies around data ownership are essential for fostering transparency, respecting patient autonomy, and ensuring that the vast potential of health data is harnessed responsibly and ethically in the years ahead.

9.2.2 Patient Rights and Control

- In today's data-driven healthcare environment, the question of patient rights and control over health data has become increasingly prominent. Patients commonly assume that they own their medical and genetic information, believing they have full authority over how it's accessed, used, and shared. After all, this data is derived from their bodies and health experiences. However, in reality, the control of health data typically lies with healthcare providers, hospitals, laboratories, or digital platforms that collect and store this information. These entities often act as de facto custodians, managing data within centralized systems that patients may find difficult to access or navigate. Legal ownership is rarely granted to the patient outright, creating a gap between perceived and actual control.

- This disconnect has given rise to a growing movement toward patient-centric data models, which prioritize individual rights, transparency, and autonomy. At the heart of this movement is the belief that patients should not be passive data subjects but active participants in the management of their own health information. Control over how, when, and with whom their data is shared—whether for treatment, research, or commercial use—should lie with the individual. This shift is not only an ethical imperative but also enhances trust and engagement between patients and healthcare systems. When patients feel they have agency over their data, they are more likely to participate in research, share information, and advocate for their health.
- One critical aspect of patient control is the right to data portability. This means individuals should be able to easily access their medical and genetic records and transfer them between different institutions, platforms, or applications without unnecessary barriers. Whether a person is changing healthcare providers, using a personal health tracking app, or enrolling in a clinical trial, they should not be forced to repeatedly provide the same information or face delays due to incompatible systems. Data portability not only enhances continuity of care but also empowers patients to seek second opinions, engage with digital health tools, or participate in personalized treatment plans.
- Regulatory frameworks like the General Data Protection Regulation (GDPR) in the EU and the Health Insurance Portability and Accountability Act (HIPAA) in the U.S. have begun to acknowledge these rights by promoting transparency, access, and individual control. However, implementation remains uneven, and technical as well as institutional resistance often hinders patients from exercising these rights effectively. Many health systems still operate with fragmented, siloed databases that limit interoperability and restrict real-time access to records. Additionally, some digital health platforms use legal loopholes in user agreements to retain ownership of the data, despite collecting it from the user directly.
- Ultimately, achieving true patient control requires a cultural and technological shift in how health data is managed. It involves building

interoperable systems, simplifying consent processes, and ensuring user-friendly tools that allow patients to manage their data confidently and securely. Patient rights are not merely about ownership—they are about empowerment, dignity, and agency in a system that has historically been provider-dominated. Moving forward, healthcare systems must centre patients not only in care delivery but in the governance of their own health information, ensuring their voices and choices are respected at every stage of data use.

9.2.3 Institutional and Corporate Claims

- In the evolving landscape of healthcare and biomedical research, institutions and corporations increasingly assert ownership over health and genetic data, raising significant ethical, legal, and practical concerns. Healthcare providers, hospitals, and academic research institutions often claim rights to the data generated during clinical encounters, diagnostic procedures, or research studies. Their rationale is that they are responsible for generating, managing, and storing the data using institutional infrastructure and expertise. For instance, a hospital conducting genetic testing may argue that the results—and even the raw genetic data—belong to the institution, not the patient, especially if the test was funded or performed as part of a clinical protocol or research initiative.
- Similarly, research institutions and biobanks that collect and analyze patient samples often include data ownership clauses in their study consent forms. Participants may unwittingly relinquish rights to their data in exchange for the opportunity to take part in a trial, without fully understanding the long-term implications. Once collected, these datasets can be stored indefinitely, reused for other studies, or even shared with third parties, sometimes without further consent from the original contributors. This creates a power imbalance where the institution holds the authority over data use, while the individual remains largely excluded from decisions concerning their own biological information.
- The rise of digital health has further complicated these dynamics. Technology companies—including app developers, wearable device manufacturers, and genomics firms—often embed broad data rights into user agreements or terms of service. For example, users of DNA testing kits or health-tracking apps may unknowingly agree to allow the company to store, analyse, and even sell their data to third parties, including pharmaceutical companies or data brokers. These user agreements are often long, opaque, and filled with legal jargon, making it easy for individuals to miss or misunderstand critical clauses. Once accepted, these contracts give companies extensive

control over how data is used, shared, and even monetized, often without any compensation or input from the user.

- This claim of ownership by institutions and corporations enables them to act as data gatekeepers, deciding not only who can access the data but also for what purpose. Whether for commercial gain, strategic partnerships, or exclusive research publications, the control of data becomes a valuable asset—sometimes more valuable than the services provided themselves. In many cases, the monetization of data becomes a significant revenue stream, especially when datasets are large, diverse, and well-structured. Companies may argue that they invest heavily in the tools and infrastructure required to collect and secure data, and therefore are entitled to the benefits derived from it.
- However, this approach raises critical ethical issues. When patients or users are excluded from the benefits generated by their data, questions of fairness, transparency, and exploitation emerge. Moreover, data collected under the pretext of care or personal use being repurposed for profit can erode trust in both the healthcare and tech industries. As data becomes more central to healthcare innovation, it is imperative to rethink and redefine ownership frameworks, ensuring they reflect not only legal authority but also ethical obligations to the individuals from whom the data originates.

9.2.4 Legal Frameworks and Variability

- The question of who owns health and genetic data is deeply influenced by the legal frameworks that govern data privacy and access across different countries and regions. These frameworks vary widely, resulting in a complex and often contradictory global landscape in which individual rights, institutional authority, and corporate control are interpreted differently depending on jurisdiction. This variability creates challenges for patients, researchers, and companies, particularly in cross-border contexts where data may be collected in one country, stored in another, and analysed in a third.
- In some jurisdictions, patients enjoy strong rights over their personal health data, including the ability to access, manage, and even delete it. These rights reflect a growing recognition that health data is not just a byproduct of care but a deeply personal asset that individuals should control. For instance, within the European Union, the General Data Protection Regulation (GDPR) stands as one of the most comprehensive data protection laws in the world. GDPR treats health and genetic data as "special category" data, deserving of heightened protections. It emphasizes the importance of informed consent, transparency, and the right to access, correct, and erase data—commonly

known as the right to be forgotten. Under GDPR, individuals must be clearly informed about how their data will be used, and consent must be freely given, specific, and revocable.

- In contrast, in other parts of the world, the legal system grants more authority to healthcare institutions, researchers, or private companies, often limiting the individual's control over their own data. For example, in the United States, the primary regulation governing medical data is the Health Insurance Portability and Accountability Act (HIPAA). HIPAA focuses on safeguarding the privacy and security of protected health information (PHI) within covered entities, such as hospitals and insurers. However, it does not recognize the patient as the legal owner of their data. Instead, it grants patients certain rights, such as accessing their records and requesting corrections, but ownership remains with the healthcare provider or institution that generated and stores the data. Furthermore, HIPAA does not apply to many consumer-facing digital health platforms and apps, leaving a gap in regulation for non-traditional data handlers.
- Adding further complexity, some countries lack specific legal protections altogether, leaving patients vulnerable to data misuse, commercial exploitation, or unauthorized access. In lower-income regions, limited regulatory oversight may result in foreign institutions collecting data with minimal consent and exporting it abroad for analysis or profit, often without benefit-sharing or transparency. This highlights the importance of establishing fair, global standards for data governance that respect individual rights while enabling ethical research and innovation.
- As health data increasingly flows across borders due to telemedicine, global research collaborations, and digital platforms, the lack of harmonized legal definitions of data ownership and privacy rights becomes more problematic. Individuals may find that their rights are drastically different depending on where their data is stored or processed. A person living in the EU might have extensive control under GDPR, while the same data handled in the U.S. or elsewhere might not be subject to comparable protections. This patchwork of laws not only creates confusion but also invites legal loopholes and inconsistent ethical practices.
- To address these challenges, international cooperation and legal harmonization are urgently needed. Global frameworks must prioritize individual control, informed consent, data portability, and redress mechanisms, while also ensuring that institutions and companies remain accountable for how they manage and profit from data. A unified approach can help build trust, facilitate ethical data sharing, and protect individuals

regardless of geographic location. Until such harmonization is achieved, navigating the legal terrain of health data ownership will remain a fragmented and contested process—posing risks to both personal privacy and the equitable advancement of medical science.

9.2.5 Data Sharing for Research and Innovation

- In the modern era of biomedical science and digital health, data sharing has become essential for advancing research, improving healthcare outcomes, and driving innovation. Access to large, diverse, and high-quality health datasets allows researchers to uncover patterns in disease progression, identify risk factors, and develop more effective treatments. For example, population-wide data is invaluable in studying chronic illnesses, tracking the spread of infectious diseases, and understanding the genetic basis of rare disorders. Furthermore, with the rise of machine learning and artificial intelligence (AI) in healthcare, large datasets are crucial for training accurate, reliable, and unbiased algorithms used in diagnostics, drug discovery, and personalized medicine.
- To protect individual privacy while enabling such progress, data shared for research is often "de-identified" or anonymized, meaning that direct identifiers like names, addresses, or social security numbers are removed. De-identification reduces the risk that individuals can be linked to their data, and in many jurisdictions, it serves as a legal safeguard that allows data to be used without explicit consent. However, in practice, re-identification remains a real and growing risk. With the increasing availability of publicly accessible datasets and powerful computational tools, it has become possible to cross-reference supposedly anonymous data with other information—such as social media or public records—to re-identify individuals, particularly in the case of genetic data, which is inherently unique.
- This growing concern emphasizes the need for ethical, transparent, and well-regulated data sharing practices. Individuals whose data may be used for research must be fully informed about how their information will be shared, who will have access to it, and for what purposes. Informed consent must be specific, meaningful, and, ideally, dynamic, allowing people to adjust their preferences over time. Blanket or vague consent undermines trust and may lead to public resistance, especially if the data is shared with commercial entities for profit-driven research. Public backlash can jeopardize valuable scientific efforts and damage the credibility of health institutions.

- Moreover, data governance systems must include strong safeguards to prevent misuse, whether intentional or accidental. This includes access controls, audit trails, strict data-sharing agreements, and ethical review by independent oversight bodies. Transparency is also critical—not just to regulators, but to the public. People deserve to know how their data contributes to science, who benefits from it, and whether results are being used for public good or private gain. Ethical data sharing frameworks should also ensure fair representation and inclusion, as underrepresentation of certain populations can result in biased research outcomes and ineffective healthcare solutions.
- Internationally, organizations like the Global Alliance for Genomics and Health (GA4GH) have proposed principles and technical standards for responsible data sharing. These aim to harmonize global research efforts while protecting participants' rights. However, enforcement and compliance depend on the commitment of governments, institutions, and companies to uphold ethical standards.
- Ultimately, the success of data sharing for research and innovation hinges on a delicate balance: enabling broad access to valuable information while respecting individual rights, preventing harm, and fostering trust. By building systems rooted in transparency, accountability, and meaningful consent, we can unlock the full potential of health data to transform medicine—without compromising the dignity or privacy of the individuals it represents.

9.2.6 Benefits of Data Sharing

- **Accelerates Medical Research and Drug Development:** One of the most significant benefits of data sharing is its ability to accelerate the pace of medical research and pharmaceutical innovation. When researchers have access to large, diverse health datasets, they can identify genetic, environmental, and lifestyle factors associated with diseases more quickly and accurately. This leads to faster identification of drug targets, biomarkers, and pathways relevant to specific conditions. For example, shared genetic data has enabled scientists to develop therapies tailored to patients with specific mutations, as seen in oncology and rare disease treatment. Furthermore, data sharing reduces duplication of efforts across institutions and promotes collaborative research, allowing findings from one study to inform and validate others. In drug development, access to real-world evidence and patient outcomes helps pharmaceutical companies design better clinical trials, select appropriate cohorts, and reduce time to market. Regulatory agencies also benefit by being able to review more comprehensive datasets, leading to faster and more informed approval decisions. Ultimately, sharing health data improves the efficiency and cost-effectiveness of research pipelines, bringing treatments to patients sooner and more safely.

- **Enables Large-Scale Studies on Disease Patterns, Treatment Efficacy, and Public Health Trends:** Health data sharing makes large-scale, population-wide studies possible, which are critical for understanding complex health dynamics. Epidemiological research relies on vast datasets to detect patterns in disease incidence, prevalence, and progression across different demographics, regions, and risk groups. For example, during pandemics or emerging health crises, shared data allows researchers and governments to track the spread of infections, evaluate containment strategies, and predict future outbreaks. Beyond infectious disease, chronic conditions like diabetes, cardiovascular disease, and cancer require longitudinal data to assess treatment effectiveness, outcomes, and health disparities. By pooling data from multiple healthcare providers or countries, researchers can achieve statistically robust results that smaller, isolated studies cannot. This collective knowledge informs clinical guidelines, public health policies, and resource allocation. Moreover, shared data supports real-world evidence—information collected outside of clinical trials—which is increasingly used by regulators and policymakers to evaluate the true impact of treatments and interventions. In this way, data sharing enhances public health preparedness, responsiveness, and equity.
- **Supports AI and Machine Learning Systems in Building Predictive and Diagnostic Models:** The development of artificial intelligence (AI) and machine learning (ML) in healthcare depends heavily on access to large, diverse, and high-quality datasets. These technologies learn by identifying patterns and correlations in data, and the accuracy of their predictions improves with the quantity and variety of information they process. For example, AI systems used in radiology require thousands of annotated medical images to accurately detect anomalies like tumours or fractures. Similarly, ML models that predict hospital readmissions, diagnose rare diseases, or forecast patient deterioration are trained using historical patient data, lab results, and clinical notes. By sharing health data across institutions, these models become more generalizable and equitable, reducing the risk of bias that often arises when algorithms are trained on limited or homogenous populations. Shared data also allows for continuous learning, enabling models to improve over time and adapt to new clinical knowledge. As a result, AI-powered tools become more reliable and effective in supporting clinicians, optimizing workflows, and personalizing

patient care. Without data sharing, the full potential of AI in transforming healthcare remains out of reach.

9.2.7 Risks of Data Sharing

- **Risk of Re-identification, Even from Anonymized Datasets:** While data anonymization and de-identification techniques are widely used to protect individuals' privacy in shared health datasets, the risk of re-identification remains a significant concern. Advances in data analytics and the availability of vast amounts of auxiliary information mean that even anonymized data can sometimes be traced back to specific individuals. For example, combining de-identified health data with publicly available databases, such as voter registries or social media profiles, can reveal a person's identity. This risk is particularly high for genetic data, which is inherently unique and difficult to fully anonymize. Re-identification could lead to serious consequences, including breaches of confidentiality, discrimination in employment or insurance, and psychological distress for individuals whose sensitive health information becomes exposed. As such, despite the use of rigorous data protection methods, the possibility that shared datasets could be compromised demands constant vigilance, updated security measures, and ethical oversight to mitigate harms.
- **Potential for Unauthorized Access, Data Breaches, and Surveillance:** The digital nature of health data sharing inherently exposes information to the risk of unauthorized access and cyberattacks. Data breaches at hospitals, research institutions, or technology companies can result in the leakage of sensitive health records to hackers, malicious actors, or the public. Such breaches may occur due to weak security protocols, insider threats, or sophisticated cyberattacks, compromising the privacy of millions of individuals. Moreover, shared data may be vulnerable to mass surveillance by governments or other entities, especially in jurisdictions with limited legal protections or oversight. This surveillance could target specific populations or be used to monitor health trends in ways that infringe on civil liberties. The fear of surveillance or misuse can deter patients from consenting to data sharing or participating in research, ultimately hindering medical progress. Therefore, robust cybersecurity, strict access controls, and transparent governance are essential to protect shared health data from these threats.
- **Data May Be Sold or Used for Purposes Not Originally Consented To, Especially by Third-Party Entities:** One of the most ethically fraught risks of health data sharing is the potential for data to be sold, traded, or repurposed by third-party entities without the informed consent of

the individuals whose information is involved. Many health datasets are shared with or sold to commercial companies, including pharmaceutical firms, insurance companies, or data brokers, often under agreements that patients are unaware of or did not explicitly approve. These third parties may use the data for marketing, product development, or other commercial objectives that diverge from the original purpose of collection. This practice not only undermines trust but raises serious questions about ownership, consent, and benefit sharing. Patients may never receive any benefits from the profits generated by their data, nor are they always informed about how their data is being used or shared. Ethical data governance frameworks must emphasize transparency, respect for consent, and restrictions on secondary uses to prevent exploitation and maintain public confidence in data sharing initiatives.

9.2.8 Informed Consent and Secondary Use

- **Informed Consent Must Address Both Primary and Secondary Uses of Data:** Informed consent is a cornerstone of ethical data sharing and protection in healthcare, requiring that individuals fully understand how their data will be collected, used, and shared. However, traditional consent models often focus solely on the primary use of data—such as treatment or a specific research study—without adequately addressing the possibility of secondary uses. Secondary uses refer to any future activities that involve the data, such as additional research projects, commercial applications, or data sharing with third parties not initially envisioned. Failing to inform patients about these possibilities can undermine trust and autonomy, leaving individuals unaware of how broadly their data may be applied. Effective informed consent must therefore be transparent and comprehensive, explicitly outlining potential secondary uses so individuals can make truly informed decisions about participation. This level of clarity helps prevent misunderstandings and ethical breaches, fostering a relationship of respect and trust between data subjects and data users.
- **Broad Consent Models Allow Flexibility but May Limit Patient Control:** To address the challenge of future, unspecified uses, many institutions have adopted broad consent models. Under broad consent, individuals agree to allow their data to be used for a wide range of future research or purposes, often described only in general terms. This approach offers valuable flexibility for researchers and institutions, enabling them to utilize datasets for multiple studies without repeatedly seeking new consent, which can be logistically complex and costly. However, broad consent can limit patient control, as individuals relinquish the right to review or approve specific

secondary uses of their data after the initial consent is given. This lack of ongoing oversight may lead to discomfort or ethical concerns, especially if data is used in ways that patients might not personally support. While broad consent can streamline research processes, it risks compromising the principles of autonomy and informed decision-making if not implemented with adequate safeguards and transparency.

- **Dynamic Consent Models Provide Granular, Ongoing Control Over Data Sharing Preferences:** An innovative alternative to broad consent is the concept of dynamic consent, which seeks to empower individuals with more granular and ongoing control over how their data is shared and used. Dynamic consent utilizes digital platforms to facilitate real-time communication between data subjects and researchers or institutions. Individuals can update their preferences, grant or revoke consent for specific uses, and receive feedback about how their data is being utilized. This approach respects patient autonomy more fully by transforming consent into a continuous, interactive process rather than a one-time transaction. Dynamic consent also builds trust by fostering transparency, engagement, and education around data use. Although dynamic consent models require investment in infrastructure and user-friendly interfaces, they offer a promising pathway to ethically responsible data sharing that balances the needs of research with the rights and preferences of individuals.

9.2.9 Commercialization of Health Data

- **Companies May Monetize Health Data for Profit:** In today's digital health ecosystem, health data has become a highly valuable commodity. Many companies—including pharmaceutical firms, insurance providers, and technology startups—leverage health and genetic data as a critical asset to drive innovation, develop new products, and optimize services. Pharmaceutical companies use large datasets to accelerate drug discovery, identify patient cohorts for clinical trials, and conduct real-world evidence studies to support regulatory approvals. Insurance companies apply data analytics to model risk profiles, personalize premiums, and detect fraud. Digital health platforms may sell anonymized or aggregated data to third parties, including advertisers or data brokers, generating significant revenue streams. This commercialization transforms personal health information into a marketable good, often without direct compensation or benefit to the individuals who provided the data. While monetization can spur innovation and improve healthcare delivery, it also raises concerns about fairness and exploitation, especially when individuals are unaware of or excluded from the financial gains.

- **Raises Ethical Questions:** The commercialization of health data brings forth profound ethical questions about ownership, equity, and justice. A central issue is whether individuals who contribute their personal and often sensitive health information should share in the financial value generated from its use. Traditional data models treat patients as mere data sources rather than stakeholders with rights to benefit from their contribution. This dynamic raises concerns about exploitation, particularly given the significant profits companies can make from aggregated health data. Advocates argue that failing to compensate individuals exacerbates inequalities, especially when vulnerable populations provide data but do not reap rewards. Moreover, the lack of transparency around how data is used and monetized can erode public trust, potentially discouraging participation in valuable research. Ethical commercialization requires mechanisms that recognize the individual's role in data creation and ensure fair benefit-sharing practices that respect their autonomy and dignity.
- **Some Propose Data Dividend Models or Cooperative Ownership Frameworks:** In response to these challenges, innovative solutions such as data dividend models and cooperative ownership frameworks have been proposed to create more equitable systems. A data dividend model envisions individuals receiving direct financial compensation or other benefits when their health data is monetized by companies. This approach treats data contributors akin to shareholders, rewarding them for the value they help generate. Cooperative ownership frameworks take this concept further by organizing data contributors into collectives or cooperatives that collectively negotiate terms of data use, control access, and share profits. These models aim to empower individuals, giving them greater agency and a tangible stake in the data economy. Implementing such frameworks requires new legal, technological, and governance structures, as well as public awareness and support. While still largely conceptual, these approaches represent a shift toward more ethical and inclusive data practices—balancing innovation with respect for individual rights and social justice.

9.2.10 Data Trusts and Governance Models

- **Emerging Frameworks Like Data Trusts Aim to Manage Data on Behalf of Contributors:** As concerns over health data ownership, privacy, and ethical use grow, new governance frameworks such as data trusts are emerging as promising solutions. A data trust is a legal and organizational structure designed to manage data assets on behalf of the individuals who contribute their information. Rather than data being controlled solely by corporations or institutions, data trusts act as fiduciaries, holding and stewarding data in the best interest of data subjects. This model allows individuals to entrust their data to a neutral third party that oversees data use, access, and sharing according to agreed-upon principles. Data trusts can enforce rules about who may use the data, for what purposes, and under what conditions, effectively protecting contributors' rights while facilitating responsible data sharing. By centralizing governance, data trusts simplify the complex landscape of data stewardship, providing a clear point of accountability and reducing risks of misuse.

- **These Models Prioritize Transparency, Public Benefit, and Collective Governance:** Data trusts are built on principles of transparency, accountability, and collective governance. They require openness about how data is collected, used, and shared, providing contributors with clear information and a voice in decision-making processes. Unlike traditional data custodianship models that often operate behind closed doors, data trusts encourage active participation from data contributors or their representatives, fostering democratic oversight. This collective governance structure ensures that decisions reflect the interests and values of the community rather than those of individual corporations or researchers alone. Moreover, data trusts are often designed to prioritize the public benefit, ensuring that data use advances health research, public health goals, and equitable innovation rather than solely commercial interests. By aligning data management with social good, these models seek to rebuild public trust and encourage greater participation in data-driven research.
- **Could Help Balance Innovation with Individual Rights:** One of the key advantages of data trusts and similar governance models is their potential to balance the competing demands of innovation and individual rights. On one hand, health data sharing drives breakthroughs in medicine, AI, and public health surveillance. On the other, it raises serious concerns about privacy, consent, and data misuse. Data trusts provide a structured framework where data can be responsibly shared to fuel innovation while simultaneously safeguarding contributors' autonomy and privacy. They can implement dynamic consent mechanisms, enforce stringent security protocols, and monitor data access in real time. This balanced approach mitigates risks associated with unrestricted data commercialization or exploitation, offering a pathway to ethical and sustainable data ecosystems. As such, data trusts represent a forward-thinking governance model that reconciles the promise of data-driven health innovation with the fundamental rights of individuals.

9.2.11 Equity and Access in Data Sharing

- **Underrepresented Groups May Be Excluded from Data Collection or Benefit Unequally from Its Use:** A critical concern in health data sharing is that underrepresented populations often face exclusion from data collection efforts or receive unequal benefits from research outcomes. Many datasets disproportionately represent populations from urban, affluent, or majority groups, leaving marginalized communities—such as ethnic minorities, rural residents, and economically disadvantaged individuals—underrepresented. This lack of representation can skew research findings, leading to healthcare innovations that are less effective or even harmful for these groups. For example, AI algorithms trained on biased data may perform poorly for certain populations, perpetuating health disparities. Moreover, when these groups are excluded, they miss out on the potential benefits of advances in precision medicine, diagnostics, and tailored treatments. Ensuring diverse participation in data collection is essential to create equitable health solutions that serve the needs of all populations and reduce systemic health inequities.
- **Ethical Data Sharing Requires Inclusivity and Respect for Cultural, Social, and Legal Diversity:** Ethical data sharing practices must go beyond mere inclusion by actively respecting the cultural, social, and legal diversity of communities involved. Different groups may have varying norms, beliefs, and expectations regarding the collection, use, and sharing of health data. For instance, some cultures have specific views on genetic material and biological samples, demanding particular consent processes or restrictions on use. Social contexts—such as historical mistrust in healthcare systems or previous exploitation—must also be acknowledged and addressed to foster genuine collaboration and consent. Furthermore, legal frameworks governing data privacy and ownership differ globally, requiring sensitive navigation when sharing data across jurisdictions. Ethical frameworks must incorporate these dimensions, ensuring that data sharing is culturally sensitive, legally compliant, and socially responsible. Doing so builds trust and fosters respectful partnerships between researchers and communities.
- **Special Care Needed for Indigenous, Rural, and Marginalized Communities:** Indigenous peoples, rural populations, and other marginalized groups require special attention and tailored protections in the context of health data sharing. Historically, these communities have often been exploited or overlooked in biomedical research, leading to mistrust and reluctance to participate. Effective engagement with these groups necessitates community-led decision-making, where representatives have

a meaningful role in governing data use and benefit-sharing. Indigenous data sovereignty, which asserts the right of Indigenous peoples to govern their own data, is a growing movement emphasizing autonomy and respect. Similarly, rural and marginalized communities may face technological barriers to participation or lack access to the infrastructure needed for data collection and consent processes. Addressing these challenges requires targeted outreach, capacity-building, and the development of culturally appropriate consent models. By prioritizing equity and justice, health data sharing can become a tool for empowerment rather than exclusion.

9.2.12 Future Considerations

- **Ongoing Debate Over Whether Data Should Be Treated as Personal Property, a Public Good, or a Human Right:** The future of health data governance is shaped by an ongoing and complex debate about the fundamental nature of data. One perspective treats health data as personal property, emphasizing individual ownership, control, and the right to monetize or restrict access. This view aligns with privacy and autonomy principles, granting individuals authority over their sensitive information. Conversely, some argue that health data should be considered a public good—a shared resource that, when pooled and analysed collectively, benefits society by accelerating medical research, improving public health, and fostering innovation. Under this framework, data sharing is seen as a collective responsibility, prioritizing accessibility over exclusive control. A third perspective frames health data access as a human right, emphasizing equitable participation and benefit, especially for vulnerable or marginalized groups. Each viewpoint carries different ethical, legal, and practical implications, influencing policy development, consent models, and governance structures. As technology and societal values evolve, balancing these perspectives will be crucial to creating fair, effective, and sustainable data ecosystems.
- **Technologies Like Blockchain and Federated Learning May Offer Secure, Decentralized Data Sharing Models:** Emerging technologies hold promise for addressing many challenges in health data sharing by enabling secure, transparent, and decentralized control over sensitive information. Blockchain technology, for instance, creates immutable, tamper-proof records of data transactions, ensuring transparency and accountability in how data is accessed and used. It also facilitates decentralized control, allowing individuals to manage permissions directly without relying on a central authority. Meanwhile, federated learning allows AI models to be trained on data that remains locally stored on users' devices or

institutional servers, without raw data ever leaving its source. This approach significantly reduces privacy risks, as data does not need to be pooled centrally. Together, these technologies can empower individuals and organizations to participate in data sharing with greater confidence, improving security while maintaining usability. However, challenges such as scalability, interoperability, and regulatory acceptance remain to be addressed before widespread adoption.

- **Legal and Ethical Frameworks Must Evolve to Support Responsible Innovation While Protecting Rights and Equity:** As data sharing technologies and practices advance, legal and ethical frameworks must adapt to keep pace, ensuring that innovation does not come at the expense of individual rights, privacy, or social justice. Current laws often lag behind technological capabilities and may not adequately address emerging concerns like cross-border data flows, secondary data use, or algorithmic bias. Future regulations should incorporate principles of transparency, accountability, inclusivity, and fairness, providing clear guidelines on consent, data ownership, and benefit-sharing. Ethical frameworks must also address potential disparities, ensuring that vulnerable populations are not disproportionately exposed to risks or excluded from benefits. Policymakers, technologists, ethicists, and affected communities need to collaborate continuously to create flexible, forward-looking governance structures. This evolution will be key to fostering public trust, encouraging responsible data sharing, and unlocking the full potential of health data for societal good.

9.3 DISCRIMINATION, STIGMATIZATION, AND EQUITY CONCERNS

9.3.1 Introduction

Predictive health technologies have rapidly advanced over the past decade, promising to revolutionize medicine by enabling earlier diagnosis, personalized treatment, and improved health outcomes. These technologies leverage vast amounts of data—from genetic information to electronic health records and social determinants of health—to forecast individual risks and guide clinical decision-making. While the potential benefits are substantial, there is a growing awareness that such tools can also unintentionally perpetuate or even exacerbate existing social inequalities and injustices. Predictive models, algorithms, and data-driven insights may reflect the biases embedded in their training data or the assumptions of their developers, resulting in unfair treatment of certain groups. For example, racial and ethnic minorities, people with disabilities, or those from lower socioeconomic backgrounds might receive inaccurate risk assessments, leading to disparities in care access, quality, and outcomes. Beyond inaccurate predictions, the very use of predictive health technologies can contribute to stigmatization—where individuals or communities are labelled or marginalized based on perceived health risks or genetic traits—further isolating vulnerable populations and undermining trust in healthcare systems. These ethical challenges require careful consideration because discrimination and stigma in healthcare not only harm individuals but also perpetuate systemic inequities that undermine public health goals. For instance, if an algorithm systematically underestimates the health risks of certain populations, those individuals may be denied necessary preventive interventions or treatments. Conversely, overestimating risks can lead to unnecessary anxiety, overtreatment, or insurance discrimination. Moreover, inequities in data collection—where some groups are underrepresented or excluded—can limit the validity of predictive models, rendering them less accurate or useful for marginalized communities. The risk of widening health disparities is especially concerning in light of social determinants of health, which are deeply intertwined with race, class, geography, and other factors. Ethical use of predictive health technologies must therefore encompass more than technical accuracy or efficiency; it must proactively address how data, models, and outcomes affect diverse populations with fairness and respect. This includes engaging affected communities in the development and evaluation of these tools, ensuring transparency about their limitations, and implementing safeguards to mitigate bias. It also involves recognizing that technology alone cannot resolve deep-rooted social inequities; instead, it must be part of broader efforts to promote justice and equity in healthcare. Ultimately, responsible deployment of predictive health technologies requires a commitment to equitable benefit-sharing, non-discrimination, and respect for human dignity, ensuring that innovations serve to reduce rather than deepen existing health disparities.

9.3.2 Genetic Discrimination

Genetic discrimination refers to the unfair treatment of individuals based on their genetic information, particularly when it reveals predispositions or risks for certain diseases or conditions. Advances in genetic testing have made it easier than ever to identify an individual's likelihood of developing illnesses such as cancer, Alzheimer's, or rare hereditary disorders long before symptoms appear. While this knowledge can empower people to take proactive health measures, it also creates significant risks of misuse. Employers, insurers, or governments may exploit genetic data to make decisions that adversely affect individuals, such as denying health insurance coverage, increasing premiums, refusing employment, or restricting access to social benefits. For example, an insurer might classify someone as a high-risk client and charge exorbitant rates or exclude coverage entirely. Employers could hesitate to hire or promote someone perceived as genetically predisposed to chronic illness or disability, fearing increased healthcare costs or absenteeism.

Similarly, governments might use genetic information for discriminatory practices or surveillance, especially in countries with weaker privacy laws or authoritarian regimes. These risks are not hypothetical; cases of genetic discrimination have been documented globally, prompting widespread concern among patients, advocacy groups, and policymakers. In response, some countries have enacted legislation to protect individuals from genetic discrimination. The United States' Genetic Information Non-discrimination Act (GINA), passed in 2008, is one of the most comprehensive laws in this area. GINA prohibits health insurers and employers from using genetic information to make coverage, pricing, or employment decisions. However, GINA's protections are limited to health insurance and employment and do not extend to life insurance, disability insurance, or long-term care insurance, leaving gaps that can be exploited. Moreover, many other countries lack equivalent laws, or their protections are unevenly enforced, leaving individuals vulnerable to discrimination. This inconsistency creates a patchwork of protections worldwide, where the risks associated with genetic discrimination vary depending on geographic and legal context.

Beyond legislation, challenges remain in implementing effective safeguards. Genetic data is often stored and shared across multiple platforms, increasing the risk of unauthorized access or breaches. Even with laws in place, individuals may hesitate to undergo genetic testing due to fear of discrimination, which can limit the benefits of personalized medicine. Addressing genetic discrimination thus requires not only robust legal frameworks but also public education, secure data management practices, and ethical guidelines that prioritize privacy and non-discrimination. Moreover, global cooperation is essential to harmonize protections, especially as genetic data increasingly crosses borders through international research collaborations and commercial testing services. Ultimately, protecting individuals from genetic discrimination is vital to ensuring that advances in genomics contribute to health equity rather than deepen existing inequalities or create new forms of social injustice.

9.3.3 Social Stigmatization

Predictive health technologies and genetic testing, while valuable for anticipating disease risks and guiding preventive care, carry the unintended consequence of social stigmatization. When individuals are labelled as "high-risk" based on their genetic profile or predictive health information, they may experience significant psychological stress, anxiety, and social exclusion. Being identified as vulnerable to certain conditions can lead to internalized fear and worry, impacting mental health and quality of life even before any symptoms manifest. This labelling can create a persistent sense of vulnerability, influencing how individuals perceive themselves and how others perceive and interact with them. For instance, someone flagged as having a genetic predisposition to a chronic illness might feel isolated or treated differently by friends, colleagues, or healthcare providers, who may inadvertently discriminate or distance themselves. Such stigma can discourage individuals from seeking testing or disclosing their health information, which undermines public health efforts and personalized medicine. Certain conditions carry particularly heavy stigma, exacerbating social exclusion and unfair treatment. Genetic predispositions linked to mental illnesses, obesity, addiction, or neurological disorders often provoke judgment and misunderstanding. These conditions are frequently surrounded by stereotypes and moral biases, with affected individuals blamed for their condition or seen as less capable or responsible. This can lead to discrimination in social settings, employment, and healthcare access, perpetuating cycles of marginalization. Moreover, stigma may not only affect the individual but also extend to their family members, who might be unfairly labelled or socially isolated based on association. Families may experience shame or secrecy, hindering open discussion and support, which are crucial for managing health challenges.

The impact of social stigmatization varies significantly across cultural and social contexts. In many cultures, illness is not only a medical issue but also carries moral, spiritual, or communal meanings. Diseases or traits perceived as curses, punishment, or moral failings can deeply affect family honour and social standing. In such societies, predictive health information revealing a genetic risk can result in ostracism, strained family relationships, or barriers to marriage and social participation. These dynamics create additional layers of complexity in addressing stigma, requiring culturally sensitive approaches that respect traditions while promoting health equity. Effective strategies to mitigate stigmatization include education campaigns to combat myths and misconceptions, fostering inclusive healthcare environments, and empowering affected individuals through support groups and counselling. By addressing social stigmatization proactively, healthcare systems can help ensure that the promise of predictive health technologies benefits all, without causing harm or deepening social divides.

9.3.4 Algorithmic Bias and Inequity

Artificial intelligence (AI) and machine learning are increasingly integrated into predictive health technologies, offering the potential to enhance diagnosis, personalize treatment, and improve risk prediction. However, a significant ethical challenge arises from algorithmic bias, which occurs when AI systems are trained on datasets that are incomplete, non-diverse, or reflect existing social prejudices. When the data used to develop these tools predominantly represent certain populations—such as urban, middle-class, or majority ethnic groups—the resulting algorithms may fail to accurately capture the health realities of marginalized communities. This leads to predictive models that produce skewed or unreliable outputs for racial minorities, rural populations, low-income groups, and other underserved segments. Consequently, these groups may receive diagnoses that are delayed or incorrect, treatments that are less effective, or risk predictions that either underestimate or exaggerate their health threats. The perpetuation of such biases not only undermines the fairness of healthcare delivery but also risks deepening longstanding health disparities. The sources of algorithmic bias are multifaceted. Biases can stem from the lack of representative data, the way data is labelled or categorized, and the assumptions embedded in algorithm design. For instance, a diagnostic tool trained primarily on images from lighter-skinned individuals may perform poorly on darker skin tones, leading to missed or erroneous diagnoses. Similarly, socioeconomic factors that affect health outcomes—such as environmental exposures, access to care, and nutrition—may be underrepresented in clinical datasets, limiting the ability of AI systems to provide equitable risk assessments. Moreover, when biased algorithms inform clinical decisions, they can inadvertently reinforce systemic inequities, disproportionately disadvantaging those already facing barriers to quality care. This raises profound concerns about justice and fairness in healthcare, highlighting the need for rigorous validation of AI tools across diverse populations before widespread implementation.

To prevent the exacerbation of disparities, it is crucial that AI developers and healthcare providers adopt proactive measures to identify, measure, and mitigate algorithmic bias. This includes collecting and incorporating diverse, high-quality data that reflect the heterogeneity of patient populations; transparently reporting model performance across demographic groups; and engaging with communities historically excluded from biomedical research. Regulatory frameworks and ethical guidelines must emphasize fairness and inclusivity as core principles, requiring ongoing monitoring and accountability. Furthermore, interdisciplinary collaboration involving data scientists, clinicians, ethicists, and patient advocates is essential to design AI systems that promote equity rather than inequality. By addressing algorithmic bias head-on, the healthcare industry can harness the transformative potential of AI while ensuring that innovations benefit all individuals, regardless of their background or circumstances.

9.3.5 Health Equity and Access Gaps

Predictive and personalized healthcare technologies hold great promise for improving patient outcomes by tailoring prevention and treatment strategies to individual genetic, environmental, and lifestyle factors. However, these advancements are often expensive and heavily dependent on sophisticated technology, which creates significant barriers for disadvantaged populations. Individuals living in low-income communities, rural areas, or developing regions may face limited or no access to the digital tools, specialized genetic testing services, and high-quality healthcare infrastructure required to benefit from these innovations. This lack of access contributes to a growing digital divide—a disparity in health outcomes linked to unequal availability and use of technology. For example, while affluent patients might receive early genetic screening and precision therapies, underserved populations often rely on standard, less personalized care, which may be less effective and contribute to ongoing health disparities. The challenges of access are multifaceted. Many underserved communities experience a shortage of healthcare providers trained in genomic medicine or predictive analytics, limiting the availability of expert care. Geographic isolation further restricts access to diagnostic facilities and advanced treatments. Economic constraints often prevent individuals from affording costly genetic tests, personalized medications, or follow-up care. Additionally, digital literacy and broadband internet access are unevenly distributed, making it difficult for some populations to engage with telemedicine platforms, mobile health applications, or online patient portals integral to modern healthcare delivery. Without deliberate interventions, these disparities risk becoming entrenched, undermining the goals of predictive health technologies to improve outcomes universally.

Achieving health equity in the era of precision medicine requires a proactive and systemic approach to inclusion. This means prioritizing the recruitment of diverse populations in genetic research and clinical trials to ensure that findings and innovations are broadly applicable. It also involves designing accessible, affordable testing services and care models that accommodate the needs and contexts of underserved communities. Public and private stakeholders must invest in expanding healthcare infrastructure, improving digital connectivity, and enhancing health literacy. Community engagement is essential to build trust, address cultural concerns, and co-create solutions that resonate with specific populations. Equitable access also demands policy initiatives that reduce financial barriers, such as insurance coverage for genetic testing and personalized therapies, and regulatory frameworks that promote fairness. Only through comprehensive and intentional efforts can predictive and personalized healthcare realize its potential as a tool for reducing, rather than exacerbating, health disparities.

9.3.6 Disparities in Genomic Research

One of the most pressing challenges in the ethical and equitable use of genomic data is the significant disparity in the representation of diverse populations within genomic research. Currently, the vast majority of genomic databases and biobanks are heavily skewed toward individuals of European descent. This imbalance stems from historical, social, and economic factors, including the concentration of research efforts and funding in Western countries and the underrepresentation or exclusion of minority and indigenous groups in scientific studies. As a result, predictive genetic models, risk assessments, and personalized treatments developed from these datasets tend to perform well for populations of European ancestry but may be less accurate or even misleading when applied to individuals from other ethnic backgrounds. This lack of diversity restricts the clinical utility and fairness of genomic medicine, perpetuating disparities in diagnosis, treatment, and health outcomes. The consequences of such underrepresentation are profound. When genomic variants specific to non-European populations are absent or under-characterized in databases, individuals from these groups face a higher risk of misdiagnosis or misclassification. For example, genetic variants that are benign in one population might be mistakenly identified as pathogenic in another, leading to unnecessary anxiety, inappropriate interventions, or missed opportunities for targeted care. Conversely, disease-associated variants that are common in underrepresented populations might be overlooked, preventing timely diagnosis or preventive measures. This gap not only undermines the scientific validity of genomic tools but also raises serious ethical concerns about justice and equity in healthcare. If genomic medicine primarily benefits a subset of the global population, it risks widening existing health disparities rather than bridging them. Addressing these disparities requires a concerted global effort to increase the inclusion of diverse populations in genomic research. This involves outreach and engagement strategies that build trust and collaboration with communities historically marginalized or wary of biomedical research due to past abuses and exploitation. It also necessitates funding initiatives and research policies that prioritize diversity and equity, encouraging the development of databases that capture the full spectrum of human genetic variation. Technological innovations, such as portable sequencing devices and decentralized data collection methods, can facilitate participation from remote or resource-limited settings. Additionally, ethical frameworks must emphasize respect for cultural values, community consent, and benefit-sharing, ensuring that genomic research does not merely extract data but contributes positively to participating populations. Ultimately, a more inclusive genomic research landscape is essential for creating predictive models and healthcare interventions that are effective, trustworthy, and just for all individuals, regardless of their ancestry or background.

9.3.7 Cultural Sensitivity and Respect

In the realm of genetics and predictive health, cultural sensitivity and respect are paramount to ensuring ethical and effective research and healthcare delivery. Different communities around the world hold diverse beliefs, values, and understandings about genetics, disease causation, and privacy, shaped by their unique cultural, spiritual, and historical contexts. For some groups, genetic conditions may carry significant moral or spiritual meanings, influencing how individuals and families perceive illness and health interventions. Others may have deep-rooted concerns about the collection and use of genetic information, often stemming from historical experiences of exploitation, discrimination, or unethical research practices. These perspectives affect willingness to participate in genetic testing, share health data, or engage with predictive health technologies. Without thoughtful adaptation, standard research and healthcare approaches risk alienating these communities, undermining trust and limiting the benefits of scientific advances.

Respecting cultural diversity requires more than superficial acknowledgment; it demands tailoring research protocols and clinical practices to align with the values, language, and lived experiences of different populations. This includes providing educational materials in local languages and dialects, using culturally appropriate metaphors and communication styles, and ensuring that consent processes are meaningful and understandable. Researchers and healthcare providers must be trained in cultural competence, developing skills to recognize and navigate cultural differences with empathy and humility. Importantly, community engagement should not be a one-way extraction of data but a genuine partnership that empowers communities to express their concerns, priorities, and preferences. Such engagement fosters mutual respect and facilitates the co-creation of research questions, ethical guidelines, and healthcare interventions that are culturally congruent.

Historical traumas and systemic discrimination have left many marginalized groups wary of biomedical research and health institutions. This legacy necessitates a heightened sensitivity and proactive efforts to rebuild trust. Transparent communication about data use, protections, and potential benefits is essential, alongside assurances that genetic information will not be used to further stigmatize or disadvantage communities. In some cases, community advisory boards or participatory governance models can provide oversight and guidance, ensuring accountability and respect for cultural norms. By integrating cultural sensitivity into every stage of genomic research and healthcare delivery, stakeholders can promote inclusivity, reduce health disparities, and enhance the relevance and acceptability of predictive health technologies. Ultimately, honouring cultural diversity strengthens the ethical foundation of precision medicine and contributes to a more just and equitable healthcare system.

9.3.8 Structural and Institutional Discrimination

Predictive health technologies, despite their promise to revolutionize medicine, risk perpetuating structural and institutional discrimination if implemented without addressing the deep-rooted inequalities embedded within healthcare systems and society at large. These tools do not exist in a vacuum; they operate within environments shaped by historical patterns of unequal healthcare funding, policy biases, and discriminatory practices that have long marginalized certain populations. For instance, communities with limited healthcare infrastructure, lower socioeconomic status, or minority racial and ethnic backgrounds often receive fewer resources and less quality care. Predictive algorithms and personalized treatments developed within such contexts may inadvertently reflect and reinforce these disparities. Rather than serving as equalizers, they can exacerbate existing inequities by favouring those already privileged with better access and support. This phenomenon underscores that technology alone cannot solve systemic health disparities; without fundamental reform, it risks entrenching them further. Structural discrimination manifests in several ways in the use of predictive tools. For example, healthcare providers serving underfunded or rural clinics may lack the resources or training to utilize advanced genomic testing or AI-driven risk assessments, leaving their patients behind. Policies governing access to personalized medicine often reflect economic or political interests that prioritize certain groups, creating barriers for others. Moreover, allocation of healthcare resources—such as insurance coverage for expensive genomic tests or targeted therapies—may be biased toward wealthier, urban populations, reinforcing cycles of disadvantage. If predictive tools are developed and deployed within these inequitable frameworks, they risk amplifying disparities in outcomes such as diagnosis accuracy, treatment effectiveness, and preventive care access. This creates a feedback loop where marginalized groups continue to suffer disproportionately despite technological advances.

Addressing structural and institutional discrimination requires ethical governance frameworks that go beyond surface-level fixes like removing bias from algorithms or ensuring diverse datasets. While these technical improvements are necessary, they are insufficient if the broader social determinants of health and systemic injustices remain unchallenged. Ethical governance must engage with the root causes of inequity—such as poverty, racism, and unequal political power—through policy reforms, resource redistribution, and inclusive decision-making processes. This includes investing in healthcare infrastructure in underserved areas, reforming insurance and reimbursement systems to ensure equitable coverage, and promoting workforce diversity and cultural competence in medicine. It also demands accountability mechanisms that monitor and address how predictive technologies impact different communities over time. Only by integrating technological innovation with structural change can we hope to harness the full potential of predictive health tools to advance health equity rather than deepen social divides.

9.3.9 Psychological Impact of Risk Labelling

The psychological impact of being labelled "high-risk" based on genetic or predictive health information is profound and often underestimated. While such labelling can be medically useful—guiding early interventions and lifestyle adjustments—it also carries emotional and social consequences that can negatively affect an individual's mental well-being, self-concept, and quality of life. For many, learning that they have a predisposition to a serious illness (such as cancer, Alzheimer's, or a mental health disorder) may trigger intense stress, anxiety, or fear about the future. This psychological burden can persist even if the actual likelihood of developing the condition is low. The label may become internalized, leading individuals to view themselves as fragile, "damaged," or perpetually ill, which can diminish their confidence and disrupt daily life. In some cases, people may become hypervigilant about their health or make drastic, unnecessary lifestyle changes out of fear. Others may adopt a sense of fatalism, believing they are destined to become ill and therefore less motivated to pursue proactive or preventive care.

The impact can be even more concerning when risk labelling occurs early in life, such as in children or adolescents. Young people who are told—or whose parents are informed—that they are genetically predisposed to certain conditions may grow up with altered perceptions of what is possible or safe for them. This may influence their educational paths, career aspirations, or participation in social and recreational activities, as families and institutions may become overly cautious or limiting. For instance, a child with a genetic risk for heart disease may be discouraged from engaging in sports, even if they are currently healthy. Additionally, early labelling can affect peer relationships, potentially leading to social exclusion, bullying, or a sense of otherness. The psychological implications are especially critical during formative years when identity, autonomy, and self-esteem are developing.

To mitigate these harms, comprehensive psychological counselling and support must accompany the process of risk disclosure. Genetic counsellors, psychologists, and other trained professionals should be involved in delivering and contextualizing predictive information, ensuring individuals and families understand the nature and limitations of risk. Counselling should be tailored to age, cultural background, and emotional readiness, and it must focus not only on conveying facts but also on supporting healthy coping strategies, decision-making, and emotional resilience. Educational materials should frame risk in a balanced way—emphasizing empowerment, not fear—and include options for preventive care and lifestyle adjustments rather than focusing solely on potential disease. Moreover, policies should guide ethical communication of predictive information in clinical, educational, and research settings, especially where minors are involved. Ultimately, predictive health technologies should be implemented with sensitivity, ensuring that information meant to help does not unintentionally harm the psychological well-being or future potential of those it seeks to serve.

9.3.10 Safeguarding Against Misuse

As predictive health technologies become more integrated into clinical practice, insurance systems, employment screening, and public health surveillance, safeguarding against their misuse is critical to protecting individual rights and promoting equity. Without robust safeguards, these tools could be exploited to deny essential services, increase surveillance, or enable discriminatory practices—intentionally or unintentionally. For example, health insurers might use predictive data to adjust premiums unfairly, or employers could screen out candidates deemed "high-risk" based on genetic or health profiles. In more extreme scenarios, governments could use predictive analytics to justify exclusionary policies, enforce social stratification, or justify unequal resource distribution. These risks underscore the need for strong regulatory frameworks that anticipate misuse and actively enforce protections against it. To address these concerns, regulatory bodies must play a proactive role in overseeing the development, deployment, and use of predictive tools. This includes ensuring that these technologies are not used as a basis for denying healthcare, education, insurance, employment, or other vital services. Laws must clearly delineate how predictive data can be collected, stored, shared, and applied, with strict penalties for misuse. Importantly, regulations must also keep pace with rapid technological advancements, avoiding outdated legal gaps that allow unethical exploitation. In addition to formal legal mechanisms, transparent and independent auditing of algorithms and decision-making systems is essential. These audits should evaluate whether predictive models operate fairly across different demographic groups, whether their decision logic is explainable, and whether unintended biases or discriminatory outcomes are present.

Crucially, the governance of predictive health technologies should be inclusive and interdisciplinary, involving a broad range of stakeholders to ensure well-rounded oversight. This includes not only data scientists and healthcare providers but also ethicists, legal experts, patient advocacy groups, and representatives from affected communities. Diverse perspectives help identify potential harms early, shape ethical guidelines, and ensure that technologies align with societal values such as autonomy, justice, and non-discrimination. Community involvement also builds trust and transparency, especially among historically marginalized groups who may be justifiably wary of technological overreach. Ultimately, safeguarding against misuse requires a multi-layered approach: strong and adaptive legal protections, rigorous technical oversight, and a commitment to participatory ethics. Only through such comprehensive and collaborative governance can society ensure that predictive health tools fulfil their promise to improve care and public health without becoming instruments of control, inequality, or harm.

9.3.11 Promoting Equity Through Design

The design and implementation of predictive health technologies must move beyond a one-size-fits-all model and instead be intentionally inclusive from the outset. Equity cannot be an afterthought or a feature added post-development—it must be embedded into the core of technological design. This involves recognizing that populations are diverse in terms of genetics, health needs, cultural values, socioeconomic status, geographic location, and access to care. When predictive tools are created primarily with data from affluent, urban, or majority populations, they often fail to serve—and may even harm—marginalized or underrepresented groups. To avoid perpetuating these disparities, developers must adopt a "design for equity" approach, which centres the needs, voices, and lived experiences of diverse populations throughout the entire life cycle of a technology—from data collection and model development to testing, deployment, and feedback loops. Equity-focused design begins with inclusive data collection. This means actively recruiting and incorporating data from populations that have historically been excluded or underrepresented in biomedical research, including racial and ethnic minorities, indigenous communities, rural populations, and individuals from low-income backgrounds. But equity also requires going beyond demographics. It involves understanding the social determinants of health, such as housing, education, and environmental exposures, and integrating these into predictive models to provide more holistic and meaningful insights. Equitable technologies should also be accessible in multiple languages, operable across different levels of digital literacy, and usable in resource-constrained environments—ensuring that no group is excluded from the benefits of innovation. To guide these efforts, equity-focused frameworks and principles should be adopted by designers, engineers, clinicians, and policymakers. These frameworks can include tools such as Health Equity Impact Assessments (HEIAs), community-based participatory research (CBPR) models, and ethical design checklists that prioritize transparency, accountability, fairness, and inclusivity. Evaluating the performance of predictive technologies across different subgroups is also critical, as it reveals hidden biases and provides opportunities for course correction. Furthermore, co-design processes involving end-users—particularly those from underserved communities—can ensure technologies are both effective and culturally relevant. Their input helps identify unintended harms and enhances trust in the technology. Ultimately, promoting equity through design is not only an ethical imperative but a practical one. Inclusive tools are more generalizable, more accurate across populations, and more likely to be adopted and sustained. As predictive health becomes increasingly central to modern medicine, embedding equity into its design and governance is essential for ensuring that the benefits of innovation are shared fairly—and that technology becomes a bridge to better health for all, not a barrier.

9.3.12 Concise Summary

Discrimination and stigma are not incidental outcomes of predictive health technologies—they are central risks that must be anticipated and addressed from the outset. As these tools become more widespread, they carry the potential to reinforce existing social and institutional inequities unless they are carefully designed, regulated, and monitored. Populations already facing systemic barriers—such as racial minorities, low-income groups, and indigenous communities—may experience further marginalization through biased algorithms, lack of access, or misapplication of genetic risk labelling. The psychological toll of being labelled "high-risk," along with the misuse of data in employment, insurance, or policy decisions, illustrates the urgent need for ethical oversight. Ensuring fairness, inclusion, and cultural sensitivity is essential not only to protect vulnerable populations but also to ensure the effectiveness and acceptance of these technologies. This requires involving diverse stakeholders, building equity-focused frameworks, and embedding cultural respect and transparency into every phase of development and deployment. A proactive, equity-cantered approach—rather than reactive fixes—can ensure that the benefits of technological progress are shared broadly and justly. Only through intentional design and ethical governance can predictive health tools truly serve as instruments for healing and progress, rather than perpetuating harm.

9.4 CULTURAL SENSITIVITY IN GENOMIC MEDICINE

9.4.1 Introduction

Genomic medicine represents a groundbreaking advancement in healthcare, offering the potential to tailor prevention, diagnosis, and treatment strategies to the unique genetic makeup of individuals. By analysing a person's genome, clinicians can predict disease risk, select more effective medications, and avoid adverse drug reactions. However, while the scientific and clinical possibilities are vast, the true success of genomic medicine hinges not only on its technical accuracy but also on its cultural acceptability and ethical integration across diverse populations. Genetics is deeply personal and often intersects with complex belief systems, social norms, and historical experiences—many of which vary significantly between communities, ethnic groups, and regions. In many cultures, beliefs about heredity, illness, and destiny are rooted in long-standing traditions, spiritual views, or religious teachings. For example, some communities may interpret genetic disorders as spiritual imbalances, ancestral consequences, or divine will—leading to hesitation or resistance toward genetic testing or interventions. Others may have concerns about privacy, family honour, or social stigma associated with inheritable conditions. Historical abuses in medical research—such as unethical sterilization programs, eugenics movements, or the exploitation of indigenous DNA—have also left legacies of mistrust that continue to influence how communities engage with genomic science. These perspectives are not barriers to be overcome but contextual realities that must be understood and respected. Therefore, cultural sensitivity is essential to ensuring that genomic medicine is not only scientifically effective but also ethically sound and socially inclusive. This involves tailoring communication strategies, consent processes, and care models to align with the cultural beliefs and preferences of different populations. It also requires building long-term trust, engaging community leaders, and co-designing solutions that reflect shared values. Without such sensitivity, there is a risk of miscommunication, non-participation, or even harm—particularly to marginalized or historically excluded groups. Conversely, culturally respectful genomic medicine fosters empowerment, autonomy, and health equity, ensuring that all individuals and communities can benefit from the transformative power of genetics. As genomic medicine continues to evolve globally, its integration must be guided by a deep commitment to respect for diversity, justice, and cultural competence.

9.4.2 Diverse Beliefs About Health and Genetics

Understanding how different cultures interpret health, illness, and genetics is essential for the ethical and effective delivery of genomic medicine. Across the globe, belief systems surrounding health and heredity vary widely, shaped by history, spirituality, religion, and traditional practices. While Western medicine tends to view genetic conditions through a biomedical lens—emphasizing DNA, inheritance patterns, and molecular causes—many communities interpret these phenomena in deeply personal, symbolic, or spiritual ways. In some cultures, illness may be seen as the result of ancestral disapproval, moral failings, imbalances in spiritual energy, or even as a test of faith. Genetic disorders may not be considered "medical" in nature at all, but rather as signs of fate, karma, or divine will. This divergence in worldview can significantly affect how individuals and families perceive genetic testing, diagnosis, and treatment. For example, in some communities, discovering a genetic predisposition to disease may bring shame to a family or negatively impact a person's marriage prospects or social standing. Others may reject genetic explanations altogether in favour of traditional healing systems or religious interpretations. This can result in hesitation or outright refusal to participate in genomic testing, counselling, or therapies, not out of ignorance, but because the interventions conflict with deeply held cultural values. Additionally, conversations about genetics and reproductive risk can be especially sensitive in cultures where discussions around illness, inheritance, or disability are taboo. Healthcare professionals and researchers must therefore approach these situations with cultural humility, empathy, and open-mindedness. Instead of dismissing non-biomedical beliefs, they should seek to understand them and engage in dialogue that respects cultural perspectives while sharing scientific information in accessible, non-threatening ways. This may involve adapting language, framing genetic risk in culturally resonant terms, and collaborating with community leaders, traditional healers, or religious figures to build trust and foster mutual understanding. The goal is not to impose one worldview over another, but to find respectful, informed pathways for shared decision-making, where patients feel heard and empowered to make choices aligned with both their health needs and cultural values. Ultimately, recognizing and respecting diverse beliefs about health and genetics is not a barrier to progress—it is a prerequisite for equitable care. Genomic medicine will only achieve its full potential when it is delivered in ways that honour the identities, beliefs, and dignity of all individuals, regardless of cultural background.

9.4.3 Historical Mistrust and Ethical Legacies

The history of genetic research and biomedical science is deeply entangled with episodes of exploitation, coercion, and unethical practices, particularly involving Indigenous peoples, African-descended populations, and other marginalized communities. This legacy has contributed to a widespread and justified mistrust of genomic medicine in many parts of the world. Historical examples such as the case of Henrietta Lacks, whose cells were taken and commercialized without her consent, or the Havasupai Tribe, whose DNA samples were used in studies far beyond what was agreed upon, serve as stark reminders of how communities have been treated as subjects rather than partners in research. These and other instances of medical colonialism, data misappropriation, and consent violations have left generational scars that continue to shape attitudes toward genetic science today. For many communities, this is not just a matter of past wrongdoing—it is an ongoing concern. Stories of non-consensual sample collection, lack of benefit-sharing, and exclusion from the advantages of medical advancements still emerge, reinforcing fears that participation in genetic research may result in harm, misuse, or exploitation. As a result, individuals from historically marginalized backgrounds may be hesitant to engage with genomic testing, participate in studies, or share genetic data. This reluctance, while often mischaracterized as resistance to science, is better understood as a protective response to historical injustice and structural inequity. To build trust and ensure ethical engagement, the genomics community must go beyond technical fixes and actively address these ethical legacies. This starts with acknowledgment—recognizing the harm done and being transparent about how past mistakes continue to influence present relationships. It also involves reparative practices, such as returning biological samples, compensating communities, sharing benefits from research outcomes, and involving community representatives in ethical oversight. Transparency in data use, clear and culturally relevant consent processes, and sustained two-way communication are critical to re-establishing trust. Moreover, long-term community partnerships, rather than transactional or one-off engagements, are essential. These should prioritize co-creation of research goals, data governance frameworks, and dissemination strategies that reflect the values and needs of the communities involved. Ethical genomic research must be rooted in respect, reciprocity, and justice—principles that demand more than compliance with regulations. They require a transformation in how the scientific community views its relationship with people, particularly those whose histories have been marked by marginalization. Only by confronting the past honestly and building truly inclusive, participatory models can genomic medicine begin to repair trust and move toward an ethically grounded future.

9.4.4 Communication and Language Barriers

Effective communication is fundamental to the ethical and successful practice of genomic medicine. However, explaining complex genetic concepts—such as inheritance patterns, mutation risks, or probabilistic outcomes—can be incredibly challenging, especially when healthcare providers and patients do not share the same language, cultural references, or levels of health literacy. Terms like "genetic predisposition," "carrier status," or "polygenic risk scores" are difficult even for well-educated individuals to fully understand. When these ideas are translated into other languages or communicated to individuals with limited formal education, the risk of misunderstanding increases significantly. Miscommunication can lead to confusion, fear, mistrust, or inappropriate healthcare decisions, undermining both the clinical value and ethical foundation of genomic interventions. Language is not merely a technical tool for translation—it is also a vessel for cultural meaning and interpretation. Certain concepts used in Western genomics may not have direct equivalents in other languages or may carry different connotations. For example, the idea of "risk" may be perceived as fate or destiny in some cultures, while words like "mutation" may carry negative moral or social implications. Thus, literal translation is not sufficient; communication strategies must be culturally adapted to ensure that the intended meaning is conveyed respectfully and clearly. Furthermore, consent processes that rely on jargon-heavy documents or fast-paced clinical explanations risk alienating patients, especially those from linguistically or culturally diverse backgrounds.

To overcome these challenges, healthcare systems and research teams must invest in culturally and linguistically appropriate communication tools and strategies. This includes the use of professional interpreters trained in medical and genetic terminology, visual aids that simplify complex ideas through culturally relevant imagery, and multilingual resources that explain genomic concepts in accessible language. Additionally, community health workers, educators, or cultural brokers can play a pivotal role in bridging communication gaps. These individuals, often trusted members of the community, can facilitate understanding, answer questions in familiar terms, and help contextualize genomic information within local belief systems and values. Moreover, communication should not be one-directional or overly clinical. Interactive, dialogue-based approaches—where patients are encouraged to ask questions, express concerns, and share their cultural perspectives—can lead to more informed, respectful, and effective care. Institutions must also continuously assess whether their communication strategies are truly inclusive, through patient feedback, community consultations, and cultural competency evaluations. Ultimately, overcoming communication and language barriers is not just a logistical task—it is a moral responsibility that ensures all individuals, regardless of background, can make truly informed choices about their genomic health and care.

9.4.5 Informed Consent in Cultural Contexts

Informed consent is a cornerstone of ethical medical practice and research, particularly in genomic medicine where participation often involves sharing deeply personal and potentially sensitive genetic information. However, the Western model of consent—centred on individual autonomy, privacy, and self-determination—may not align with the values and decision-making norms of all cultures. In many Indigenous, African, Asian, and Pacific communities, health decisions are not made by individuals in isolation, but rather through collective processes that involve families, elders, or community leaders. This reflects a worldview in which health, identity, and responsibility are seen as shared, rather than personal, matters. In such contexts, seeking consent from a single individual without broader consultation may be perceived as inappropriate, disrespectful, or even invalid. For example, in some Indigenous cultures, providing genetic material is not merely a biological act—it may carry spiritual, ancestral, or communal significance, and thus requires discussion with tribal leaders or cultural authorities. Similarly, in many patriarchal or family-centric societies, decisions about genetic testing may rest with heads of households or involve the extended family. Failure to acknowledge these dynamics can result in community backlash, withdrawal from research participation, or long-term damage to trust. Therefore, informed consent processes must be adapted to fit the cultural context while still upholding ethical principles like transparency, voluntariness, and comprehension. This does not mean compromising on ethics, but rather broadening the ethical lens to include cultural norms around decision-making. Engaging with communities early in the planning process—before recruitment begins—can help determine the most respectful and appropriate ways to seek consent. In some cases, it may be necessary to first secure community-level or collective consent, followed by individual-level consent that is fully informed and voluntary. This layered approach honours both the individual's rights and the community's values.

Culturally sensitive consent also requires clear, non-technical communication, translated into local languages and conveyed through trusted intermediaries. It may involve multiple conversations rather than a single signature on a form. Importantly, respect for collective decision-making should never override the rights of individuals to opt out or to withdraw from participation. Ethical genomic engagement lies in finding a balance—where respect for cultural traditions enhances, rather than undermines, informed and autonomous decision-making. Ultimately, recognizing and adapting to cultural norms in consent practices is not a logistical obstacle, but a fundamental aspect of ethical inclusion in genomic medicine. By honouring diverse ways of knowing and deciding, the field can build more respectful, trustworthy, and equitable relationships with the communities it seeks to serve.

9.4.6 Perceptions of Genetic Testing

Genetic testing, while increasingly seen as a valuable tool in modern medicine, can evoke a wide range of emotional, cultural, and social responses—many of which are shaped by longstanding beliefs, taboos, and communal values. In some cultures, the idea of testing for genetic conditions is closely tied to fears of curses, bad luck, divine punishment, or ancestral displeasure. Rather than being viewed as a scientific inquiry, the act of uncovering a genetic risk may be perceived as "inviting" illness or uncovering something that is best left unknown. These beliefs can generate anxiety, reluctance, or outright rejection of testing, regardless of medical advice. Additionally, genetic results may carry social consequences that extend beyond the individual, especially in close-knit communities where family reputation and honour are paramount. A diagnosis or predisposition to a genetic condition could bring shame to the family, affect sibling relationships, or even impact marriage prospects—particularly in cultures where arranged marriages are common and health history is scrutinized. For women, in particular, a genetic finding might raise fears of being blamed for infertility, congenital conditions in offspring, or future burdens on the family. These social stigmas and gendered consequences can result in silence, denial, or refusal to share or even learn one's own genetic information.

Fear of discrimination—by employers, insurers, or the wider community—is also prevalent, especially in societies where legal protections are weak or mistrust in institutions is high. Individuals may worry that their genetic information could be used against them, either now or in the future. These fears, while sometimes based on hypothetical risks, are very real to those who have experienced past discrimination or medical exploitation. In some cases, people who undergo testing choose not to receive their results or avoid disclosing them to others, even healthcare providers, due to fear of judgment or misuse. To address these concerns, it is essential to provide clear, culturally sensitive explanations about what genetic testing is, what it can and cannot reveal, and how the information will be used and protected. Healthcare providers and counsellors must emphasize privacy protections, voluntary participation, and the individual's right to decline or withdraw. Framing genetic testing as a tool for empowerment and future planning, rather than prediction or punishment, can help reframe narratives around fear and stigma. Engaging trusted community leaders, patient advocates, and culturally competent counsellors can also be highly effective in demystifying the process and encouraging informed, autonomous decisions. Ultimately, understanding and respecting local perceptions of genetic testing is critical to making genomic medicine more acceptable, inclusive, and beneficial for all.

9.4.7 Impact on Family and Community

In many cultures around the world, health is viewed not solely as an individual concern but as a shared responsibility that extends to the family and even the wider community. This collective perspective fundamentally shapes how genetic information is perceived, disclosed, and acted upon. When a person receives a diagnosis or learns of a genetic risk factor, the implications often ripple beyond their personal health to influence the wellbeing and decision-making of family members and, in some cases, entire communities. For example, genetic findings can affect important family decisions regarding marriage prospects, childbearing, caregiving responsibilities, and inheritance, creating a complex web of social and ethical considerations that genomic services must thoughtfully navigate. In many traditional societies, family members—parents, siblings, spouses, and elders—play a central role in interpreting health information and determining subsequent actions. A genetic diagnosis in one individual might prompt relatives to seek testing themselves, alter reproductive choices, or adjust caregiving plans. Conversely, stigma or fears around genetic conditions may lead families to conceal such information to protect collective honour or prevent social exclusion. These dynamic highlights how genomic data is rarely 'private' in the Western individualistic sense, but is instead often deeply embedded within family systems and cultural contexts. Healthcare providers and genetic counsellors must be sensitive to these realities by acknowledging the social fabric within which genetic information exists. This means expanding conversations beyond the individual patient to include, with consent, appropriate family members or community representatives. It also requires awareness that the emotional and ethical burden of genetic risk can be shared collectively, with decisions sometimes made in consultation or through communal consensus. In some cases, this approach can foster stronger support networks and more informed family planning, but it also raises important questions about autonomy, confidentiality, and the potential for coercion or discrimination within families. Moreover, genomic services should recognize that the social consequences of genetic information may extend to broader community dynamics, particularly in small or tight-knit groups. For instance, in some Indigenous or tribal societies, the revelation of hereditary risks could affect communal resource allocation, leadership roles, or cultural practices. Addressing these implications requires collaboration with community leaders and culturally competent engagement to ensure that genetic services are respectful, inclusive, and beneficial at both individual and collective levels. Ultimately, the interconnectedness of individuals, families, and communities in health-related decisions underscores the need for culturally informed, context-specific approaches to genomic medicine. By considering these broader social dimensions, healthcare providers can better support patients and their families, minimize harm, and promote ethical, equitable genomic care that honours both individual rights and collective values.

9.4.8 Cultural Competence in Healthcare Providers

Cultural competence among healthcare providers is essential for delivering effective, respectful, and ethical genomic medicine, particularly in increasingly diverse societies. At its core, cultural competence involves the ability of clinicians, genetic counsellors, and other healthcare professionals to understand, appreciate, and respond appropriately to the cultural beliefs, values, and practices of their patients. This competence goes far beyond simply acquiring factual knowledge about different cultures; it requires ongoing self-reflection, awareness of personal biases, and a commitment to adapting one's approach to meet the unique needs of each patient. Healthcare providers must recognize that their own cultural perspectives inevitably shape how they interpret medical information and interact with patients. Without this awareness, unconscious biases may influence clinical judgment, communication, and decision-making, potentially leading to misunderstandings or inequitable care. For example, assumptions about a patient's education level, language skills, or health beliefs may result in oversimplified explanations, missed questions, or a failure to explore cultural factors influencing health behaviours. Therefore, training programs should encourage providers to critically examine their own attitudes and preconceptions, fostering humility and openness.

Effective cultural competence also means mastering respectful listening skills. This involves creating a safe and nonjudgmental environment where patients feel comfortable sharing their concerns, beliefs, and preferences. Providers should actively listen for cultural cues and be willing to ask sensitive questions in a tactful manner. They must acknowledge that patients may prioritize different health outcomes or interpret genetic information through a cultural lens that differs from biomedical models. Recognizing and validating these perspectives can enhance trust and patient engagement. Adapting communication styles is another key component of cultural competence. This may include using plain language, avoiding jargon, incorporating culturally relevant metaphors, and utilizing translators or cultural mediators when needed. Visual aids, storytelling, and community-based education strategies can also improve comprehension and acceptance of genomic concepts. Providers should be flexible and patient, understanding that some patients may require more time or repeated discussions to process complex information, especially when it intersects with deeply held cultural values. Importantly, cultural competence is not a one-time achievement but an ongoing process of learning and adaptation. Healthcare institutions can support this through continuous education, mentorship, and reflective practice opportunities. Policies and protocols should also be designed to promote cultural sensitivity, such as including diverse patient voices in program development and evaluation. In sum, developing cultural competence in healthcare providers is critical to bridging the gap between advanced genomic science and diverse patient communities. It ensures that genomic medicine is not only scientifically sound but also ethically grounded, culturally respectful, and accessible to all. This commitment to cultural competence ultimately improves patient outcomes, strengthens trust in healthcare systems, and contributes to more equitable health care delivery worldwide.

9.4.9 Inclusivity in Genomic Research

Inclusivity in genomic research is a critical factor in ensuring that the benefits of genomic medicine are equitably distributed across all populations. Historically, most genomic databases and studies have been overwhelmingly populated by individuals of European descent, resulting in predictive models, risk assessments, and treatment guidelines that may not be accurate or relevant for underrepresented groups such as Indigenous peoples, African, Asian, Latin American, and other minority populations. This lack of diversity in genomic data creates significant gaps in our understanding of genetic variation and disease predisposition across different ancestries, potentially leading to misdiagnosis, ineffective treatments, and health disparities. Addressing this imbalance requires intentional and culturally sensitive strategies to encourage participation from diverse communities in genomic research. Simply inviting individuals to participate without acknowledging and respecting their unique cultural contexts, histories, and concerns is unlikely to yield meaningful engagement. Many marginalized communities have valid reasons to be cautious or mistrustful of genetic research, often stemming from past exploitation, unethical practices, or concerns about misuse of genetic information. For example, Indigenous groups may worry about loss of control over their genetic heritage, while other populations may fear discrimination or stigmatization. Therefore, researchers must develop collaborative partnerships that prioritize transparency, mutual respect, and shared decision-making. Engaging community leaders, health advocates, and culturally competent intermediaries helps build trust and fosters open dialogue about the goals, risks, and benefits of genomic studies. Researchers should also be clear about data governance, privacy protections, and how research findings will be shared with communities. Consent processes should be adapted to respect cultural norms, ensuring that participation is fully informed and voluntary. Inclusivity also means addressing practical barriers such as language differences, literacy levels, and accessibility. Providing educational resources tailored to diverse audiences and designing studies that accommodate varying socioeconomic circumstances can improve recruitment and retention of participants from underserved populations. Moreover, funding agencies and policymakers should prioritize resources to support inclusive research initiatives and incentivize diversity in genomic science. By enhancing inclusivity in genomic research, the field can generate more comprehensive and representative genetic databases, improving the accuracy and generalizability of predictive models and therapeutic interventions. This, in turn, helps reduce health disparities and ensures that advances in genomic medicine benefit all populations, rather than exacerbating existing inequities. Ultimately, fostering inclusivity is not just a scientific imperative but an ethical one—grounded in the principles of justice, equity, and respect for human dignity.

9.4.10 Indigenous Knowledge and Sovereignty

Indigenous communities possess unique and deeply rooted worldviews that integrate health, land, ancestry, and genetics into a holistic framework. These perspectives often differ significantly from Western biomedical models, emphasizing the interconnectedness of people, environment, and spirituality. Recognizing and respecting Indigenous knowledge systems is essential when engaging in genomic research involving Indigenous populations. Central to this respect is the principle of data sovereignty, which asserts that Indigenous communities have the inherent right to govern the collection, storage, access, and use of their genetic data. Unlike conventional research paradigms where data is controlled by institutions or researchers, Indigenous data sovereignty requires that communities maintain decision-making authority over their genetic information to protect cultural integrity, privacy, and self-determination. This approach helps address historical injustices where Indigenous peoples' genetic materials were collected without consent or used in ways that undermined their rights and dignity. Data sovereignty frameworks emphasize transparency, accountability, and reciprocity, ensuring that research benefits are shared and aligned with community priorities. Indigenous-led or community-partnered research models have demonstrated greater success in building trust, fostering ethical collaboration, and producing outcomes that are culturally relevant and socially responsible. These models incorporate community governance structures, such as advisory councils or research committees, to guide all phases of genomic studies from design to dissemination. Ultimately, honouring Indigenous knowledge and sovereignty in genomic research is not only an ethical imperative but also enriches scientific understanding by integrating diverse perspectives and values. It promotes a more equitable, respectful, and inclusive future for genomic medicine, where Indigenous communities are active partners rather than passive subjects. This shift supports both the preservation of Indigenous cultural heritage and the advancement of health equity.

9.4.11 Role of Religion and Spirituality

Religion and spirituality play a significant role in shaping how individuals and communities perceive health, illness, and medical interventions, including those involving genetics. Many religious traditions offer frameworks for understanding human life, suffering, and destiny that can influence attitudes toward genetic testing, diagnosis, and treatment. For example, some faiths may view genetic conditions as part of a divine plan or spiritual journey, and therefore may approach genetic interventions with caution or reluctance. Concepts such as fate, karma, or the sanctity of life can deeply affect decisions about reproductive choices, prenatal testing, and gene editing technologies. Respecting these beliefs is essential for healthcare providers when discussing genomic medicine with patients. Sensitivity to religious and spiritual perspectives helps build trust and facilitates more meaningful, patient-centred communication. It allows providers to navigate complex ethical concerns that patients might have, such as fears of "playing God," interfering with natural destiny, or violating moral principles. Additionally, religious leaders or spiritual counsellors often serve as important sources of guidance and support within communities, and involving them in discussions around genetic healthcare can enhance acceptance and understanding. Moreover, religion and spirituality can offer coping mechanisms and hope for patients facing genetic risks or diagnoses, emphasizing compassion, resilience, and community solidarity. Healthcare systems must therefore create space for patients' spiritual needs and beliefs, integrating them respectfully into care plans without compromising medical ethics or scientific integrity. By acknowledging the diverse religious landscapes and their impact on genomic medicine, healthcare providers can offer more culturally congruent and ethically sensitive care, ultimately improving patient satisfaction and health outcomes.

9.4.12 Building Trust Through Engagement

Building trust with diverse communities is fundamental to the successful integration of genomic medicine into healthcare, and this process requires sustained, long-term engagement rather than one-off or short-term outreach efforts. Trust cannot be rushed or assumed; it must be nurtured through ongoing dialogue, transparency, and a genuine commitment to understanding and addressing community concerns. This means moving beyond transactional interactions to establish meaningful partnerships where communities feel valued and heard. Trust is strengthened when researchers and healthcare providers demonstrate respect for cultural values, histories, and lived experiences, especially in communities that may have faced historical marginalization or exploitation. One effective strategy for fostering trust is partnering with trusted cultural leaders, faith-based organizations, and grassroots community groups. These entities often hold significant influence and credibility within their communities and can act as bridges between medical institutions and individuals. Involving these partners early and consistently in the development and implementation of genomic programs helps ensure that interventions are culturally appropriate and ethically sound. It also facilitates the dissemination of accurate information and counters misinformation, which can be a significant barrier to acceptance. Moreover, the co-creation of policies, educational materials, and consent processes with community input enhances their relevance, clarity, and respectfulness. When communities actively participate in shaping research agendas, data governance frameworks, and healthcare practices, they are more likely to trust the process and outcomes. This participatory approach empowers communities, promotes transparency, and fosters a sense of shared ownership and responsibility. Ultimately, building trust through sustained engagement not only improves participation and adherence to genomic medicine but also contributes to health equity by ensuring that the benefits of genomic advances are accessible and acceptable to all populations. It is a cornerstone of ethical and effective healthcare innovation that honours diversity and promotes social justice.

9.5 ETHICAL USE OF AI IN PATIENT CARE

9.5.1 Introduction

Artificial Intelligence (AI) is becoming an integral part of modern healthcare, transforming how patient care is delivered through advanced capabilities in diagnosis, treatment planning, risk prediction, and optimizing clinical workflows. By analysing vast amounts of data quickly and accurately, AI systems can assist healthcare professionals in making more informed decisions, improving the precision and efficiency of medical care. However, despite its many benefits, the integration of AI into healthcare introduces complex ethical challenges that must be thoughtfully addressed. These challenges include concerns about maintaining patient privacy, avoiding algorithmic biases, ensuring transparency in AI decision-making, and safeguarding against errors that could harm patients. Ethical AI in healthcare demands that technologies are developed and deployed with a commitment to upholding human dignity, ensuring fairness and equity in care, and maintaining patient safety. Furthermore, accountability mechanisms must be established to monitor AI systems' performance and address any unintended consequences. As AI continues to evolve, it is essential that ethical principles guide its use to promote trust, protect vulnerable populations, and enhance the overall quality of healthcare delivery.

9.5.2 Benefits of AI in Patient Care

Artificial Intelligence (AI) has brought significant advancements to patient care by enhancing diagnostic accuracy, particularly in areas such as medical imaging and pathology. AI algorithms can analyse complex patterns in images and test results with remarkable precision, often detecting subtle abnormalities that may be missed by human eyes. This capability leads to earlier and more accurate diagnoses, improving patient outcomes. Additionally, AI enables personalized treatment by leveraging vast datasets to tailor therapies according to an individual's genetic profile, lifestyle, and medical history. Data-driven decision-making supports clinicians in selecting the most effective interventions while minimizing side effects. AI also helps reduce human error, which is a common cause of medical mistakes, by providing consistent and evidence-based recommendations. Beyond clinical care, AI optimizes hospital operations by streamlining scheduling, resource allocation, and patient monitoring, enhancing overall efficiency. Furthermore, AI-powered chatbots and telemedicine platforms expand access to healthcare services, especially for patients in remote or underserved areas. These technologies facilitate timely medical advice, symptom checking, and follow-up care, bridging gaps caused by geographic and socioeconomic barriers. Together, these benefits highlight AI's transformative potential to improve both the quality and accessibility of healthcare.

9.5.3 Transparency and Explainability

One of the major challenges in integrating Artificial Intelligence (AI) into healthcare is the limited transparency of many AI systems, particularly those based on deep learning models. These systems often function as "black boxes," meaning their internal decision-making processes are complex and difficult for humans to interpret. This lack of interpretability poses significant ethical concerns because both patients and healthcare providers may struggle to understand how AI arrives at its conclusions or recommendations. Without clear insight into the reasoning behind AI outputs, trust in these technologies can be undermined, and accountability becomes harder to enforce. Transparency is critical in healthcare, where decisions can have profound impacts on patient wellbeing and safety. To address these concerns, the development and deployment of explainable AI (XAI) have become essential. Explainable AI strives to make the decision-making process of AI systems more understandable by providing clear, comprehensible explanations that can be communicated to clinicians and patients alike. This allows healthcare providers to critically evaluate AI suggestions, incorporate them appropriately into clinical judgment, and engage patients in shared decision-making. Ultimately, promoting transparency and explainability is vital for ethical AI use, fostering trust, improving outcomes, and ensuring responsible integration of AI technologies into patient care.

9.5.4 Patient Autonomy and Consent

Patient autonomy is a foundational principle in healthcare ethics, emphasizing the right of individuals to make informed decisions about their own care. As Artificial Intelligence (AI) becomes increasingly involved in diagnosis, treatment recommendations, and care management, it is crucial that AI supports rather than supplants this autonomy. Patients must be fully informed when AI technologies play a role in their healthcare process, including clear explanations of what the AI system does, how it influences clinical decisions, and any inherent limitations it may have. Transparency about AI's involvement empowers patients to understand and question their care pathways, fostering trust and collaboration between patients and healthcare providers. Informed consent processes should be updated to explicitly disclose the use of AI, detailing its potential benefits, risks, and available alternatives to AI-guided interventions. This ensures patients retain control over their health decisions and are not unknowingly subjected to automated or opaque decision-making. Moreover, clinicians must remain accountable for integrating AI recommendations responsibly and respecting patient preferences. Upholding patient autonomy in the era of AI not only protects individual rights but also enhances ethical standards, patient satisfaction, and shared decision-making in clinical practice.

9.5.5 Data Privacy and Security

Artificial Intelligence (AI) systems in healthcare depend heavily on large volumes of sensitive patient data to train algorithms and provide accurate, personalized insights. This reliance raises significant concerns about data privacy and security, as health information is among the most personal and confidential types of data. The risk of data breaches, unauthorized access, or the re-identification of de-identified datasets poses serious threats to patient confidentiality and trust. To mitigate these risks, healthcare organizations and AI developers must implement robust data protection measures, including encryption, secure storage, and strict access controls. Compliance with legal and regulatory frameworks such as the

General Data Protection Regulation (GDPR) in the European Union and the Health Insurance Portability and Accountability Act (HIPAA) in the United States is critical to ensure data is handled responsibly. Beyond legal compliance, patients must retain clear rights over how their data is collected, shared, and used, with informed consent processes that explain these aspects transparently. Empowering patients with control over their data fosters trust and respects their autonomy. Additionally, ongoing monitoring, auditing, and updating of security protocols are necessary to keep pace with evolving cyber threats. Ensuring data privacy and security is foundational to ethical AI implementation and maintaining the integrity of patient care.

9.5.6 Bias and Fairness

Artificial Intelligence (AI) systems in healthcare are only as unbiased as the data on which they are trained. Unfortunately, many training datasets reflect historical inequalities and systemic biases related to race, gender, socioeconomic status, and other factors. When these biases are embedded in AI models, the technology risks perpetuating and even amplifying disparities in care. For example, biased algorithms may lead to misdiagnoses, inappropriate treatment recommendations, or under-treatment for marginalized populations, thereby exacerbating existing health inequities. Addressing these concerns requires rigorous and ongoing efforts, including regular auditing of AI models to detect and correct biases before deployment. It also demands the incorporation of diverse and representative datasets that encompass the broad spectrum of patient demographics and health conditions. Employing fairness metrics during model development helps quantify and reduce disparities in performance across different groups. Additionally, transparency about potential biases allows clinicians and patients to understand the limitations of AI tools. By actively mitigating bias and promoting fairness, AI can contribute to more equitable healthcare outcomes and restore trust among all patient communities.

9.5.7 Accountability and Responsibility

The integration of Artificial Intelligence (AI) into healthcare raises complex questions about accountability and responsibility, especially when errors or harm occur. Unlike traditional medical tools, AI systems involve multiple stakeholders, including developers, healthcare providers, and institutions, making it challenging to pinpoint liability in cases of malfunction or adverse outcomes. Ethical frameworks must establish clear guidelines that define the roles and responsibilities of each party involved, ensuring that accountability does not become obscured by technological complexity. Human oversight remains essential; AI should function as an assistive technology that supports clinical judgment rather than replacing it. Healthcare providers must critically evaluate AI recommendations and retain ultimate decision-making authority to safeguard patient well-being. Institutions are responsible for implementing robust policies around AI use, including training, validation, and continuous monitoring. Developers, meanwhile, have a duty to design transparent, reliable, and well-tested systems. By clarifying these accountability structures, the healthcare ecosystem can promote trust, encourage responsible innovation, and protect patients from preventable harm.

9.5.8 Professional Integrity and Trust

The growing reliance on Artificial Intelligence (AI) in healthcare presents challenges related to professional integrity and the trust patients place in their clinicians. While AI can enhance diagnostic accuracy and streamline care, over-dependence on automated systems risks undermining the expertise and critical judgment that healthcare professionals bring to patient care. It is vital that clinicians remain the central decision-makers, interpreting AI outputs within the broader context of individual patient histories, values, and preferences. The human touch—marked by empathy, nuanced communication, and compassionate understanding—is irreplaceable and fundamental to building trust between patients and providers. Patients often seek reassurance and emotional support that AI cannot provide, underscoring the importance of maintaining meaningful clinician-patient relationships. Upholding professional integrity means clinicians must be transparent about AI's role, limitations, and uncertainties, fostering informed consent and shared decision-making. Ultimately, balancing technological innovation with human-centred care will strengthen patient confidence, improve outcomes, and preserve the core values of medicine.

9.5.9 Equity and Access

The promise of Artificial Intelligence (AI) in healthcare is immense, yet its benefits are not evenly distributed across all populations and regions. Many AI tools require advanced infrastructure, including high-speed internet, powerful computing resources, and skilled personnel, which are often lacking in resource-poor or rural healthcare settings. This disparity creates a digital divide where marginalized communities may be excluded from the advantages of AI-driven diagnostics, personalized treatments, and telemedicine services. Additionally, limited digital literacy among patients and providers can hinder effective use of AI technologies, further compounding inequities. To ensure that AI contributes to reducing health disparities rather than exacerbating them, developers and policymakers must prioritize inclusive design principles that consider diverse user needs and contexts from the outset. Efforts should focus on expanding access through affordable technologies, user-friendly interfaces, and capacity-building initiatives. Furthermore, equitable deployment requires policy interventions and funding models that support underserved areas. By fostering fairness in access and usability, AI can become a powerful tool to enhance healthcare for all, bridging gaps rather than widening them.

9.5.10 Informed Clinical Decision Support

Artificial Intelligence (AI) has become an invaluable tool in assisting healthcare professionals with clinical decision-making, offering data-driven insights that can enhance treatment planning and patient management. However, while AI can analyse vast datasets and generate recommendations, it should not replace the nuanced judgment of clinicians who consider the unique circumstances, values, and preferences of each patient. Ethical use of AI in clinical settings means that AI tools act as supportive aids—providing suggestions, risk assessments, or diagnostic probabilities—rather than prescriptive mandates that dictate care pathways. This approach ensures that healthcare providers remain the ultimate decision-makers, integrating AI outputs with their medical expertise, patient histories, and cultural or social contexts. Additionally, respecting patient autonomy means that clinicians should engage patients in shared decision-making, transparently discussing how AI recommendations inform but do not determine treatment options. This collaborative process promotes trust, supports personalized care, and helps avoid overreliance on automated systems that may overlook individual complexities. By balancing AI assistance with human judgment and patient input, healthcare can achieve more ethical, effective, and compassionate outcomes.

9.5.11 Continuous Monitoring and Evaluation

The deployment of Artificial Intelligence (AI) in healthcare is not a one-time event but an ongoing process that requires continuous monitoring and evaluation. AI models must be regularly updated to reflect new medical knowledge, changing patient populations, and evolving clinical practices. Without regular oversight, AI systems risk becoming outdated, less accurate, or even harmful if they fail to adapt to new data or environments. Continuous performance monitoring ensures that AI tools maintain their safety, effectiveness, and relevance over time. This includes tracking key metrics such as accuracy, bias, and unintended consequences, with prompt intervention if issues arise. Ethical AI stewardship also involves managing the entire lifespan of AI systems, which includes responsibly decommissioning or replacing models that no longer meet safety or ethical standards. Independent review boards or ethics committees can play a crucial role in overseeing these processes, providing external validation, and ensuring accountability. These bodies bring together diverse expertise to scrutinize AI performance, assess risks, and recommend improvements. By embedding continuous evaluation into AI governance, healthcare organizations can uphold patient safety, maintain trust, and ensure AI remains a beneficial tool in clinical care.

9.5.12 Regulatory and Ethical Guidelines

The rapid integration of Artificial Intelligence (AI) into healthcare demands that regulatory frameworks evolve to address the unique challenges posed by these emerging technologies. Traditional healthcare regulations often fall short in managing AI's complexity, such as algorithmic opacity, adaptive learning, and data-driven decision-making. In response, several initiatives have begun to shape the landscape of AI governance. The European Union's AI Act aims to establish comprehensive rules that ensure AI systems are safe, transparent, and respect fundamental rights. Similarly, the World Health Organization (WHO) has issued guidelines emphasizing ethical principles like human-centred design, accountability, and inclusivity in AI deployment. In the United States, the Food and Drug Administration (FDA) is developing frameworks to evaluate and monitor AI-based medical devices, balancing innovation with patient safety. Effective ethical governance requires a proactive and flexible approach that can adapt to technological advances while safeguarding public trust. This governance must be multidisciplinary, involving ethicists, legal experts, clinicians, technologists, and patient representatives to ensure diverse perspectives are incorporated. By fostering collaboration and transparency, regulatory bodies can create standards that promote responsible AI development and use, protect patient rights, and enhance the quality and equity of healthcare outcomes worldwide.

10 Chapter HEALTH ECONOMICS AND REIMBURSEMENT MODELS

10.0 INTRODUCTION: AN OVERVIEW

The delivery of modern healthcare is increasingly shaped by the interplay between medical innovation, financial sustainability, and equitable access. As healthcare systems worldwide grapple with rising costs, aging populations, chronic disease burdens, and technological advancements, health economics has emerged as a critical discipline to evaluate how resources are allocated, how value is defined, and how care is financed. Health economics provides a framework to assess the efficiency, cost-effectiveness, and impact of medical interventions, informing decisions that affect patients, providers, payers, and policymakers alike. At its core, health economics seeks to answer fundamental questions: What healthcare services should be provided? Who should receive them? How should they be paid for? And how can limited resources be used to achieve the greatest possible health outcomes? By applying economic principles to these questions, health economists aim to guide policies that balance quality, access, and cost—often referred to as the "iron triangle" of healthcare. From evaluating the price of pharmaceuticals to analysing the benefits of early diagnostics, health economics plays a pivotal role in shaping the future of healthcare delivery. One of the most complex and evolving aspects of health economics is the reimbursement model—the way healthcare providers are compensated for the services they deliver. Traditional fee-for-service (FFS) systems have long dominated, incentivizing volume over value. However, the limitations of this model—such as overuse of procedures, fragmented care, and inefficiencies—have led to a global shift toward value-based care, where reimbursement is tied to patient outcomes and quality metrics rather than the quantity of services rendered (Fig. 1).

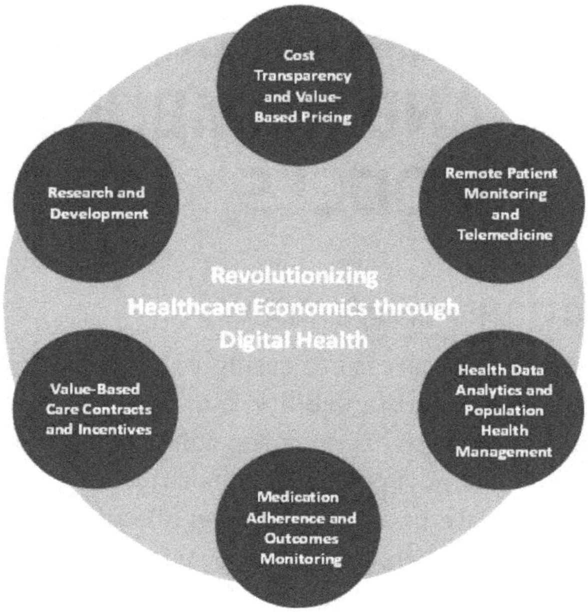

Fig. 1 Healthcare economics through digital health

New reimbursement frameworks are being tested and implemented, including bundled payments, capitation, pay-for-performance (P4P), accountable care organizations (ACOs), and outcome-based contracts. These models aim to encourage more coordinated, efficient, and patient-centred care, aligning financial incentives with long-term health improvements. At the same time, they introduce new challenges: how to measure outcomes fairly, how to manage risk among providers, and how to ensure that cost control does not compromise care quality or access. The emergence of digital health, telemedicine, artificial intelligence (AI), and precision medicine further complicates the economics of care. These innovations offer the potential for more proactive, personalized, and scalable healthcare, but also raise questions about affordability, reimbursement, and return on investment. As predictive tools and genomics become more integrated into routine care, health systems must determine how to equitably reimburse services that may prevent disease years before symptoms arise—a challenge for both insurers and governments. Globally, health systems vary widely in their structure, financing, and reimbursement strategies. While some countries rely heavily on public funding and universal coverage models, others depend on private insurers, employer-based plans, or out-of-pocket payments. These differences impact not only how care is delivered and funded, but also how innovation is adopted, how pricing is negotiated, and how equitable access is ensured. Understanding these variations is essential for developing sustainable and context-appropriate reimbursement models that serve the needs of diverse populations. In the context of constrained budgets, healthcare innovations must now demonstrate not just clinical effectiveness but also economic value—often quantified through tools like cost-utility analysis, quality-adjusted life years (QALYs), and incremental cost-effectiveness ratios (ICERs). These methods help decision-makers evaluate trade-offs and prioritize interventions that deliver the most value for money.

Moreover, reimbursement decisions are not only economic but also ethical and political. Choices about what to fund, and for whom, often reflect broader societal values about fairness, solidarity, and the right to health. As a result, transparent and inclusive decision-making processes are vital to maintain public trust and legitimacy.

10.1 COST-EFFECTIVENESS OF PERSONALIZED INTERVENTIONS

Personalized interventions in healthcare refer to treatments and prevention strategies tailored to an individual's genetic, environmental, and lifestyle factors. These approaches aim to improve outcomes by targeting therapies more precisely than traditional "one-size-fits-all" methods. However, personalized interventions often involve advanced diagnostics, genetic testing, and novel therapeutics that can be costly. Evaluating their cost-effectiveness is critical to determining their value in healthcare systems, ensuring that resources are allocated efficiently while maximizing patient benefit.

10.1.1 Clinical Benefits and Outcome Improvements

Personalized interventions represent a transformative advancement in healthcare, offering significant clinical benefits and improvements in patient outcomes. By tailoring treatments to the unique genetic, molecular, and environmental profiles of individual patients, personalized medicine enhances treatment efficacy while simultaneously reducing the risk of adverse effects. One prominent example of this approach is pharmacogenomics, which enables clinicians to select medications that are optimally suited to a patient's genetic makeup. This precision reduces the traditional trial-and-error method of prescribing, thereby minimizing the likelihood of ineffective treatments and harmful side effects. As a result, patients experience faster therapeutic responses and improved overall safety. Moreover, personalized medicine facilitates the early identification of disease risks through genetic screening and molecular diagnostics. By detecting predispositions to conditions such as cardiovascular diseases, certain cancers, and metabolic disorders at an early stage, healthcare providers can implement preventive strategies tailored specifically to the patient's risk profile. These preventive interventions might include lifestyle modifications, targeted surveillance, or prophylactic therapies, which collectively reduce the incidence and severity of disease. Consequently, early interventions can delay or even prevent disease onset, improving quality of life and extending patient longevity.

Importantly, these clinical advantages translate into substantial reductions in healthcare utilization, such as fewer hospital admissions, decreased need for intensive treatments, and lowered rates of disease complications. Over time, these improvements contribute to significant cost savings for healthcare systems, despite the initially higher costs associated with genetic testing and personalized care. However, quantifying the true impact of personalized interventions on clinical outcomes and cost-effectiveness remains crucial. Rigorous clinical studies and health economic analyses are needed to evaluate whether the benefits in terms of enhanced health outcomes and reduced adverse events sufficiently offset the upfront investments. Personalized medicine holds immense promise for improving patient outcomes through more precise, effective, and safer therapeutic approaches. The integration of genomic data into clinical decision-making not only elevates the standard of care but also supports a shift from reactive to proactive healthcare. As personalized interventions become more accessible and affordable, their widespread adoption could revolutionize disease management, ultimately resulting in healthier populations and more sustainable healthcare systems.

10.1.2 Cost Components of Personalized Medicine

The cost-effectiveness of personalized medicine hinges on a complex interplay of multiple cost components that must be carefully considered in economic evaluations. A major upfront expense is the price of genetic testing and biomarker analyses, which often involve advanced technologies such as next-generation sequencing, microarrays, or mass spectrometry. These sophisticated platforms require highly specialized personnel and stringent quality control processes, driving costs higher compared to conventional diagnostic tests. Furthermore, the sheer volume and complexity of data generated demand robust bioinformatics infrastructure to ensure accurate interpretation, adding to overall expenditure. In addition to diagnostic costs, personalized therapeutics themselves frequently come with premium price tags. Targeted biologic drugs, such as monoclonal antibodies designed to interact with specific molecular pathways, and gene therapies that directly modify genetic material, often represent cutting-edge innovations with high research and development investments reflected in their pricing. These therapies may offer superior efficacy and fewer side effects but can significantly increase initial treatment costs relative to standard, one-size-fits-all medications.

Healthcare systems must also allocate resources to build the necessary infrastructure for personalized medicine implementation. This includes investment in electronic health record systems capable of integrating genomic data, secure data storage solutions, and analytical platforms that support clinical decision-making. Clinician training is another critical cost factor, as providers need to acquire specialized knowledge to interpret genetic results accurately and apply them appropriately in patient care. Ongoing education ensures that the workforce remains proficient as personalized medicine evolves. Beyond direct costs, indirect expenses associated with patient monitoring and long-term follow-up care are also significant. Personalized interventions often require more intensive surveillance to evaluate therapeutic responses and manage potential side effects. However, these costs may be offset by savings generated from avoiding ineffective treatments, reducing hospitalizations, and preventing complications. For example, by identifying non-responders early, clinicians can discontinue costly therapies that would otherwise offer no benefit, thereby optimizing resource utilization. Ultimately, comprehensive economic evaluations must encompass all these cost dimensions—upfront diagnostic and therapeutic expenses, infrastructure and training investments, and ongoing care costs—balanced against the potential financial benefits accrued through improved clinical outcomes and healthcare efficiencies. Only through such holistic assessments can the true value and sustainability of personalized medicine be determined, guiding policy decisions and resource allocation in healthcare systems worldwide.

10.1.3 Economic Evaluation Methods

Economic evaluation methods are essential tools for assessing the value of personalized medicine interventions and guiding healthcare decision-making. Among the most commonly employed approaches are cost-effectiveness analysis (CEA), cost-utility analysis (CUA), and budget impact analysis (BIA), each serving distinct purposes in evaluating the financial and clinical implications of new healthcare technologies. Cost-effectiveness analysis (CEA) focuses on comparing the costs and health outcomes of personalized interventions relative to standard or conventional care. This method quantifies health benefits often in terms of natural units such as life years gained, disease cases prevented, or symptom-free days. One widely accepted metric used within CEA is the cost per quality-adjusted life year (QALY) gained, which integrates both the quantity and quality of life into a single measure. By calculating the incremental cost-effectiveness ratio (ICER), CEA helps policymakers determine whether a personalized treatment offers sufficient clinical benefits to justify its additional costs compared to existing alternatives.

Cost-utility analysis (CUA) extends beyond CEA by incorporating patient preferences and quality of life considerations into the evaluation framework. This approach uses utilities derived from patient-reported outcomes or preference-based instruments to weigh different health states, recognizing that the impact of a disease or treatment may vary significantly between individuals. CUA thereby provides a more patient-centred assessment, capturing not only survival gains but also improvements in functional status, symptom relief, and overall well-being that personalized medicine may deliver. Budget impact analysis (BIA) complements

CEA and CUA by addressing the financial feasibility and affordability of integrating personalized interventions on a broader scale within healthcare systems. BIA evaluates the short- to medium-term effects on healthcare budgets by estimating changes in expenditure related to drug acquisition, diagnostics, healthcare utilization, and other relevant costs. This analysis is critical for payers and healthcare providers as they plan resource allocation, reimbursement strategies, and policy frameworks needed to support sustainable adoption of personalized medicine. For these economic evaluations to be robust and credible, they must be grounded in high-quality clinical evidence derived from randomized controlled trials, observational studies, and real-world data. Furthermore, long-term impacts should be considered through modelling techniques that project outcomes beyond the immediate trial periods, capturing the full trajectory of disease progression, treatment response, and healthcare utilization over time. Sensitivity analyses are often conducted to account for uncertainties in data and assumptions, ensuring that conclusions remain valid under varying scenarios (Fig. 2).

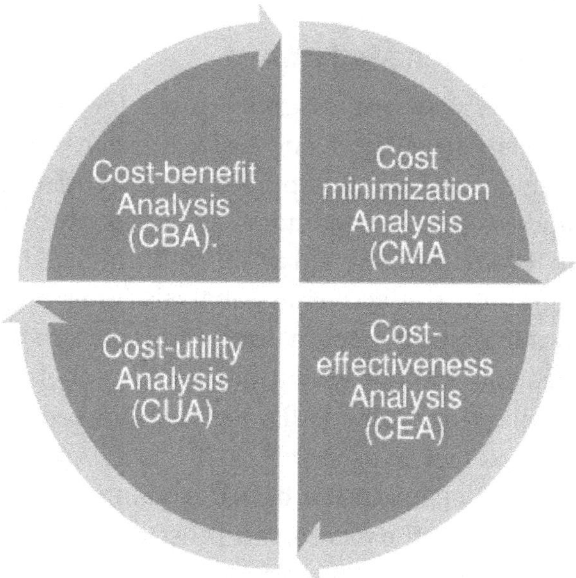

Fig. 2 Types of economic evaluation

10.1.4 Challenges in Measuring Cost-Effectiveness

Evaluating the cost-effectiveness of personalized interventions presents several significant challenges that complicate economic analyses and decision-making processes. One primary difficulty stems from data limitations. Many personalized medicine studies involve relatively small patient cohorts due to the highly specific nature of genetic or biomarker-defined subpopulations. These small sample sizes can restrict the statistical power of studies and limit the generalizability of results to broader patient groups. Additionally, clinical trials and observational studies often have short follow-up periods, which may not capture the full spectrum of long-term benefits, risks, and costs associated with personalized treatments. As a result, projecting long-term outcomes requires modelling techniques that depend heavily on assumptions and extrapolations, potentially introducing uncertainty into economic evaluations.

Another major challenge is the inherent heterogeneity in patient responses to personalized therapies. Variability in genetic, environmental, and lifestyle factors means that outcomes can differ widely even among patients with similar risk profiles. This heterogeneity complicates efforts to generate average estimates of cost-effectiveness that apply across diverse populations. It also raises the question of how to value benefits in patients who experience exceptional responses versus those with minimal improvements, making standardized economic comparisons difficult. Moreover, the value of personalized interventions often transcends measurable clinical endpoints. Psychological and emotional benefits, such as the reassurance gained from knowing one's genetic risk or the empowerment derived from tailored care plans, are important but notoriously difficult to quantify. These intangible benefits can enhance patient satisfaction, adherence, and overall well-being, yet they are seldom incorporated into traditional cost-effectiveness frameworks, which focus primarily on clinical outcomes and direct costs. Ethical and social considerations further complicate the evaluation of personalized medicine's value. Issues such as equitable access to expensive genetic testing and advanced therapies influence societal perceptions of fairness and justice. Disparities in availability could exacerbate existing health inequalities, raise concerns that go beyond economic metrics. While these factors profoundly affect the acceptability and implementation of personalized interventions, they are not easily captured or weighted in conventional economic models.

10.1.5 Health System Implications

Integrating personalized medicine into routine healthcare delivery presents both opportunities and challenges that require careful consideration by health systems, payers, and policymakers. The adoption of personalized interventions necessitates thoughtful allocation of limited healthcare resources to ensure that innovative technologies deliver meaningful clinical benefits without compromising financial sustainability. Decision-makers must rigorously evaluate which personalized approaches provide sufficient value—balancing improved patient outcomes against their often-substantial costs. Cost-effectiveness evidence plays a crucial role in guiding reimbursement policies and prioritizing healthcare services, helping to identify interventions that warrant coverage and integration into standard practice. Personalized medicine has the potential to fundamentally reshape cost structures within health systems. By enabling more precise diagnosis and targeted treatment, it can reduce the use of ineffective therapies, thereby avoiding unnecessary expenditures. Furthermore, early identification of disease risk and timely intervention may prevent costly complications and reduce hospital admissions. Over time, these improvements can lead to significant system-wide savings and enhance the overall efficiency of care delivery. However, realizing these long-term benefits requires substantial upfront investments in technology, infrastructure, and workforce training to support personalized approaches effectively.

Equitable access to personalized medicine remains a critical concern for health systems worldwide. The high costs associated with genetic testing, biomarker analyses, and targeted therapies can limit availability to certain populations, exacerbating existing healthcare disparities. Policymakers must therefore consider strategies to ensure that advances in personalized medicine do not disproportionately benefit only those with greater financial means or geographic access. This may include negotiating pricing agreements, expanding insurance coverage, and investing in outreach programs to underserved communities. Moreover, the integration of personalized medicine demands ongoing adaptation within healthcare delivery models. Clinicians need to be equipped with the skills and tools to interpret complex genetic data and incorporate it into patient care effectively. Health systems must develop robust data management capabilities to handle large volumes of genomic and clinical information while maintaining patient privacy and security. Collaboration across multidisciplinary teams, including genetic counsellors, pharmacists, and IT specialists, is essential to realize the full potential of personalized interventions. The successful incorporation of personalized medicine into health systems depends on striking a balance between fostering innovation and maintaining affordability. Policymakers and payers must leverage evidence-based frameworks to make informed decisions, ensuring that personalized interventions enhance patient outcomes while promoting equity and sustainability. With strategic planning and investment, personalized medicine can become an integral component of modern healthcare, improve quality of care and optimize resource utilization on a broad scale.

10.1.6 Future Perspectives

Looking ahead, the future of personalized medicine is poised for transformative growth driven by rapid technological advancements and evolving healthcare paradigms. One of the most significant factors shaping this future is the continual decline in the costs of genome sequencing and other molecular diagnostic technologies. As these technologies become more affordable and accessible, the widespread implementation of personalized interventions will become increasingly feasible, lowering barriers to entry for healthcare systems worldwide. This democratization of genomic data will empower clinicians to make more informed, precise treatment decisions across a broader range of conditions. Alongside technological progress, improvements in data analytics and artificial intelligence are expected to revolutionize how personalized medicine is applied and evaluated. Enhanced computational tools will enable more sophisticated integration of diverse data sources, including genomic information, electronic health records, and real-world evidence, offering a more comprehensive understanding of patient outcomes. The incorporation of patient-reported outcomes into economic models will further refine assessments by capturing dimensions of health and quality of life that traditional clinical endpoints may overlook. These advances will improve the accuracy, relevance, and patient-centeredness of cost-effectiveness analyses, facilitating better-informed healthcare decisions.

Achieving the full potential of personalized medicine will require robust collaboration among stakeholders, including healthcare providers, pharmaceutical and diagnostic industries, payers, and regulatory agencies. These partnerships are essential to develop sustainable frameworks that balance innovation incentives with affordability, ensuring that personalized therapies deliver maximum clinical and economic value. Joint efforts can also drive standardization in data collection, sharing, and interpretation, fostering transparency and reproducibility in both clinical and economic evaluations. Furthermore, as personalized medicine matures, ethical considerations such as equitable access and patient privacy will remain central to its development and implementation. Policymakers will need to craft policies that promote inclusivity and protect sensitive genetic information, thereby building public trust and acceptance. Addressing these social dimensions is critical for ensuring that advances in personalized care benefit diverse populations without exacerbating health disparities. Ultimately, cost-effective personalized medicine holds the promise to fundamentally transform healthcare delivery. By tailoring interventions to the unique characteristics of each patient, it can improve clinical outcomes, enhance quality of life, and optimize resource utilization. As technology continues to evolve and economic evaluation methods become more sophisticated, personalized medicine is set to become a cornerstone of modern, value-based healthcare systems that strive to balance innovation with fiscal responsibility.

10.2 VALUE-BASED HEALTHCARE AND OUTCOME-BASED PRICING

Value-Based Healthcare (VBHC) represents a paradigm shift in healthcare delivery, moving away from the traditional fee-for-service model that prioritizes the volume of care provided towards a system that emphasizes the quality, effectiveness, and overall value of care. At its core, VBHC seeks to maximize patient outcomes while controlling or reducing healthcare costs, thereby ensuring that every dollar spent contributes meaningfully to improving health and well-being. This approach aligns the interests of patients, providers, and payers by focusing on results rather than procedures, promoting a more patient-centred and sustainable healthcare system. Unlike conventional healthcare models where providers are reimbursed based on the quantity of services rendered—such as tests, visits, or procedures—VBHC rewards clinicians and healthcare organizations for achieving measurable improvements in patient health. This focus encourages the adoption of best practices, care coordination, and prevention strategies that reduce complications, hospital readmissions, and unnecessary interventions. By centring care around outcomes that matter most to patients, including survival, functional status, quality of life, and patient satisfaction, VBHC fosters a holistic and efficient approach to managing health. Complementing VBHC, Outcome-Based Pricing (OBP) is an innovative reimbursement strategy that ties the price of treatments or medical interventions directly to the health outcomes they deliver. Pharmaceutical companies and device manufacturers are motivated to invest in treatments that provide clear, demonstrable benefits, while payers gain assurance that expenditures correlate with meaningful patient outcomes. This alignment drives competition toward value rather than volume and encourages providers to adopt evidence-based practices and patient monitoring systems to track effectiveness in real time (Fig. 3).

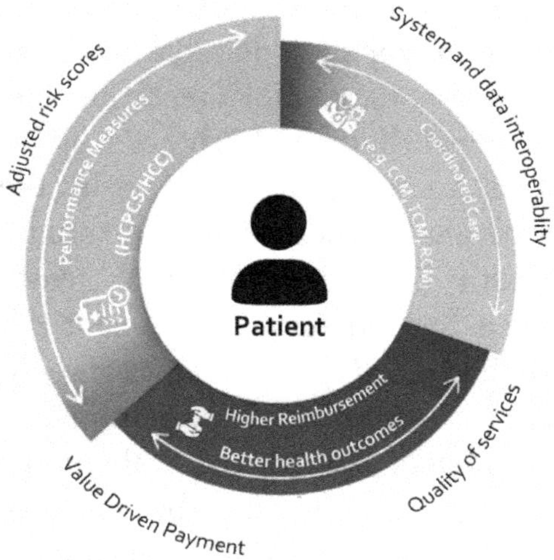

Fig. 3 Value based care model

Implementing VBHC and OBP requires robust data infrastructure and measurement frameworks. Reliable, standardized outcome metrics must be developed and systematically collected to accurately assess the impact of interventions on patient health. This often involves integrating electronic health records, patient registries, and real-world data sources, along with patient-reported outcomes that capture the lived experience of illness and recovery. Such data enable ongoing evaluation, benchmarking, and adjustment of care pathways and pricing agreements, fostering a dynamic system responsive to evolving clinical evidence and patient needs. Moreover, VBHC and OBP models promote collaboration among all healthcare stakeholders. Providers, payers, patients, and industry partners must work together to define meaningful outcomes, establish fair pricing mechanisms, and design care delivery models that support sustained improvements. This collective effort helps overcome traditional silos in healthcare, encourages innovation in care coordination, and supports shared decision-making grounded in transparent evidence. However, transitioning to VBHC and OBP is not without challenges. Healthcare systems must address complexities related to outcome measurement, data privacy, regulatory frameworks, and equitable access to ensure that value-based models benefit diverse patient populations.

10.2.1 Concept of Value in Healthcare

In Value-Based Healthcare (VBHC), the concept of value is fundamentally redefined as the health outcomes achieved for every dollar spent. This represents a crucial departure from traditional healthcare models that emphasize inputs such as the volume of procedures, diagnostic tests, or office visits, regardless of their impact on patient well-being. Instead, VBHC places measurable improvements in patient health, quality of life, and functional status at the centre of care delivery. By prioritizing outcomes that matter most to patients, such as symptom relief, enhanced mobility, and overall life satisfaction, VBHC ensures that healthcare resources are directed toward interventions that truly make a difference. This patient-centric approach encourages the reduction of unnecessary or low-value procedures that do not contribute meaningfully to health improvements, thereby minimizing waste and potential harm. It fosters more efficient use of healthcare resources by focusing on interventions with proven effectiveness, ultimately enhancing both clinical outcomes and economic sustainability. By aligning incentives with value rather than volume, VBHC motivates providers to innovate, coordinate care, and engage patients actively in their treatment plans. Moreover, emphasizing value promotes transparency and accountability in healthcare, enabling stakeholders—including patients, providers, and payers—to make informed decisions based on robust outcome data. The shift toward measuring and rewarding value has the potential to improve patient satisfaction, increase trust in the healthcare system, and drive continuous quality improvement. In essence, VBHC transforms healthcare delivery into a system were maximizing meaningful health outcomes relative to cost becomes the guiding principle, fostering better care for patients and more sustainable health systems overall.

10.2.2 Outcome Measurement and Metrics

The successful implementation of Value-Based Healthcare (VBHC) hinges on the rigorous and systematic measurement of health outcomes that truly reflect the effectiveness of care. These outcomes encompass a broad range of indicators, including clinical metrics such as survival rates, disease remission, complication rates, and functional recovery. Equally important are patient-reported outcomes, which capture the patient's perspective on quality of life, symptom burden, mental well-being, and overall satisfaction with care. Incorporating these subjective measures ensures that healthcare improvements align with what patient's value most, providing a holistic picture of health beyond traditional clinical endpoints. In addition to clinical and patient-centred metrics, economic indicators play a vital role in assessing value within VBHC. Metrics such as hospital readmission rates, length of stay, emergency department visits, and total cost of care offer insight into the efficiency and sustainability of healthcare delivery. By combining these diverse data points, VBHC frameworks can evaluate not only whether treatments improve health but also whether they do so in a cost-effective manner.

Reliable data collection methods and standardized outcome metrics are fundamental to enabling meaningful comparisons across providers, institutions, and treatment modalities. Standardization promotes transparency, allowing stakeholders to benchmark performance, identify best practices, and drive continuous improvement. Moreover, robust outcome measurement supports outcome-based payment models by providing the objective evidence necessary to link reimbursement to clinical success and patient benefit. Advances in health information technology, including electronic health records, patient registries, and wearable devices, are increasingly facilitating real-time and comprehensive outcome tracking. These tools empower providers to monitor progress, adjust care plans dynamically, and engage patients actively in their health journeys. Ultimately, effective outcome measurement and metrics are the backbone of VBHC, ensuring that healthcare systems can deliver high-quality, patient-centred care while maximizing value.

10.2.3 Outcome-Based Pricing Models

Outcome-Based Pricing (OBP) models represent an innovative approach to healthcare reimbursement, where payment for medical interventions is directly linked to the achievement of predefined clinical outcomes. Unlike traditional pricing models that reimburse providers or manufacturers based solely on volume or list prices, OBP structures financial agreements so that payments depend on real-world therapeutic success. For instance, a pharmaceutical company may receive full reimbursement only if a medication demonstrably reduces hospital admissions, improves survival rates, or achieves other agreed-upon health benchmarks. If the treatment fails to deliver these results, the payment may be reduced, deferred, or subject to refund.

This results-oriented payment mechanism aligns financial incentives across stakeholders, fostering a shared commitment to maximizing patient benefit. It encourages manufacturers to develop and bring to market therapies that provide meaningful, measurable improvements in health outcomes rather than incremental or uncertain benefits. Simultaneously, payers—such as insurers and government programs—can mitigate financial risks associated with high-cost treatments by linking expenditures to actual clinical effectiveness. OBP also drives innovation in treatment development and post-market surveillance, as manufacturers invest more in patient selection, adherence strategies, and long-term outcome monitoring to ensure their products meet agreed standards. Furthermore, this model incentivizes collaboration between manufacturers, providers, and payers to define relevant outcomes, develop robust measurement systems, and establish transparent reporting mechanisms.

While promising, implementing OBP models requires overcoming challenges such as defining appropriate, measurable outcomes, managing data collection, and negotiating complex contracts. Nonetheless, as healthcare systems increasingly prioritize value over volume, outcome-based pricing stands as a critical tool to promote accountability, improve patient care, and optimize resource allocation in modern medicine.

10.2.4 Benefits of Outcome-Based Pricing

Outcome-Based Pricing (OBP) offers numerous benefits that contribute to a more accountable, efficient, and patient-centred healthcare system. By linking payments directly to the achievement of real-world clinical outcomes, OBP promotes accountability among manufacturers and providers, ensuring that financial rewards are tied to actual health improvements rather than merely the volume of services or products delivered. This focus on results helps reduce wasteful spending on ineffective or marginally beneficial treatments, allowing healthcare funds to be allocated more judiciously and directed toward therapies that truly enhance patient well-being. For patients, OBP can increase access to innovative and potentially life-changing therapies by mitigating payer concerns about the financial risks associated with high-cost treatments. Knowing that reimbursement is contingent upon demonstrable benefits encourages payers to support coverage of novel interventions that might otherwise be limited due to uncertain outcomes. This model also fosters greater transparency about treatment effectiveness, empowering patients and clinicians to make more informed decisions based on evidence of what works best. From the perspective of providers and manufacturers, OBP creates powerful incentives for continuous improvement and innovation.

Drug developers and device makers are motivated to invest in rigorous clinical research, optimize patient selection, and enhance adherence strategies to ensure their products deliver measurable benefits. Healthcare providers, in turn, are encouraged to adopt best practices, focus on coordinated care, and monitor patient progress closely to meet outcome targets. This alignment of incentives helps drive a culture of quality improvement across the healthcare ecosystem. Moreover, OBP can facilitate better collaboration among stakeholders by fostering shared risk and reward arrangements. This collaborative environment supports the development of more effective treatments, streamlined care pathways, and improved patient experiences. In sum, outcome-based pricing is a transformative approach that aligns financial incentives with patient-centred outcomes, promoting sustainable healthcare delivery and maximizing value for all involved.

10.2.5 Challenges and Limitations

Implementing Value-Based Healthcare (VBHC) and Outcome-Based Pricing (OBP) presents a range of complex challenges and limitations that must be addressed to realize their full potential. One of the foremost difficulties lies in consistently and fairly measuring health outcomes across diverse patient populations, diseases, and clinical settings. Variability in patient characteristics, comorbidities, and social determinants of health can significantly influence outcomes, making it challenging to establish standardized metrics that accurately reflect provider performance without penalizing those who treat more complex cases. Defining appropriate clinical endpoints and evaluation timelines further complicates implementation. Different diseases and interventions require distinct outcome measures—while survival rates may be paramount in oncology, quality of life or symptom control might be more relevant in chronic conditions. Moreover, the timeframe over which outcomes should be assessed varies; some treatments demonstrate benefits quickly, whereas others require long-term follow-up, adding uncertainty to payment models tied to outcomes. Robust data collection infrastructure and interoperability are critical enablers for VBHC and OBP, yet many healthcare systems struggle with fragmented electronic health records, inconsistent documentation practices, and limited capacity for integrating diverse data sources. Without reliable, comprehensive data, it becomes difficult to monitor outcomes accurately, track progress, or verify that agreed-upon benchmarks have been met. Investment in health IT and data governance is essential but can be costly and time-consuming. Negotiating outcome-based contracts introduces additional complexity. These agreements must clearly define outcome measures, payment terms, and risk-sharing arrangements, often requiring lengthy negotiations among manufacturers, payers, and providers. Legal and regulatory frameworks may not yet be fully adapted to support such innovative contracting models, leading to uncertainty and reluctance among stakeholders. Finally, there is inherent uncertainty in attributing outcomes solely to the interventions being evaluated. Patient adherence, variations in clinical practice, and external factors such as socioeconomic status or environmental influences can impact results beyond the control of providers or manufacturers. This uncertainty complicates the design of fair payment models and may necessitate risk adjustment or shared risk mechanisms to ensure equitable compensation. Despite these challenges, ongoing advancements in data analytics, standardized outcome sets, and collaborative stakeholder engagement are helping to overcome barriers. Addressing these limitations is crucial to unlocking the promise of VBHC and OBP as transformative models that improve patient care while promoting financial sustainability.

10.2.6 Policy and Regulatory Considerations

Policymakers play a pivotal role in advancing the adoption and effective implementation of Value-Based Healthcare (VBHC) and Outcome-Based Pricing (OBP) by creating an enabling environment that promotes transparency, data sharing, and alignment of incentives across the healthcare ecosystem. To support this transformation, regulatory frameworks must evolve to accommodate innovative contracting models that link reimbursement to patient outcomes, while simultaneously safeguarding patient rights and privacy. Clear policies are needed to govern the collection, use, and sharing of health data, ensuring interoperability and minimizing barriers to information exchange among providers, payers, and manufacturers. Regulatory agencies must also provide guidance on the design and approval of outcome-based contracts, helping to standardize outcome definitions, measurement methodologies, and reporting requirements. This regulatory clarity can reduce uncertainty and encourage broader participation by payers and providers in VBHC initiatives. Furthermore, patient protections remain paramount; regulations must ensure that outcome-based models do not inadvertently restrict access to care or impose undue burdens on vulnerable populations.

Equitable access and non-discrimination should be embedded in all VBHC policies to avoid exacerbating existing healthcare disparities. Reimbursement policies represent a critical area for adaptation. Traditional fee-for-service payment systems often do not support outcome-based agreements, necessitating reforms that enable flexible payment structures aligned with clinical performance. Policymakers should incentivize value-driven care by encouraging public and private payers to adopt OBP models and provide guidance on risk-sharing arrangements. Pilot programs and demonstration projects can serve as valuable tools to test and refine these models before broader implementation. Moreover, fostering collaboration among all stakeholders—including patients, providers, payers, manufacturers, and regulators—is essential for the success of VBHC and OBP. Policymakers can facilitate forums for dialogue, data sharing platforms, and partnerships that promote shared learning and innovation. Engaging patients in the design and evaluation of value-based programs ensures that care models remain patient-centred and responsive to real-world needs. Comprehensive policy and regulatory support are crucial to overcoming barriers and enabling a sustainable shift toward value-based healthcare. By promoting transparency, protecting patients, and adapting reimbursement frameworks, policymakers can help transform healthcare systems into models that prioritize outcomes, efficiency, and equity.

10.2.7 Future Directions

Looking ahead, technological advancements are poised to significantly accelerate the adoption and impact of Value-Based Healthcare (VBHC) and Outcome-Based Pricing (OBP). Innovations such as sophisticated electronic health records (EHRs), interoperable data systems, and artificial intelligence (AI)-driven analytics are enhancing the ability to collect, track, and analyse patient outcomes in real time. These tools enable more accurate, timely, and comprehensive measurement of health indicators, facilitating dynamic adjustments to care plans and more precise assessment of treatment effectiveness. AI algorithms can identify patterns and predict patient risks, supporting proactive interventions that improve outcomes and reduce costs. Simultaneously, increasing patient engagement and shared decision-making are critical components of the future VBHC landscape. Empowering patients to actively participate in their care decisions ensures that treatment plans align with individual preferences, values, and lifestyles, thereby enhancing satisfaction and adherence. Tools such as patient portals, mobile health applications, and digital communication platforms are making it easier for patients to access information, monitor their health, and communicate with providers, fostering a more collaborative care environment.

Expanding pilot programs and demonstration projects around the world provides valuable insights into effective strategies, challenges, and best practices in implementing VBHC and OBP models. Sharing these learnings across healthcare systems, payers, and providers accelerates the diffusion of successful approaches and helps to refine outcome measures, contracting mechanisms, and care delivery innovations. This iterative process builds a robust evidence base to support wider adoption. Over time, the integration of technology, patient-centred care, and data-driven decision-making has the potential to transform healthcare systems into sustainable models that prioritize value over volume. VBHC and OBP can incentivize continuous innovation, improve population health outcomes, and optimize resource utilization, ultimately creating healthcare ecosystems that are both financially viable and deeply responsive to patient needs. This transformation promises a future where quality, efficiency, and equity coexist, reshaping the delivery of care for generations to come.

10.3 INSURANCE MODELS AND ACCESS BARRIERS

Insurance models are fundamental determinants of access to healthcare services, playing a critical role in shaping who receives care, what type of care is available, and how quickly it can be accessed. In the context of personalized medicine and advanced medical interventions, insurance coverage often dictates whether patients can benefit from cutting-edge diagnostics, targeted therapies, or innovative treatment modalities. The structure of insurance plans—including coverage limits, formularies, and prior authorization requirements—directly impacts patients' ability to obtain these services in a timely and equitable manner. Despite the potential for insurance to facilitate access, significant barriers persist that limit patient entry into personalized healthcare. Coverage gaps remain a primary obstacle; many insurance policies do not fully cover the costs of genetic testing, biomarker analysis, or novel therapies, leaving patients with substantial out-of-pocket expenses. High deductibles, copayments, and coinsurance further exacerbate financial burdens, discouraging patients from seeking or adhering to recommended treatments. Moreover, systemic inequalities within insurance models can widen disparities in access. Individuals from lower socioeconomic backgrounds, marginalized communities, or rural areas are more likely to be uninsured or underinsured, facing reduced options and lower quality of care. These disparities are compounded by complex administrative processes, such as prior authorization hurdles and limited provider networks, which can delay or deny access to essential personalized services.

Additionally, insurance models vary widely across public and private sectors, creating inconsistencies in coverage policies and reimbursement rates for innovative treatments. This variability complicates navigation for patients and providers alike, often requiring extensive coordination and advocacy to secure necessary care. Addressing these access barriers requires policy interventions that promote comprehensive coverage of personalized medicine, reduce financial burdens on patients, and ensure equitable access across populations. Enhancing transparency in insurance benefits, streamlining authorization procedures, and expanding provider networks are vital steps toward removing obstacles. Ultimately, aligning insurance models with the goals of personalized, value-based care is essential to achieving broad access, improving health outcomes, and reducing disparities in healthcare delivery.

10.3.1 Types of Insurance Models

Healthcare insurance systems around the world exhibit considerable diversity, encompassing public insurance programs, private insurance plans, and hybrid or universal coverage models. Public insurance schemes, such as Medicare and Medicaid in the United States, provide coverage primarily for specific populations—elderly, low-income, or disabled individuals—and are often funded and administered by government entities. These programs typically have defined formularies, coverage criteria, and reimbursement policies that influence patient access to personalized treatments, sometimes limiting availability based on cost-effectiveness assessments or regulatory guidelines. Private insurance, which includes employer-sponsored plans and individual market policies, generally offers a broader range of coverage options but varies widely in terms of premiums, deductibles, copayments, and out-of-pocket maximums. Private plans may provide more flexible access to innovative therapies, yet high cost-sharing requirements can pose significant barriers, especially for expensive personalized interventions. Provider networks within private insurance can also affect access, as restricted networks may limit patients' ability to see specialists who deliver advanced care. Mixed or universal coverage models, found in many countries with national health systems, strive to balance equity and efficiency by providing comprehensive coverage to all citizens. These models often integrate public funding with private delivery mechanisms and may incorporate value-based reimbursement approaches to manage costs while promoting access to personalized medicine. However, the scope and speed of adopting new technologies and treatments within these systems can vary depending on policy priorities and budget constraints. Each insurance model's unique rules for coverage, reimbursement, and patient cost-sharing critically shape the accessibility and affordability of personalized treatments. Understanding these differences is essential for designing policies and interventions that expand access and reduce disparities in healthcare.

10.3.2 Coverage Limitations

Many insurance plans impose significant limitations on coverage for newer, personalized interventions, including genetic testing, targeted therapies, and advanced diagnostic tools. These cutting-edge services are often categorized as experimental, investigational, or non-essential due to their relatively recent emergence and evolving evidence base. As a result, insurers may deny coverage outright or impose stringent restrictions such as prior authorizations, narrow eligibility criteria, or caps on the number of tests or treatments reimbursed. Such limitations create financial barriers for patients seeking access to personalized medicine, frequently resulting in out-of-pocket expenses that many cannot afford. The lack of standardized coverage policies across insurers further complicates access. Variability in decision-making criteria and inconsistent application of clinical guidelines lead to confusion among patients and providers, who may struggle to navigate complex authorization processes. This inconsistency also contributes to delays in care, as approvals can take weeks or months, adversely affecting timely diagnosis and treatment initiation. Moreover, evolving evidence on the clinical utility and cost-effectiveness of personalized interventions often lags behind policy updates, creating a gap between technological innovation and insurance reimbursement. Without clear, evidence-based coverage guidelines, payers may be hesitant to broadly cover these services, slowing the integration of personalized medicine into routine care. Addressing these coverage limitations requires the development of transparent, consistent policies that reflect the growing clinical value of personalized interventions. Enhanced collaboration among insurers, clinicians, and researchers to establish standardized coverage criteria and real-world evidence generation is critical to reducing barriers, improving access, and ensuring equitable patient care.

10.3.3 Cost-Sharing and Financial Barriers

Even when insurance coverage for personalized medicine and advanced healthcare interventions is available, patients often face significant financial barriers due to cost-sharing mechanisms such as deductibles, copayments, and coinsurance. These out-of-pocket expenses can be substantial, particularly for high-cost therapies like targeted biologics, gene therapies, or comprehensive genetic testing. For many patients, especially those in low-income or underinsured populations, these costs may be prohibitive, effectively limiting access to treatments that could improve or even save their lives. High cost-sharing requirements can discourage patients from pursuing recommended personalized care, leading to delays in diagnosis, treatment initiation, or adherence. This financial strain not only impacts individual health outcomes but also exacerbates existing disparities, as vulnerable populations are disproportionately affected by affordability challenges. Consequently, there is a risk of widening the gap in healthcare quality and outcomes between socioeconomically advantaged and disadvantaged groups. Moreover, cost-related nonadherence can increase overall healthcare expenditures by contributing to disease progression, avoidable hospitalizations, and complications. Patients may forgo essential follow-up appointments, diagnostic tests, or medication refills due to financial concerns, undermining the effectiveness of personalized interventions. Addressing these financial barriers requires innovative insurance design strategies, such as reducing or eliminating cost-sharing for high-value personalized therapies, implementing income-based subsidies, and expanding patient assistance programs. Policymakers and payers must consider affordability as a critical component of access to personalized care to ensure equitable utilization and maximize the clinical and economic benefits of precision medicine.

10.3.4 Prior Authorization and Administrative Hurdles

Insurance plans frequently mandate prior authorization for advanced, high-cost, or personalized interventions, creating significant administrative complexity that can hinder timely patient access. This process requires healthcare providers to submit detailed documentation and justification to insurers before treatments like genetic testing, targeted therapies, or novel diagnostics are approved for coverage. While intended to ensure appropriate use and cost control, prior authorization often results in prolonged delays—sometimes lasting days or weeks—that can postpone critical diagnosis and treatment initiation, adversely affecting patient outcomes. The administrative burden associated with prior authorization frustrates both patients and providers. Patients face uncertainty and anxiety while awaiting approvals, and providers must dedicate substantial time and resources to manage paperwork, follow-ups, and appeals. This additional workload can detract from direct patient care, contribute to provider burnout, and reduce overall system efficiency. These challenges are amplified in underserved or resource-limited settings, where staff shortages and limited expertise make it difficult to navigate complex authorization requirements. Patients in these contexts may experience disproportionately long delays or outright denials, further exacerbating healthcare disparities. Moreover, inconsistent criteria across insurers add confusion, complicating care coordination and planning. Streamlining prior authorization processes through standardized criteria, electronic submissions, and real-time decision support can alleviate these barriers. Policymakers and payers should also consider exemptions or expedited pathways for high-value personalized interventions to minimize administrative friction while maintaining oversight. Ultimately, reducing administrative hurdles is crucial to enhancing access, improving patient experiences, and supporting the efficient delivery of personalized care.

10.3.5 Impact on Health Equity

Access barriers within insurance models disproportionately affect vulnerable and marginalized populations, including racial and ethnic minorities, rural residents, individuals with lower socioeconomic status, and those with disabilities. These groups often face systemic challenges that limit their ability to obtain comprehensive insurance coverage, leading to significant disparities in access to personalized medicine and advanced healthcare interventions. Insurance disparities manifest in various ways, such as lower enrolment rates in private insurance plans, higher rates of underinsurance, and greater reliance on public insurance programs that may have more restrictive coverage policies for cutting-edge treatments. The unequal availability of personalized medicine exacerbates existing health inequities by limiting access to early diagnostics, targeted therapies, and preventive care that could improve outcomes for historically underserved populations. For example, lack of coverage or high out-of-pocket costs may deter these groups from utilizing genetic testing or novel therapeutics, perpetuating disparities in disease detection and treatment efficacy. Moreover, insurance-related barriers can lead to delays in care, fragmented treatment pathways, and poorer health outcomes, reinforcing cycles of disadvantage. Structural factors such as employment type, geographic location, and broader social determinants of health further compound these challenges. Individuals employed in part-time, gig, or informal sectors often lack employer-sponsored insurance or access to affordable coverage options. Rural residents face additional hurdles due to limited provider networks, fewer specialists trained in personalized medicine, and inadequate healthcare infrastructure. Social determinants—including education, income, housing stability, and transportation—impact individuals' ability to navigate complex insurance systems and adhere to personalized treatment regimens. Addressing health equity requires multifaceted interventions aimed at expanding insurance coverage, reducing financial barriers, and ensuring culturally competent care tailored to diverse populations. Policymakers must prioritize equitable insurance reforms that broaden access to personalized interventions and support targeted outreach to vulnerable groups. Strengthening community health resources, enhancing telemedicine capabilities, and integrating social support services are also essential strategies to mitigate disparities. Ultimately, achieving health equity in personalized medicine depends on dismantling systemic insurance barriers and fostering inclusive healthcare systems that serve all populations fairly.

10.3.6 Innovations in Insurance Design

In response to persistent access barriers and rising healthcare costs, some insurers are pioneering innovative insurance designs aimed at improving access to personalized medicine and enhancing overall care quality. One notable approach is Value-Based Insurance Design (VBID), which strategically lowers or eliminates patient cost-sharing—such as copayments and deductibles—for high-value services that have proven clinical effectiveness. By reducing financial burdens on patients for essential personalized interventions like genetic testing, targeted therapies, and chronic disease management, VBID encourages greater utilization of these services and supports better health outcomes. Additionally, several insurers are developing programs that offer tailored benefits specifically for individuals with chronic conditions or identified genetic risks. These initiatives focus on preventive care and early intervention, leveraging personalized data to create customized care plans that address patients' unique needs. Such targeted coverage promotes proactive management of diseases, potentially reducing costly complications and hospitalizations in the long term. Flexible insurance plans that provide broader provider networks and integrated care pathways further help reduce access barriers. By expanding the choice of specialists and facilities experienced in delivering personalized treatments, these plans improve timely access to high-quality care. Integrated care models also facilitate coordination among multidisciplinary teams, enhancing patient experience and clinical effectiveness. Moreover, some insurers are embracing digital health tools and telemedicine within their coverage to reach underserved populations and streamline care delivery. These innovations can bridge geographic and socioeconomic gaps, making personalized healthcare more accessible and convenient. Collectively, these innovative insurance designs represent important steps toward aligning financial incentives with value-driven care. By focusing on affordability, customization, and integrated support, insurers can play a crucial role in expanding access to personalized medicine and fostering more equitable healthcare systems.

10.3.7 Role of Policy and Regulation

Government policies and regulations play a pivotal role in shaping the landscape of insurance coverage, affordability, and consumer protections, thereby directly influencing access to personalized medicine and advanced healthcare interventions. Legislative mandates that require insurance plans to cover essential services—such as specific genetic tests, targeted therapies, and preventive screenings—help establish a baseline of standardized access across populations. These mandates reduce variability among insurers and ensure that critical personalized healthcare options are not excluded due to cost or perceived novelty. Subsidies and financial assistance programs, including Medicaid expansion and premium tax credits offered through insurance marketplaces, are vital tools to increase insurance uptake and reduce the prevalence of underinsurance, particularly among low-income and vulnerable groups. By making coverage more affordable and accessible, these policy measures enable more patients to benefit from personalized interventions that might otherwise be financially out of reach. Regulatory frameworks also serve to protect consumers from unfair practices such as discriminatory coverage denials or excessive cost-sharing. Protections against pre-existing condition exclusions, coverage rescissions, and surprise billing help create a more equitable insurance environment that supports sustained access to necessary care. Ongoing policy reforms continue to grapple with balancing the need to incentivize medical innovation with the imperative of equitable access. This includes efforts to streamline coverage approval processes, promote transparency in pricing and outcomes, and encourage value-based payment models that reward effective, personalized care. Policymakers are increasingly recognizing the importance of integrating real-world evidence and patient-centred outcomes into coverage decisions to ensure that policies remain responsive to evolving healthcare technologies and patient needs. Ultimately, robust policy and regulatory frameworks are essential for creating a healthcare system where personalized medicine can thrive—delivering high-quality, affordable, and equitable care for all individuals regardless of socioeconomic status or geographic location.

10.3.8 Future Directions

As personalized healthcare continues to advance rapidly, insurance models must evolve proactively to ensure broad, equitable access to these transformative interventions. One critical future direction is enhancing transparency in coverage decisions, enabling patients and providers to better understand what services are covered, under what conditions, and how to navigate the approval processes. Clear, accessible information can reduce confusion, build trust, and empower informed decision-making. Streamlining prior authorization and other administrative requirements is also essential to minimize delays and administrative burdens that currently impede timely access to personalized diagnostics and treatments. Leveraging technology such as electronic prior authorization systems and standardized clinical criteria can accelerate approvals and reduce provider workload. In addition to financial barriers, non-financial obstacles like social determinants of health—housing instability, transportation challenges, and limited health literacy—play a significant role in limiting access to personalized care. Insurance models that integrate social support services, either directly or through partnerships with community organizations, can help address these factors. Providing care navigation, language assistance, and patient education tailored to diverse populations will improve adherence and outcomes. Collaborative efforts among payers, healthcare providers, policymakers, and patient advocates are crucial to designing and implementing insurance frameworks that are both inclusive and sustainable. These stakeholders must work together to develop flexible benefit designs, equitable reimbursement policies, and value-based approaches that reward innovation while maintaining affordability. Ultimately, by fostering adaptive insurance models that respond to scientific progress and patient needs holistically, the healthcare system can unlock the full potential of personalized medicine—ensuring that its benefits reach all individuals, regardless of socioeconomic status or geographic location, and contribute to improved population health on a broad scale.

10.4 ECONOMIC EVALUATION OF GENOMIC TESTING

Genomic testing has fundamentally transformed personalized medicine by facilitating more precise diagnosis, prognosis, and individualized treatment strategies. As these tests become increasingly integrated into clinical practice, understanding their economic impact is crucial for sustainable healthcare delivery. Economic evaluations of genomic testing systematically assess both the direct and indirect costs involved—such as test expenses, downstream healthcare savings, and productivity changes—alongside clinical outcomes like improved patient survival and quality of life. These analyses employ methodologies like cost-effectiveness, cost-utility, and cost-benefit assessments to provide comprehensive insights. By quantifying the value for money, economic evaluations help policymakers and healthcare providers prioritize interventions that maximize health benefits within budget constraints. Additionally, they highlight areas where genomic testing may reduce unnecessary treatments and hospitalizations, potentially lowering overall healthcare expenditure. Balancing innovation with affordability ensures equitable access to genomic technologies while optimizing resource allocation. Consequently, economic evaluations play a pivotal role in guiding investment decisions, reimbursement policies, and the integration of genomic testing into routine care pathways.

10.4.1 Types of Economic Evaluations

Several methodologies are used to assess genomic testing economically:

- **Cost-Effectiveness Analysis (CEA):** CEA compares the relative costs and health outcomes of genomic testing against standard care, often measuring outcomes in terms of quality-adjusted life years (QALYs) or life years gained. This method helps determine whether the additional health benefits of genomic testing justify its higher costs. By quantifying both the economic investment and clinical effectiveness, CEA supports healthcare decision-makers in prioritizing interventions that deliver the greatest value. It is particularly useful for assessing new technologies where clinical benefits are measurable but costs are substantial. This approach can guide reimbursement decisions and optimize allocation of limited healthcare resources.
- **Cost-Benefit Analysis (CBA):** CBA translates both the costs and outcomes of genomic testing into monetary values, enabling a direct comparison of net benefits or losses. This comprehensive approach assesses whether the financial gains, such as reduced hospital admissions or increased productivity, outweigh the costs of testing and follow-up care. By assigning dollar values to health outcomes, CBA provides a clear metric for decision-makers focused on maximizing economic efficiency. It is especially valuable when comparing genomic testing to other healthcare investments with diverse outcomes. Ultimately, CBA helps determine if genomic testing offers a positive return on investment within broader health and societal contexts.
- **Cost-Utility Analysis (CUA):** CUA extends beyond traditional cost-effectiveness by incorporating patient preferences and quality of life into the evaluation framework. It quantifies outcomes using metrics like QALYs that reflect both the length and quality of life gained through genomic testing. This patient-centred approach captures the subjective benefits of personalized medicine, including improved wellbeing and reduced anxiety. By balancing costs against these nuanced outcomes, CUA provides a richer understanding of value from the patient's perspective. It supports decisions that not only enhance survival but also improve overall life satisfaction and functional status, which are critical in chronic or complex conditions.

- **Budget Impact Analysis (BIA):** BIA estimates the short- and medium-term financial consequences of adopting genomic testing within a specific healthcare system or budget. Unlike other analyses focused on cost-effectiveness, BIA addresses affordability by projecting the total expenditure impact over a defined time horizon. It accounts for factors such as the number of eligible patients, test uptake rates, and downstream cost savings from improved clinical management. This analysis helps healthcare payers anticipate budgetary pressures and plan resource allocation effectively. By providing a realistic financial forecast, BIA supports the sustainable integration of genomic technologies without compromising other healthcare priorities.

10.4.2 Direct Costs Considered

Economic evaluations of genomic testing rigorously incorporate a range of direct costs associated with the testing process and subsequent clinical management. These costs begin with the price of the genomic test itself, which can vary significantly depending on the technology used—ranging from targeted single-gene tests to more comprehensive approaches like multi-gene panels, whole-exome sequencing, or whole-genome sequencing. Beyond the initial test cost, evaluations also consider expenses related to follow-up diagnostic procedures required to confirm or further investigate findings. Genetic counselling services, an essential component for interpreting results and guiding patients, add to the overall direct costs. Additionally, treatment modifications prompted by genomic findings, such as targeted therapies or preventive interventions, contribute to expenditure. Continuous monitoring and long-term patient management based on test outcomes also represent ongoing costs. The healthcare setting—whether inpatient, outpatient, or specialized clinics—further influences cost variability due to differences in resource utilization and pricing structures. Accurate accounting of these direct costs is crucial for assessing the economic viability and budget impact of integrating genomic testing into routine clinical practice. Such detailed cost consideration enables stakeholders to understand the financial commitments involved and to plan accordingly for sustainable implementation.

10.4.3 Indirect and Downstream Costs

In addition to direct expenses, economic evaluations of genomic testing take into account indirect costs that impact patients and society. These include patient-related factors such as time spent undergoing testing and counselling, travel expenses to healthcare facilities, and productivity losses due to time off work or reduced functional capacity. Such costs can be substantial, especially when testing requires multiple visits or specialized centres far from the patient's home. Furthermore, downstream costs and savings play a critical role in the overall economic assessment. Early and more precise genomic-based interventions often lead to avoidance of ineffective or unnecessary treatments, thereby reducing medication costs and adverse effects. Preventing complications or disease progression through timely, targeted therapy can also decrease hospital admissions and emergency care expenses. These downstream effects can generate significant long-term savings that offset the initial investment in testing. By capturing both indirect and downstream financial impacts, evaluations provide a more comprehensive understanding of the true economic value of genomic testing across the entire patient care pathway.

10.4.4 Clinical Utility and Impact on Outcomes

The clinical utility of genomic testing—the extent to which it meaningfully improves patient health outcomes—is a central consideration in economic evaluations. Tests that enable more precise and personalized treatment plans can lead to better-targeted therapies, reducing exposure to ineffective or harmful medications. Early disease detection through genomic insights facilitates timely interventions, which can slow or prevent disease progression and improve prognosis. Additionally, genomic risk stratification helps identify patients at higher risk who may benefit from intensified monitoring or preventive measures, thereby minimizing adverse events. These improvements in clinical management can translate into significant reductions in morbidity and mortality, directly enhancing patient quality of life. Moreover, by optimizing healthcare utilization—such as fewer hospitalizations, emergency visits, or invasive procedures—genomic testing may offset its upfront costs over time. Therefore, demonstrating clear clinical utility is essential not only for patient benefit but also for supporting the cost-effectiveness and broader adoption of genomic technologies within healthcare systems.

10.4.5 Challenges in Economic Evaluation:

- **Uncertain Evidence:** The limited availability of robust, long-term clinical data on genomic testing's benefits and potential risks makes it difficult to produce precise cost-effectiveness estimates. As many genomic applications are relatively new, evidence on patient outcomes, durability of benefits, and unintended consequences is still evolving. This uncertainty can lead to wide variations in economic models and impact confidence in decision-making.

- **Rapid Technological Change:** Genomic technologies are advancing at a rapid pace, with frequent introduction of new testing methods, improved accuracy, and reduced costs. This swift innovation cycle often outpaces the timelines required for thorough economic evaluations, leading to assessments that may quickly become outdated or fail to capture the latest improvements in clinical utility or cost savings.

- **Population Heterogeneity:** Patients differ widely in genetics, disease characteristics, and response to genomic-guided interventions. This heterogeneity means that the benefits and cost-effectiveness of genomic testing can vary significantly across subgroups, challenging the generalizability of economic results. Tailored evaluations may be needed to accurately assess value within specific populations.
- **Ethical and Social Considerations:** Certain benefits of genomic testing, such as psychological reassurance, informed family planning, or reduced uncertainty about disease risk, are inherently subjective and difficult to quantify economically. Incorporating these ethical and social dimensions into traditional cost-effectiveness frameworks remains a complex challenge, yet they are vital for a holistic assessment of genomic testing's value.

10.4.6 Health System Perspectives

Economic evaluations of genomic testing can yield different conclusions depending on the perspective adopted, as each stakeholder values costs and benefits differently. From the payer perspective—such as insurance companies or government health programs—the focus tends to be on direct healthcare costs and short- to medium-term budget impact. Payers prioritize interventions that demonstrate clear cost savings or cost-effectiveness within their coverage period to ensure sustainable spending. In contrast, the provider perspective, including hospitals and clinicians, often emphasizes clinical outcomes, workflow implications, and resource utilization, considering how genomic testing affects patient management, staff time, and operational efficiency. From the patient perspective, evaluations highlight out-of-pocket expenses, quality of life improvements, and psychosocial benefits such as reduced anxiety or increased empowerment through personalized care. Meanwhile, the societal perspective offers the broadest view by incorporating not only healthcare costs but also wider economic and social factors. This includes productivity gains from patients returning to work sooner, decreased absenteeism, and reduced burden on caregivers and families. Societal evaluations also consider intangible benefits like improved population health and long-term economic growth. The choice of perspective influences which costs and outcomes are included in the analysis and, ultimately, the perceived value of genomic testing. Recognizing these varied viewpoints is essential for balanced decision-making and for developing policies that reflect the interests of all stakeholders within the health ecosystem.

10.4.6 Reimbursement and Coverage Decisions

Economic evaluations play a critical role in shaping insurance coverage and reimbursement policies for genomic testing. When cost-effectiveness analyses demonstrate clear clinical benefits and acceptable costs relative to health outcomes, payers are more likely to approve funding, facilitating broader patient access to these innovative tests. Conversely, if evaluations reveal uncertain or unfavourable economic value, reimbursement may be restricted, limiting the availability of genomic testing in routine care. Transparent, evidence-based decision-making frameworks are essential to ensure that coverage policies are fair, consistent, and aligned with the best available data. Such frameworks help balance innovation with affordability, preventing unsustainable spending while encouraging adoption of technologies that truly improve patient outcomes. Additionally, ongoing data collection and re-evaluation enable policies to adapt as new evidence and technologies emerge. Ultimately, integrating economic evidence into reimbursement decisions supports a sustainable healthcare system that maximizes value for patients and society.

10.4.7 Future Directions

The future of economic evaluation in genomic testing is poised for significant advancement, driven by improvements in data analytics and the increased availability of real-world evidence. Leveraging large-scale clinical and genomic databases will enable more accurate and dynamic assessments of cost-effectiveness, reflecting diverse patient experiences and long-term outcomes beyond controlled trial settings. Emerging personalized cost-effectiveness models, which integrate individual risk profiles, genetic variability, and patient preferences, promise to enhance the precision and relevance of economic evaluations. These tailored approaches will better capture heterogeneity in patient responses and optimize decision-making at the individual level. Additionally, future evaluations are likely to incorporate ethical and equity considerations more explicitly, addressing disparities in access and outcomes to ensure that genomic testing benefits are distributed fairly across populations. By embedding social values and fairness into economic frameworks, evaluations will align more closely with societal priorities. Together, these developments will support more informed, equitable, and sustainable integration of genomic technologies into healthcare systems worldwide.

10.5 HEALTH TECHNOLOGY ASSESSMENT IN PERSONALIZED MEDICINE

Health Technology Assessment (HTA) is a comprehensive, multidisciplinary process designed to systematically evaluate the wide-ranging implications of health interventions or technologies. In the context of personalized medicine, HTA becomes particularly vital due to the complex nature of genomic and biomarker-driven innovations. It encompasses not only clinical effectiveness but also economic value, organizational impact, ethical considerations, and social consequences. By integrating evidence from clinical trials, real-world data, economic analyses, and patient perspectives, HTA provides a robust framework to assess whether new personalized technologies genuinely improve health outcomes and do so in a cost-effective manner. This ensures that healthcare systems adopt innovations that offer meaningful benefits without exacerbating inequalities or straining resources. HTA also evaluates practical feasibility, including infrastructure needs, workforce training, and integration into existing care pathways, which are critical for the successful implementation of personalized approaches. Ethical dimensions—such as informed consent, data privacy, and equitable access—are scrutinized to uphold patient rights and societal values. Moreover, HTA supports decision-makers by synthesizing complex information into actionable recommendations for policymakers, payers, clinicians, and patients. In an era of rapid technological advancement, HTA helps balance innovation with affordability, guiding sustainable investment in personalized medicine. Ultimately, HTA serves as a bridge between cutting-edge science and real-world healthcare, ensuring that personalized interventions translate into improved health outcomes, better quality of life, and equitable access for diverse patient populations.

10.5.1 Scope and Objectives of HTA

Health Technology Assessment (HTA) aims to provide comprehensive, evidence-based information to policymakers, healthcare providers, and payers regarding personalized medicine technologies. It evaluates multiple dimensions including the clinical effectiveness, safety profile, economic implications, and broader societal impacts of these interventions. The primary objective is to guide informed decision-making around the adoption, reimbursement, and clinical use of innovative genomic and biomarker-driven tools. HTA seeks to balance the promise of cutting-edge personalized therapies with the practical realities of healthcare sustainability, ensuring that new technologies deliver meaningful health improvements without imposing unsustainable costs. By synthesizing data from clinical trials, real-world studies, and economic analyses, HTA offers a rigorous framework to assess value. It also anticipates potential challenges in implementation, resource allocation, and equity. Through its multidisciplinary approach, HTA supports healthcare systems in prioritizing interventions that improve patient outcomes efficiently and equitably. Ultimately, the scope of HTA extends beyond technical assessment to include ethical, organizational, and societal considerations critical for responsible innovation in personalized medicine.

10.5.2 Assessment of Clinical Effectiveness

Within HTA, a thorough evaluation of clinical effectiveness is fundamental. This involves assessing the clinical validity—how accurately a genomic or biomarker test identifies or predicts a clinical condition—and clinical utility, which measures the impact of test results on patient management and health outcomes. HTA reviews evidence from randomized controlled trials, observational studies, and real-world data sources to compare personalized interventions with existing standard care. This includes targeted therapies, companion diagnostics, and genetic tests, determining whether they lead to improved survival rates, reduced morbidity, or enhanced quality of life. The assessment also considers the strength, consistency, and applicability of the data across different populations and healthcare settings. Identifying gaps in evidence and areas of uncertainty is key to guiding further research and ensuring responsible clinical adoption. Ultimately, by validating both accuracy and meaningful clinical benefit, HTA ensures that personalized medicine technologies provide tangible improvements in patient care rather than incremental or unproven advantages.

10.5.3 Economic Evaluation within HTA

Economic evaluation is a cornerstone of HTA, providing critical insight into the value for money of personalized medicine interventions. This includes cost-effectiveness analysis, which compares the costs and health outcomes—often measured in quality-adjusted life years (QALYs)—of genomic tests or targeted therapies against standard treatment options. Budget impact analysis estimates the financial implications of adopting these technologies at a system level, helping payers anticipate changes in expenditure over time. HTA also examines resource utilization, including hospital stays, outpatient visits, medication use, and long-term care costs that may be influenced by personalized approaches. Importantly, economic evaluations extend beyond upfront costs, factoring in potential savings from reduced adverse events, improved disease management, and avoided complications. By integrating these analyses, HTA supports decisions that optimize healthcare spending while enhancing patient outcomes. Transparency in assumptions, data sources, and modelling techniques is essential to build trust among stakeholders and facilitate evidence-based reimbursement and coverage policies (Fig. 4) .

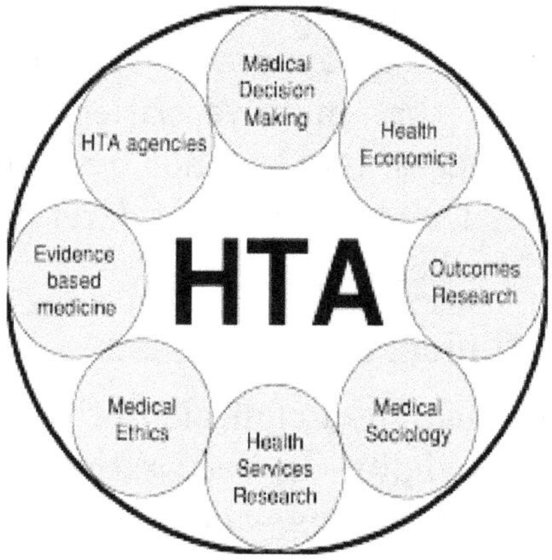

Fig. 4 Health technology assessment

10.5.4 Ethical, Legal, and Social Implications (ELSI)

HTA frameworks rigorously incorporate the ethical, legal, and social implications (ELSI) of personalized medicine technologies to ensure that innovation aligns with societal values and respects individual rights. This involves addressing critical issues such as patient privacy, informed consent processes, and data ownership in the context of genomic information, which is uniquely sensitive and potentially identifiable. Equity of access is a major concern, as disparities in availability of genomic tests or therapies could exacerbate existing health inequalities across socioeconomic or demographic groups. HTA also considers the risk of genetic discrimination in employment or insurance based on test results. Furthermore, the psychosocial impact on patients and families, including anxiety or stigma, is examined to provide a holistic view of the technology's consequences. By embedding ELSI considerations, HTA promotes ethical stewardship and fosters public trust, which are essential for the responsible deployment of personalized medicine in clinical practice.

10.5.5 Organizational and Implementation Considerations

A critical component of HTA is evaluating the readiness of healthcare systems to integrate personalized medicine technologies effectively. This includes assessing infrastructure needs such as advanced laboratory facilities, bioinformatics platforms, and data management systems essential for handling complex genomic information. Workforce capacity and training are pivotal, as clinicians, genetic counsellors, and support staff require specialized skills to interpret test results and communicate them to patients. HTA also examines potential changes to clinical workflows, ensuring that genomic testing fits seamlessly into existing care pathways without causing delays or inefficiencies. Consideration of reimbursement mechanisms and regulatory requirements further informs implementation feasibility. Identifying barriers and facilitators within healthcare organizations enables proactive strategies to support adoption, minimize disruption, and maximize clinical benefit. By addressing these organizational challenges, HTA helps ensure that personalized medicine innovations translate from research settings into routine, scalable healthcare delivery.

10.5.6 Stakeholder Engagement

Effective HTA processes rely on meaningful engagement with a broad range of stakeholders to ensure that assessments are comprehensive, relevant, and trustworthy. Patients and patient advocacy groups provide critical insights into lived experiences, preferences, and priorities, helping to centre evaluations around real-world needs and outcomes. Clinicians contribute expertise on clinical applicability, practical challenges, and potential benefits or harms of personalized interventions. Payers and insurers offer perspectives on budget constraints, reimbursement policies, and health system sustainability. Industry representatives share information on technology development, market trends, and innovation pathways. Ethicists and legal experts guide considerations of societal values, patient rights, and regulatory frameworks. Engaging these diverse groups promotes transparency and inclusivity, fostering mutual understanding and trust. It also enhances the quality and acceptability of HTA recommendations, facilitating smoother adoption and broader support for personalized medicine technologies. Structured stakeholder involvement is thus a cornerstone for robust and socially responsive health technology assessments.

10.5.7 Challenges Specific to Personalized Medicine HTA

Health Technology Assessment (HTA) in personalized medicine faces unique challenges due to the rapid pace of innovation. Genomic and multi-omics technologies evolve quickly, often outstripping the time required to generate robust clinical evidence and complete thorough assessments. This fast development cycle complicates decision-making and risks rendering HTA findings outdated shortly after publication. The complexity of data adds another layer of difficulty; integrating diverse biological information such as genomics, proteomics, metabolomics, and other biomarkers requires sophisticated analytical methods, which can be resource-intensive and introduce uncertainty in interpretation. Additionally, personalized interventions typically benefit specific patient subgroups defined by genetic or molecular profiles, making it challenging to generalize results across broader populations or healthcare settings. This heterogeneity demands tailored assessments and complicates the development of universal reimbursement policies. Finally, the evidence base in personalized medicine is highly dynamic, with ongoing discoveries, improved technologies, and evolving clinical guidelines necessitating adaptive HTA frameworks. These must be flexible enough to incorporate new data continuously and update recommendations accordingly, ensuring relevance and responsiveness in a rapidly changing landscape.

- **Rapid Innovation:** Fast-paced development of genomic tools can outstrip evidence generation and HTA processes.
- **Complexity of Data:** Integrating multi-omics data and biomarkers complicates assessment.
- **Heterogeneity of Patient Populations:** Personalized interventions may benefit only specific subgroups, challenging generalization of results.
- **Dynamic Evidence Base:** Continuous updates in technology and knowledge require adaptive HTA approaches.

10.5.8 International Variability

Health Technology Assessment (HTA) methods and regulatory requirements differ considerably across countries and regions, leading to variability in how personalized medicine technologies are evaluated, approved, and reimbursed. These differences stem from diverse healthcare system structures, funding mechanisms, cultural values, and policy priorities. As a result, access to genomic tests, targeted therapies, and other personalized interventions can vary widely between high-income and low- or middle-income countries, as well as among different healthcare settings within the same country. This variability poses challenges for manufacturers, payers, and clinicians, complicating market entry and limiting the global reach of innovations. To address these issues, international harmonization efforts and collaborative initiatives have emerged, aiming to standardize HTA methodologies, share best practices, and promote alignment in evidence requirements. Organizations such as the International Network of Agencies for Health Technology Assessment (INAHTA) and the European Network for Health Technology Assessment (EUnetHTA) facilitate cross-border cooperation and knowledge exchange. Such collaborations help streamline assessments, reduce duplication of efforts, and accelerate the adoption of effective personalized medicine technologies worldwide. Ultimately, fostering international consistency enhances equity in access, supports innovation, and optimizes resource use across diverse healthcare systems.

10.5.9 Future Directions

The future of Health Technology Assessment (HTA) in personalized medicine is increasingly shaped by advancements in data science and evolving healthcare priorities. Emerging HTA models are beginning to incorporate real-world data analytics, leveraging large-scale health databases, electronic health records, and patient registries to generate timely, relevant evidence on clinical effectiveness and safety outside controlled trial settings. Machine learning and artificial intelligence tools are being integrated to analyse complex multi-omics data, identify patterns, and predict treatment responses, thereby enhancing the precision and depth of assessments. Additionally, patient-reported outcomes are gaining prominence in HTA, capturing quality of life, symptom burden, and treatment preferences directly from patients to ensure that evaluations reflect real-world experiences and priorities. These innovations enable a more holistic understanding of personalized medicine's value, beyond traditional clinical and economic metrics. Furthermore, there is a growing shift toward continuous and iterative HTA processes that adapt dynamically as new evidence and technologies emerge. This flexible approach allows timely updates to recommendations, ensuring assessments remain relevant amid rapid scientific progress and changing clinical practice. By embracing these future directions, HTA can better support sustainable, patient-centred integration of personalized medicine into healthcare systems worldwide.

11 Chapter

REGULATORY LANDSCAPE AND CLINICAL IMPLEMENTATION

11.0 INTRODUCTION: AN OVERVIEW

The regulatory landscape and clinical implementation of personalized medicine represent critical and intertwined domains that influence the successful translation of genomic and biomarker-driven innovations from research laboratories to routine patient care. Personalized medicine, characterized by the tailoring of healthcare decisions and treatments to individual genetic, environmental, and lifestyle factors, holds great promise for improving health outcomes, enhancing treatment efficacy, and reducing adverse effects. However, realizing this potential requires navigating a complex framework of regulations designed to ensure the safety, effectiveness, quality, and ethical use of emerging technologies. These regulations encompass a broad range of components, including the approval and oversight of genomic tests, companion diagnostics, targeted therapies, and digital health tools that support personalized care. Regulatory bodies across different countries have developed distinct pathways, guidelines, and standards that reflect their unique legal systems, healthcare infrastructures, and societal values. This diversity creates challenges for developers and healthcare providers in achieving global harmonization and timely patient access. Beyond regulatory approval, the clinical implementation of personalized medicine involves practical considerations such as integration into healthcare workflows, provider education, reimbursement mechanisms, and patient engagement. Effective implementation is essential to ensure that genomic technologies are not only available but also appropriately utilized to inform diagnosis, prognosis, and treatment decisions. It requires multidisciplinary collaboration among clinicians, laboratorians, genetic counsellors, payers, and policymakers, supported by robust infrastructure for data management, interpretation, and sharing. Moreover, clinical implementation must address barriers related to cost, health equity, data privacy, and ethical concerns to foster trust and maximize benefits across diverse populations (Fig. 1).

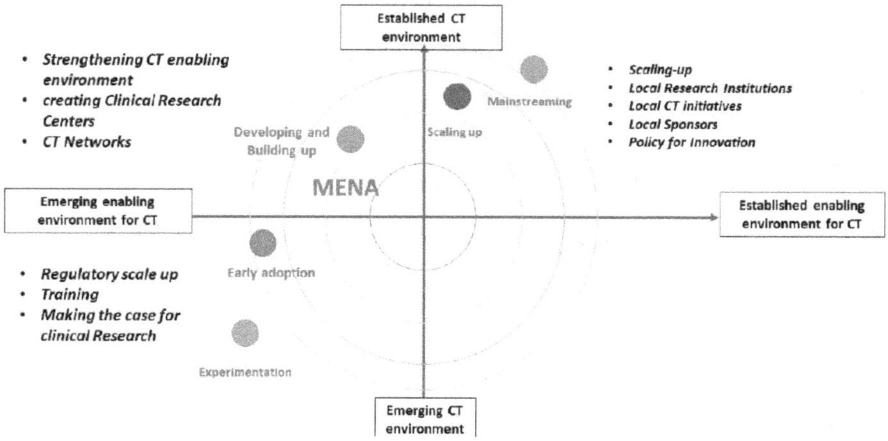

Fig. 1Regulatory framework and sustainable capacity development

This chapter provides a comprehensive overview of the regulatory environment governing personalized medicine, highlighting the evolving frameworks that govern the development, validation, and commercialization of genomic tests and associated therapies. It explores the pathways for regulatory approval, quality assurance, and post-market surveillance, emphasizing the role of international harmonization efforts in facilitating innovation while safeguarding public health. Additionally, the chapter examines key factors influencing clinical adoption, including clinical guidelines, healthcare system readiness, reimbursement policies, and the importance of stakeholder engagement. Emerging trends such as adaptive regulatory models, real-world evidence integration, and digital health innovations are also discussed, reflecting ongoing efforts to align regulatory processes with the fast pace of scientific discovery. Ultimately, understanding the regulatory landscape and clinical implementation strategies is vital for all stakeholders involved in personalized medicine—from researchers and industry developers to clinicians and patients. It ensures that advancements in genomics and precision therapeutics translate into improved patient care in a manner that is safe, effective, ethical, and sustainable.

11.1 GLOBAL REGULATORY FRAMEWORKS (FDA, EMA, PMDA)

Global regulatory agencies play an essential role in overseeing the safety, efficacy, and quality of medical products, and their responsibilities have expanded significantly with the rise of personalized medicine. As genomic testing, biomarker-driven therapies, and AI-assisted diagnostics become central to clinical decision-making, regulators are adapting their frameworks to accommodate these complex and evolving technologies. Among the leading authorities, the U.S. Food and Drug Administration (FDA), the European Medicines Agency (EMA), and Japan's Pharmaceuticals and Medical Devices Agency (PMDA) are at the forefront of shaping global regulatory standards. The FDA has been a pioneer in regulating personalized medicine through initiatives like the Precision Medicine Initiative and its established guidance for companion diagnostics, next-generation sequencing (NGS), and AI-based tools. It employs a risk-based approach and has introduced expedited review pathways such as Breakthrough Device and Fast Track designations to accelerate access to promising innovations. The EMA similarly emphasizes scientific rigor and early stakeholder engagement, using adaptive pathways and parallel scientific advice to support timely approvals for advanced therapies and diagnostics within the European Union. The PMDA in Japan has made significant strides in integrating personalized medicine into its regulatory agenda, promoting innovation through early consultation systems and accelerated approval mechanisms, particularly for regenerative and cell-based therapies. Despite differences in regulatory structure and policy priorities, all three agencies share common objectives: safeguarding public health, fostering innovation, ensuring patient access to effective treatments, and supporting international harmonization. Collaborative efforts like the International Council for Harmonisation of Technical Requirements for Pharmaceuticals for Human Use (ICH) and the International Medical Device Regulators Forum (IMDRF) aim to streamline global regulatory processes and reduce redundancies. As personalized medicine continues to evolve, these regulatory bodies are working toward more flexible, data-driven, and patient-centred approaches to support safe and equitable implementation worldwide.

11.1.1 U.S. Food and Drug Administration (FDA)

The FDA oversees the regulation of pharmaceuticals, medical devices, biologics, and genetic tests in the United States. It has developed specific pathways for personalized medicine, including:

- **Regulatory Pathways:** The FDA utilizes established regulatory pathways such as Investigational New Drug (IND) applications for pharmaceuticals and Premarket Approval (PMA) or 510(k) clearances for medical devices. In the era of personalized medicine, these pathways have been adapted to account for new modalities, including gene therapies, cell-based products, and companion diagnostics. Companion diagnostics, in particular, must demonstrate a clear linkage between the diagnostic result and the effectiveness or safety of a corresponding therapy. The FDA works closely with sponsors to ensure co-development of drugs and diagnostics. Flexibility has been introduced to streamline approvals when safety and efficacy are well established. Additionally, the agency encourages early dialogue and submission of comprehensive genomic and biomarker data. This adaptive approach allows faster evaluation of breakthrough therapies that address unmet medical needs in targeted patient populations.

- **Precision Medicine Initiative:** Launched in 2015, the Precision Medicine Initiative (PMI) signalled a transformative shift in the FDA's approach to healthcare, emphasizing individualized treatment strategies based on genetic, environmental, and lifestyle differences. This initiative has driven regulatory reforms aimed at accelerating the development and approval of precision therapies. It supports data sharing, biobanking, and the integration of genomic information into clinical research and regulatory submissions. The initiative has also helped foster collaboration between public and private stakeholders, advancing the development of more effective, patient-centred treatments. The FDA, as a key agency in PMI, developed new frameworks for evaluating complex biomarkers, adaptive clinical trials, and real-world data. As a result, the regulatory process has become more responsive to innovations in precision therapeutics and diagnostics.
- **Guidance on Genomic Data:** Recognizing the growing role of genomics in medicine, the FDA has issued several guidance documents on the appropriate use, interpretation, and validation of genomic data in drug development and regulatory submissions. These documents aim to standardize the use of next-generation sequencing (NGS), pharmacogenomics, and biomarker-based strategies to ensure reliability and reproducibility. Guidance includes recommendations for data quality, bioinformatics pipelines, variant classification, and analytical validation. The FDA also encourages the use of genomic data to identify subpopulations for targeted therapies and supports master protocols that integrate genomics into clinical trials. This regulatory clarity helps industry stakeholders align with best practices and accelerates the safe adoption of personalized therapies in clinical practice.
- **Digital Health and AI Regulation:** As software and algorithms become increasingly central to personalized care, the FDA has established frameworks for regulating digital health tools, including Software as a Medical Device (SaMD). The agency evaluates AI and machine learning (AI/ML)-based technologies through a risk-based approach, considering factors such as transparency, explainability, and the potential for adaptive learning. Its Digital Health Centre of Excellence leads efforts to ensure that digital tools are safe, effective, and appropriately validated. The FDA has also released discussion papers and guidance on the regulatory oversight of AI/ML products that evolve post-market. Continuous learning algorithms, in particular, pose regulatory challenges, prompting the development of the "Predetermined Change Control Plan" to manage future updates. These policies aim to promote innovation while maintaining robust safeguards.

- **Post-market Surveillance:** Post-market surveillance is a vital aspect of the FDA's approach to regulating personalized medicine, ensuring ongoing safety and effectiveness once products reach the market. For high-risk or novel therapies—such as gene therapies or AI-driven diagnostics—the FDA emphasizes the use of real-world evidence (RWE) collected from electronic health records, registries, and patient-reported outcomes. Manufacturers may be required to conduct post-approval studies or submit periodic safety updates. This ongoing data collection supports early detection of adverse events, long-term risk assessment, and iterative improvements in product performance. The Sentinel Initiative and other real-world data platforms further strengthen the agency's capacity for active surveillance. These strategies allow the FDA to maintain regulatory oversight in a rapidly evolving scientific and technological environment (Table-1).

Table:1 The key aspects of the FDA's approach to personalized medicine

Regulatory Focus	FDA Approach
Regulatory Pathways	Uses traditional IND and PMA pathways, adapted for gene therapies and companion diagnostics.
Precision Medicine Initiative	Launched to accelerate development and regulatory support for tailored, individualized treatments.
Guidance on Genomic Data	Provides guidance on NGS, biomarker validation, and use of genomic data in drug submissions.
Digital Health & AI Regulation	Regulates SaMD; applies risk-based framework for AI/ML tools with focus on transparency and safety.
Post-market Surveillance	Utilizes real-world evidence and post-approval monitoring, especially for high-risk personalized therapies.

11.1.2 European Medicines Agency (EMA)

The EMA serves as the central regulatory body for the European Union member states, coordinating evaluation and supervision of medicines.

Centralized Marketing Authorization: The EMA offers a centralized marketing authorization procedure, allowing pharmaceutical companies to obtain a single approval that is valid across all European Union (EU) member states. This streamlined process enhances efficiency and consistency, making it easier for innovative personalized medicine products to enter multiple markets simultaneously. The centralized route is mandatory for certain product categories, including advanced therapies and medicines developed using biotechnology, which are often central to personalized medicine. This approach reduces regulatory duplication, accelerates patient access to new treatments, and promotes uniform safety and efficacy standards across Europe.

- **Adaptive Pathways:** To keep pace with rapidly advancing science, the EMA has developed adaptive pathways that allow for flexible, stepwise marketing authorization, particularly for therapies that address unmet medical needs. This regulatory model enables early access to promising personalized treatments based on initial data, with additional evidence generated post-approval. Adaptive pathways are especially useful for rare diseases or targeted therapies supported by biomarker data. The iterative process fosters earlier patient benefit while maintaining rigorous safety oversight. It also encourages closer collaboration among regulators, developers, HTA bodies, and patient groups throughout the product lifecycle.
- **Pharmacogenomics and Biomarkers:** EMA has made substantial efforts to integrate pharmacogenomics and biomarker data into regulatory decision-making, recognizing their essential role in stratified and personalized medicine. The agency provides scientific advice and guidance on incorporating biomarker validation into clinical trial design, companion diagnostic development, and patient selection. Biomarkers are assessed not only for diagnostic utility but also for their ability to predict efficacy, safety, or disease progression. Through these measures, the EMA supports more precise and individualized approaches to treatment, reducing trial inefficiencies and enhancing therapeutic outcomes.
- **Health Technology Assessment (HTA) Alignment:** Understanding the need for coherence between regulatory approval and reimbursement decisions, the EMA collaborates with Health Technology Assessment (HTA) bodies across Europe. This cooperation aims to align evidence requirements and accelerate access to personalized medicine therapies. Joint scientific consultations and early dialogue mechanisms allow developers to obtain feedback from both regulators and HTA agencies, promoting efficient trial design and robust value demonstration. Such alignment improves the likelihood of rapid adoption into national healthcare systems and ensures that both clinical and economic considerations are addressed early in development.
- **Digital Health Regulations:** The European Union's Medical Device Regulation (MDR) and In Vitro Diagnostic Regulation (IVDR) have significantly impacted the approval pathways for digital health solutions, including genomic tests and AI-driven tools. These regulations emphasize clinical evidence, performance validation, cybersecurity, and post-market surveillance, raising the bar for compliance. For personalized medicine, this means higher standards for companion diagnostics, NGS panels, and AI software used in clinical decision support. The EMA works in coordination

with other EU regulatory bodies to ensure these digital technologies are safe, effective, and appropriately integrated into healthcare systems.

11.1.3 Pharmaceuticals and Medical Devices Agency (PMDA) - Japan

The Pharmaceuticals and Medical Devices Agency (PMDA) is Japan's key regulatory authority responsible for ensuring the safety, efficacy, and quality of pharmaceuticals, medical devices, and regenerative medicine products. Operating under the Ministry of Health, Labour and Welfare (MHLW), the PMDA plays a central role in the approval, post-marketing surveillance, and risk management of medical products. Over the years, the agency has significantly evolved to keep pace with scientific advances and healthcare needs. One of its major areas of focus is now personalized medicine, which tailors' treatments based on individual genetic, environmental, and lifestyle factors. The PMDA actively collaborates with academic institutions, healthcare professionals, and international regulatory bodies to streamline the development and approval of precision therapies. It also emphasizes regulatory science to ensure timely access to innovative treatments without compromising patient safety. The agency supports accelerated pathways for breakthrough therapies and orphan drugs. Through initiatives like the Sakigake Designation System, the PMDA promotes early development and fast-track approval of innovative products. Its patient-centric approach aims to improve outcomes while fostering innovation in the medical field.

- **Regulatory Innovation:** The PMDA is at the forefront of regulatory innovation, particularly in the area of regenerative medicine and advanced therapies. It offers accelerated review pathways designed to bring cutting-edge treatments to patients more quickly while maintaining rigorous safety and efficacy standards. The Sakigake Designation System is a notable initiative that supports early engagement between developers and regulators, encouraging innovation in Japan. This system allows priority consultation and shortened review periods for products with high potential. By facilitating fast-track approvals, the PMDA enables quicker access to life-saving therapies, especially for rare and serious conditions. The agency is also adapting its regulatory frameworks to accommodate gene and cell therapies, where traditional models may not be suitable. Continuous improvement of regulatory science underpins these efforts, helping the PMDA balance innovation and patient protection. Through proactive dialogue with stakeholders and adaptive regulatory models, the PMDA is shaping a more responsive and forward-looking review process that keeps pace with technological advances in healthcare.
- **Collaborative Research:** The PMDA places a strong emphasis on collaborative research to drive the advancement of personalized medicine.

It actively engages with academic institutions, industry stakeholders, and research organizations to develop scientific knowledge and regulatory approaches for new therapies. These collaborations aim to bridge the gap between innovation and regulation, ensuring that cutting-edge science is supported by sound policy. The PMDA also promotes joint studies to better understand biomarkers, pharmacogenomics, and individualized treatment strategies. By fostering an ecosystem of cooperation, it enables smoother clinical translation of research into therapeutic options. Involvement in cross-sector consortia and advisory boards allows the agency to stay ahead of emerging trends in personalized healthcare. Collaborative data-sharing initiatives further help in the development of evidence-based regulatory decisions. This approach not only accelerates the development pipeline but also ensures alignment with global best practices. Through such partnerships, the PMDA contributes to a robust infrastructure for the future of precision medicine in Japan and beyond.

- **Guidance on Companion Diagnostics:** Recognizing the critical role of diagnostics in personalized medicine, the PMDA has developed comprehensive regulatory guidance for companion diagnostics (CDx). These are tests that help identify patients most likely to benefit from specific drugs, making them essential to targeted therapy development. The PMDA requires the simultaneous development and approval of CDx and their corresponding therapeutic agents. This co-development strategy ensures clinical relevance and accurate patient selection during trials. The agency provides early-stage consultation and review support to drug and diagnostic developers to streamline the process. Regulatory frameworks include clear pathways for validation, analytical performance, and clinical utility of diagnostics. By setting high standards, the PMDA ensures that only robust and reliable diagnostic tools are brought to market. It also addresses the unique challenges of CDx, such as handling updates and changes post-approval. This guidance promotes safe and effective integration of diagnostics into clinical practice. Through these efforts, the PMDA plays a pivotal role in the successful implementation of personalized treatment approaches in Japan.

- **Post-market Risk Management:** The PMDA emphasizes a comprehensive approach to post-market risk management, especially for personalized medical products. Recognizing that risks may not be fully evident during clinical trials, the agency enforces strict post-marketing surveillance requirements. It monitors adverse events and safety signals through mandatory reporting systems and real-world data collection. For high-risk or novel therapies, the PMDA may require Risk Management Plans (RMPs), including educational programs and usage restrictions. Patient registries and long-term follow-up studies are encouraged to assess ongoing efficacy and safety. The agency also collaborates with healthcare professionals and institutions to ensure timely detection of any emerging issues. Real-time monitoring enables quicker intervention, which is especially crucial for gene therapies and other advanced treatments. The PMDA continually updates its risk management strategies to reflect evolving knowledge and post-market evidence. Its proactive stance helps maintain public trust and minimizes harm. Overall, the agency's vigilant post-market oversight is a cornerstone of safe personalized healthcare in Japan.

- **Global Harmonization:** The PMDA is a strong advocate for global harmonization in regulatory science, contributing actively to initiatives such as the International Council for Harmonisation (ICH). Through its participation, the agency aligns Japan's regulatory standards with global best practices, ensuring consistency in the development, approval, and monitoring of medical products. This harmonization facilitates international clinical trials and the mutual recognition of data, which is particularly important for personalized medicine and rare diseases. The PMDA also engages with other regulatory agencies through the International Pharmaceutical Regulators Programme (IPRP) and bilateral collaborations. These efforts help reduce duplication, improve efficiency, and accelerate access to innovative therapies worldwide. By contributing to global guideline development on topics like genomics, biomarkers, and advanced therapies, the PMDA helps shape the international regulatory landscape. It also adapts global recommendations into its domestic framework to support Japanese industry competitiveness. This global perspective enhances patient access to high-quality, innovative healthcare solutions. Ultimately, the PMDA's commitment to harmonization supports both regulatory excellence and public health on an international scale.

11.1.4 Comparison and Harmonization Efforts

Although the FDA (United States), EMA (European Union), and PMDA (Japan) operate within different legal, organizational, and cultural frameworks, they share a common commitment to ensuring the safety and efficacy of medical products. Each agency has distinct regulatory pathways and approval mechanisms, but increasing global collaboration is bridging these differences. Through participation in international bodies such as the International Council for Harmonisation (ICH) and the International Medical Device Regulators Forum (IMDRF), these agencies work toward harmonizing technical requirements and regulatory standards. These efforts reduce redundancies in clinical trials and streamline submissions for multinational companies. Shared guidelines on topics like clinical trial design, good manufacturing practices (GMP), and pharmacovigilance enhance global consistency. Harmonization supports the efficient development and faster approval of personalized medicines, including gene and cell therapies. Cross-agency collaboration also improves post-market safety surveillance and scientific knowledge exchange. As innovation accelerates, such partnerships are crucial for ensuring timely patient access to cutting-edge treatments worldwide. These harmonization initiatives ultimately contribute to improved global health outcomes.

Challenges and Trends:

- **Rapid Innovation Pace:** The rapid evolution of science and technology—particularly in genomics, artificial intelligence (AI), and cell and gene therapies—poses both opportunities and challenges for regulatory agencies worldwide. Regulatory bodies like the FDA, EMA, and PMDA are under constant pressure to modernize frameworks that were originally designed for traditional pharmaceuticals. These agencies are investing heavily in regulatory science to understand and evaluate the safety and effectiveness of increasingly complex innovations. For instance, AI-driven diagnostics and personalized therapies based on individual genetic profiles require novel assessment tools. Adaptive regulatory approaches, such as rolling reviews and conditional approvals, are being adopted to accelerate timelines. Agencies are also creating specialized task forces and expert panels to assess emerging technologies in real time. The aim is to strike a balance between rigorous oversight and enabling timely patient access. Continuous training for regulators and dynamic policy updates are essential to remain aligned with the frontiers of medical innovation. This responsiveness ensures that regulatory systems remain relevant and resilient in the face of ongoing technological disruption.
- **Data Integration:** Modern personalized medicine relies heavily on integrating complex and diverse data types, including genomics, proteomics, metabolomics, and real-world evidence (RWE). Regulatory agencies are working to develop robust frameworks that can incorporate this multidimensional data into decision-making processes. Traditional clinical trial data alone is no longer sufficient to assess the efficacy and safety of individualized therapies. To this end, regulators are exploring new analytical tools and data infrastructure to manage, standardize, and interpret high-throughput omics data. Real-world data from electronic health records, patient registries, and wearable devices also provides valuable insights into treatment performance in diverse populations. These

data sources, however, raise challenges in terms of data quality, privacy, and interoperability. Agencies like the PMDA and FDA are piloting initiatives to use RWE in approval and post-market surveillance decisions. Collaborative efforts with industry, academia, and international bodies help define data standards and methodologies. Successfully integrating these data streams supports more precise, evidence-based regulatory decisions and promotes the advancement of personalized healthcare.

- **Balancing Innovation and Safety:** Striking the right balance between rapid innovation and patient safety remains a core challenge for regulatory authorities. As the demand for faster access to groundbreaking therapies grows, so too does the need for rigorous safety assessments. Personalized medicine products, such as gene therapies or biomarker-driven treatments, often target small populations, limiting the size of clinical trials and increasing uncertainty at the time of approval. To address this, regulators are employing flexible approval mechanisms like conditional authorizations, fast-track designations, and risk-sharing models. These approaches allow earlier access while requiring ongoing data collection and monitoring. Post-market surveillance becomes critical in this context, with tools like Risk Management Plans and real-world data playing a central role. Agencies must also ensure transparency and informed consent in the face of evolving risk-benefit profiles. Regular updates to guidance documents and stakeholder consultations help maintain accountability. Ultimately, regulators must facilitate innovation while ensuring that new therapies meet acceptable standards of quality, efficacy, and safety for patients.
- **Global Access and Equity:** As personalized medicine continues to evolve, ensuring global access and equity becomes increasingly important. While high-income countries benefit from advanced regulatory systems and infrastructure, many low- and middle-income countries face barriers to accessing personalized therapies. These disparities arise from limited regulatory capacity, lack of trained personnel, inadequate data systems, and affordability challenges. Regulatory harmonization efforts led by international bodies like ICH and WHO help to bridge these gaps by promoting global standards and capacity building. Initiatives such as regulatory reliance and work-sharing allow resource-constrained agencies to leverage the assessments of established authorities like the FDA or EMA. However, beyond harmonization, equitable access also requires addressing pricing, intellectual property, and distribution challenges. Personalized treatments, often tailored for small populations, can be prohibitively expensive and logistically complex to deliver. To promote global equity, regulators, governments, and industry must collaborate to ensure that

innovative therapies are not limited to a privileged few. Supporting inclusive regulatory policies is essential to achieving health equity in the era of precision medicine.

11.2 REGULATORY APPROVAL OF COMPANION DIAGNOSTICS

Companion diagnostics (CDx) are in vitro diagnostic tools developed to identify patients who are likely to respond to a specific therapeutic product or are at heightened risk of adverse effects. These tests are essential for enabling precision medicine, as they guide clinicians in selecting the most appropriate and effective treatment based on individual patient profiles. Regulatory agencies such as the FDA, EMA, and PMDA require that CDx undergo a rigorous review process, often in parallel with the therapeutic drug it supports. Approval hinges on demonstrating analytical validity (accuracy and reproducibility), clinical validity (relevance to the target patient population), and clinical utility (impact on treatment outcomes). Co-development of the drug and diagnostic is encouraged to ensure timely availability of both products upon market entry. Agencies provide guidance documents to streamline submissions and clarify performance expectations. In some regions, CDx is classified as a high-risk medical device, warranting additional oversight. Post-market monitoring is also critical to ensure ongoing safety and effectiveness in real-world use. The successful approval of CDx fosters more personalized, effective, and safer treatment strategies.

11.2.1 Definition and Importance

Companion diagnostics (CDx) are specialized in vitro diagnostic (IVD) devices that play a critical role in the delivery of personalized medicine. These tests are designed to generate essential information about a patient's biological profile, which determines whether a specific therapeutic product is safe and effective for them. Typically, CDx identify biomarkers such as genetic mutations (e.g., EGFR, BRCA), protein expression levels (e.g., HER2), or other molecular signatures that directly influence treatment decisions. By stratifying patients into subgroups, CDx ensure that therapies are administered only to those who are most likely to benefit, while avoiding unnecessary exposure in non-responders or those at risk of severe adverse effects. The use of CDx is especially prominent in oncology, where tumor profiling helps tailor treatment to individual genetic alterations. For instance, drugs targeting ALK or ROS1 mutations in lung cancer depend on CDx to determine eligibility. Similarly, in rare diseases and infectious diseases, CDx supports accurate patient selection, aiding in the effective deployment of high-cost or high-risk therapies. Their role is expanding as more treatments are developed with a precision medicine approach.Regulatory authorities emphasize the co-development of CDx alongside the therapeutic drug, ensuring both products are evaluated and approved in tandem. This alignment supports simultaneous market access, enhancing clinical decision-making at the point of care. Moreover, CDx contribute to cost-effective healthcare by avoiding trial-and-error prescribing, reducing adverse events, and improving overall treatment outcomes. In clinical trials, CDx can enrich patient selection, increasing the likelihood of demonstrating therapeutic benefit. Beyond efficacy and safety, CDx also drive innovation in biomarker discovery and translational research, bridging laboratory science with clinical application. As technologies like next-generation sequencing (NGS) and AI-driven diagnostics advance, CDx are becoming increasingly complex and informative. Their growing importance highlights the need for robust regulatory oversight, interdisciplinary collaboration, and continued investment in diagnostic innovation. Ultimately, CDx are indispensable tools in the move toward more precise, personalized, and predictive healthcare models worldwide.

11.2.2 Regulatory Pathways

Companion diagnostics (CDx) are subject to stringent regulatory oversight due to their direct impact on critical treatment decisions and patient safety. Regulatory agencies require rigorous evaluation to ensure that these tests demonstrate high levels of analytical validity, clinical validity, and clinical utility before approval. Because CDx guide the use of specific therapeutics, inaccuracies can lead to ineffective treatment or harmful side effects, making regulatory scrutiny essential. Typically, CDx undergo a premarket approval (PMA) or equivalent process, classified as high-risk medical devices in many jurisdictions. Regulators often mandate the co-development and simultaneous review of the CDx and the associated drug or biologic to ensure coordinated availability. Early and ongoing communication between diagnostic developers, pharmaceutical companies, and regulators is encouraged to streamline approvals. Post-market surveillance is also critical to monitor performance in real-world settings. Agencies provide clear guidance and frameworks to help developers navigate regulatory requirements while promoting innovation. This rigorous oversight safeguards patient outcomes and reinforces trust in personalized medicine.

The approval processes vary by region but generally require:

- **Analytical Validation:** Analytical validation is a fundamental step in the regulatory evaluation of companion diagnostics, focusing on the test's technical performance. This process demonstrates the assay's ability to accurately, precisely, and reliably detect the intended biomarker in clinical samples. Parameters assessed include sensitivity (the ability to detect even low levels of the biomarker), specificity (the ability to distinguish the biomarker from similar molecules), reproducibility (consistent results across different runs, operators, and laboratories), and robustness (stability under varying conditions). The test must perform reliably with relevant sample types, such as blood, tissue biopsies, or saliva, reflecting real-world clinical settings. Rigorous validation ensures that measurement errors are minimized, preventing false positives or negatives that could misguide treatment decisions. Standardized protocols and quality control measures are often employed to maintain consistency. Analytical validation also addresses the limits of detection and quantification, cross-reactivity, and potential interferences. Regulators require comprehensive documentation of these performance characteristics to grant approval. Ultimately, robust analytical validation forms the foundation for trust in the diagnostic's reliability and accuracy in clinical practice.

- **Clinical Validation:** Clinical validation establishes the scientific link between the biomarker detected by the companion diagnostic and relevant clinical outcomes, such as treatment response, disease progression, or adverse events. This step confirms that the presence, absence, or level of the biomarker reliably predicts how patients will respond to the corresponding therapeutic intervention. Clinical validation typically involves retrospective or prospective studies correlating biomarker status with efficacy or safety endpoints in well-characterized patient populations. Statistical rigor and appropriate study design are crucial to avoid bias and ensure reproducibility. In oncology, for example, clinical validation might demonstrate that patients with a particular genetic mutation experience better survival or tumour shrinkage when treated with a targeted therapy. The strength of this association supports the test's use in selecting patients likely to benefit. Regulators require clear evidence that the biomarker's predictive value is clinically meaningful and consistent across different cohorts. Without strong clinical validation, the utility of the diagnostic remains uncertain. Therefore, this stage bridges laboratory findings with practical therapeutic implications, reinforcing the diagnostic's role in guiding personalized treatment decisions.
- **Clinical Utility:** Clinical utility refers to the evidence that the use of the companion diagnostic in routine healthcare improves patient management and outcomes compared to not using the test. This includes demonstrating that the diagnostic leads to better therapeutic choices, reduces unnecessary treatments, minimizes adverse effects, or improves survival and quality of life. Clinical utility is often shown through prospective clinical trials or real-world studies assessing the impact of biomarker-guided therapy on patient health. This evidence may encompass improved progression-free survival, reduced hospitalizations, or cost-effectiveness analyses showing optimized resource use. Importantly, clinical utility addresses the practical

value of the test beyond its analytical and clinical validity, focusing on tangible benefits for patients and healthcare systems. Regulators and payers increasingly require this data to support approval and reimbursement decisions. Without demonstrated clinical utility, even a highly accurate test may struggle to justify its routine clinical use. Thus, establishing clinical utility is vital to integrating companion diagnostics into standard care, ensuring they translate into meaningful improvements in personalized medicine and patient-centered healthcare.

11.2.3 U.S. Food and Drug Administration (FDA)

- The FDA classifies companion diagnostics as high-risk medical devices (Class III) requiring Premarket Approval (PMA).
- The agency often reviews the drug and its companion diagnostic simultaneously or in a coordinated manner to ensure aligned labelling.
- FDA guidance emphasizes co-development and co-approval strategies, where the diagnostic and therapeutic product undergo concurrent clinical trials.
- Post-market surveillance is important to monitor ongoing performance and emerging data.
- Examples include HER2 testing for trastuzumab (Herceptin) and EGFR mutation testing for osimertinib.

11.2.4 European Medicines Agency (EMA)

- In the EU, companion diagnostics fall under the In Vitro Diagnostic Regulation (IVDR), which came into full effect in 2022.
- The IVDR introduces stricter requirements for clinical evidence, performance evaluation, and conformity assessment.
- Companion diagnostics are classified as Class C devices, requiring involvement of a notified body for certification.
- EMA coordinates with notified bodies and medicinal authorities to ensure that diagnostics and therapeutics are harmonized.
- The IVDR mandates enhanced transparency and post-market surveillance, increasing patient safety.

11.2.5 Pharmaceuticals and Medical Devices Agency (PMDA) - Japan

- PMDA regulates companion diagnostics as medical devices with approval required before market launch.
- Japan encourages early engagement with PMDA for co-development of diagnostics and therapeutics.

- PMDA has guidelines outlining requirements for analytical and clinical validation tailored to Japan's healthcare system.
- Collaborative efforts with FDA and EMA facilitate alignment and faster approvals for global companies.

11.2.6 Challenges in Regulatory Approval

- **Co-Development Complexity:** The co-development of companion diagnostics alongside therapeutic drugs presents significant logistical and scientific challenges. Coordinating clinical trials to simultaneously generate robust data for both the drug and the diagnostic requires meticulous planning and cross-disciplinary collaboration. Timing is critical, as delays in diagnostic development can stall drug approvals, and vice versa. Differences in development timelines, trial designs, and regulatory submission processes add layers of complexity. Additionally, aligning the data requirements and expectations of multiple regulatory authorities can complicate global development strategies. Communication between pharmaceutical companies, diagnostic developers, and regulators must be seamless to address issues promptly. Ensuring synchronized approval of both products is essential to avoid gaps that could hinder patient access. These challenges necessitate early and ongoing dialogue, flexible trial designs, and integrated regulatory strategies to facilitate efficient co-development pathways.
- **Evolving Technologies:** Rapid technological advancements in genomics, multiplex testing, and next-generation sequencing continuously reshape the landscape of companion diagnostics. While these innovations offer unprecedented precision and depth of biological insight, they also complicate regulatory validation and standardization processes. Multiplex assays that detect multiple biomarkers simultaneously challenge traditional single-analyte test frameworks, requiring new approaches for analytical and clinical validation. The sheer volume and complexity of data generated necessitate sophisticated bioinformatics and data interpretation tools, raising questions about reproducibility and consistency. Moreover, evolving platforms and continuous software updates demand flexible regulatory models that can adapt without compromising patient safety. Regulators and developers must work together to establish clear guidelines that accommodate these technologies while ensuring rigorous quality controls. Keeping pace with innovation while maintaining robust standards remains a delicate balance in companion diagnostic regulation.
- **Global Harmonization:** Differences in regulatory requirements across regions pose a significant barrier to the efficient global development and

approval of companion diagnostics. Variability in submission formats, data expectations, risk classifications, and approval timelines can result in duplicated efforts and delayed market entry. Companies often must tailor applications to meet the specific demands of agencies like the FDA, EMA, and PMDA, increasing costs and complexity. These disparities hinder timely patient access to critical diagnostics and associated therapies worldwide. International harmonization initiatives, such as those led by the International Council for Harmonisation (ICH) and the International Medical Device Regulators Forum (IMDRF), aim to align standards and foster mutual recognition. However, complete convergence remains a work in progress, requiring ongoing cooperation and dialogue. Streamlining regulatory pathways through harmonization will enhance innovation, reduce duplication, and improve equitable access to personalized medicine on a global scale.

- **Clinical Utility Evidence:** Demonstrating the clinical utility of companion diagnostics—evidence that their use improves patient outcomes—is often one of the most demanding regulatory hurdles. Unlike analytical and clinical validation, which focus on test performance and predictive value, clinical utility requires proof that the diagnostic positively influences treatment decisions and health outcomes. Gathering this evidence typically involves prospective, well-controlled clinical trials or extensive real-world studies, which can be costly and time-consuming. Long-term follow-up is often necessary to assess survival benefits, quality of life improvements, or reductions in adverse events. The heterogeneity of patient populations and evolving treatment landscapes add complexity to study design and interpretation. Regulators and payers increasingly require robust clinical utility data to justify approval and reimbursement. This demand places significant pressure on developers to design rigorous studies that conclusively demonstrate the practical benefits of companion diagnostics, ensuring they translate into real-world value for patients and healthcare systems.

11.2.7 Emerging Trends

- **Digital Companion Diagnostics:** The rise of digital companion diagnostics, which integrate artificial intelligence (AI) and advanced software algorithms, is transforming personalized medicine. These tools analyse complex biological and clinical data to provide predictive insights that guide treatment decisions. However, the integration of AI introduces new regulatory challenges, including ensuring algorithm transparency, validation of software performance, and managing continuous updates or learning systems. Regulators are adapting frameworks to assess both the diagnostic device and the underlying software, focusing on data integrity, cybersecurity, and patient privacy. Digital diagnostics require ongoing monitoring post-approval to detect changes in performance over time. As AI-driven diagnostics evolve rapidly, regulators face the challenge of balancing innovation with rigorous oversight to protect patient safety. The development of international guidelines and harmonized standards is underway to address these complexities. This trend highlights the growing intersection of healthcare, data science, and regulation in the era of precision medicine.

- **Real-World Evidence:** Real-world evidence (RWE), derived from data collected outside traditional clinical trials—such as electronic health records, patient registries, and wearable devices—is playing an increasingly vital role in regulatory decision-making for companion diagnostics. RWE complements clinical trial data by providing insights into how diagnostics perform across diverse populations and routine clinical settings. It helps to monitor long-term safety and effectiveness, supports label expansions, and may expedite approvals through adaptive regulatory pathways. However, incorporating RWE raises challenges related to data quality, standardization, and potential biases. Regulators are developing guidance on how to systematically collect, analyse, and interpret RWE to ensure it meets scientific rigor. Collaborative initiatives between agencies, industry, and academia promote best practices for leveraging real-world data. The use of RWE enhances the evidence base for companion diagnostics, supporting more informed, patient-centric regulatory decisions and ultimately improving healthcare outcomes.
- **Adaptive Licensing:** Adaptive licensing, also known as progressive or conditional approval, is an innovative regulatory approach designed to accelerate patient access to promising companion diagnostics and associated therapies. This flexible pathway allows for initial approval based on limited but compelling data, with the condition that additional evidence is gathered post-market. It supports a stepwise evaluation, where the diagnostic's use can expand as more data become available, reducing the time patients wait for novel treatments. Adaptive licensing requires robust post-approval monitoring systems and risk management plans to promptly identify and mitigate safety concerns. Regulators engage in early dialogue with developers to define clear data generation milestones and approval conditions. This approach balances the urgent need for innovation with patient safety and evidence quality. It is particularly valuable in areas of high unmet medical need, such as rare diseases and oncology. Adaptive

licensing reflects a shift towards more dynamic, evidence-based regulatory models aligned with the rapid pace of medical innovation.

Regulatory approval of companion diagnostics is a critical step in the personalized medicine pathway. It ensures that diagnostic tests are reliable and clinically meaningful, enabling precise treatment decisions that improve patient outcomes. Coordinated efforts among global regulators continue to evolve frameworks that keep pace with technological innovation while safeguarding public health.

11.3 CLINICAL GUIDELINES AND STANDARDIZATION

Clinical guidelines and standardization are foundational to the successful integration of personalized medicine and companion diagnostics into everyday healthcare. These evidence-based protocols synthesize the latest scientific research and clinical trial data to provide clear recommendations on how to interpret biomarker or genomic test results accurately. By guiding clinicians on patient selection, treatment choices, and monitoring strategies, guidelines help ensure that personalized therapies are used effectively and safely. Standardization efforts establish consistent procedures for specimen collection, assay performance, result reporting, and data interpretation, reducing variability and enhancing diagnostic reliability across laboratories and healthcare institutions. This uniformity is critical for maintaining patient trust and facilitating seamless care transitions, especially in complex healthcare systems. Professional societies, regulatory agencies, and international consortia collaborate to develop, update, and disseminate these guidelines, reflecting advances in technology and emerging clinical evidence. Moreover, standardized reporting formats improve communication between laboratories, clinicians, and patients, supporting informed decision-making. Clinical guidelines also address ethical considerations, such as informed consent and genetic counselling, which are integral to personalized medicine. By fostering best practices and minimizing disparities in care delivery, guidelines and standardization contribute to equitable access to precision diagnostics and treatments. Ultimately, these frameworks enhance patient outcomes, optimize resource utilization, and support the widespread adoption of innovative healthcare solutions worldwide.

11.3.1 Purpose and Importance

- **Consistency in Care:** Standardized clinical guidelines play a crucial role in minimizing variability in how genetic and genomic information is applied in patient care. By providing clear, uniform protocols, these guidelines help ensure that patients receive the same level of high-quality care regardless of geographic location, healthcare setting, or provider expertise. This consistency is particularly important in personalized medicine, where complex biomarker data can be interpreted differently without established standards. Standardization helps reduce disparities in treatment decisions and outcomes by fostering equitable access to precision diagnostics and targeted therapies. Moreover, it supports seamless communication and collaboration among multidisciplinary care teams. When healthcare providers follow consistent guidelines, patients benefit from predictable, evidence-based care pathways that optimize therapeutic effectiveness and safety. Ultimately, this reduces clinical uncertainty and builds trust between patients and healthcare systems.

- **Evidence-Based Practice:** Clinical guidelines serve as essential tools to translate the rapidly expanding body of scientific knowledge into practical recommendations for healthcare providers. By systematically reviewing and synthesizing the latest research, including clinical trial data and real-world evidence, guidelines distill complex information into actionable best practices. This helps clinicians keep pace with the fast-evolving fields of genomics, biomarker discovery, and personalized therapeutics. Evidence-based guidelines support informed decision-making, reducing reliance on anecdotal experience or outdated practices. They also facilitate the integration of novel diagnostic tools and treatment options into standard care. By grounding clinical decisions in robust evidence, these guidelines improve the quality and consistency of care delivery. They also provide a framework for ongoing education, enabling providers to stay current with emerging innovations and evolving treatment paradigms.
- **Improved Patient Outcomes:** Following validated clinical guidelines significantly enhances patient outcomes by ensuring accurate diagnosis, appropriate treatment selection, and avoidance of unnecessary or harmful interventions. Guidelines enable clinicians to interpret genetic and biomarker test results within a structured framework that links molecular findings to specific therapeutic strategies. This precision reduces the risk of administering ineffective or toxic treatments, thereby improving efficacy and patient safety. Moreover, standardized protocols often include recommendations for monitoring and follow-up, supporting early detection of adverse events or disease progression. Improved diagnostic accuracy and tailored therapies contribute to better survival rates, quality of life, and overall patient satisfaction. By optimizing resource utilization and minimizing trial-and-error approaches, guidelines also reduce healthcare costs. Thus, adherence to clinical guidelines is instrumental in translating scientific advances into tangible health benefits for patients.
- **Facilitation of Regulatory Compliance:** Adherence to established clinical guidelines plays a pivotal role in supporting compliance with regulatory

requirements and reimbursement policies. Regulatory agencies and payers often reference these guidelines when evaluating the appropriateness of diagnostic tests and therapies for approval and coverage. Following evidence-based protocols helps healthcare providers demonstrate that personalized medicine interventions meet recognized standards of care. This alignment facilitates smoother regulatory reviews and expedites patient access to innovative treatments. Additionally, compliance with guidelines can protect clinicians and institutions from legal or reimbursement challenges related to off-label or unsupported use of diagnostics and therapeutics. Guidelines also guide documentation practices, ensuring thorough and consistent reporting of clinical decisions and outcomes. By integrating regulatory expectations with clinical practice, guidelines serve as essential tools for harmonizing patient care, policy adherence, and healthcare system sustainability.

11.3.2 Development of Clinical Guidelines

- **Multidisciplinary Collaboration:** The development of clinical guidelines for personalized medicine and companion diagnostics relies on extensive multidisciplinary collaboration. Experts from diverse fields—including geneticists, oncologists, pathologists, pharmacologists, bioinformaticians, ethicists, and patient advocates—contribute their specialized knowledge and perspectives. This collaborative approach ensures that guidelines address the scientific, clinical, ethical, and patient-centred aspects of care comprehensively. By incorporating diverse expertise, guidelines are better equipped to balance complex considerations such as diagnostic accuracy, therapeutic efficacy, patient safety, and ethical implications like informed consent and data privacy. Inclusion of patient representatives ensures that the guidelines reflect patient values and preferences, promoting shared decision-making. This broad engagement fosters consensus-building and enhances the credibility, relevance, and acceptance of the final recommendations within the clinical community.
- **Systematic Review of Evidence:** A rigorous and systematic review of the available scientific evidence forms the backbone of guideline development. This process involves evaluating data from clinical trials, observational studies, meta-analyses, and real-world evidence to assess the safety, effectiveness, and clinical utility of genomic tests and targeted therapies. Evidence is critically appraised for methodological quality, bias, and relevance to specific patient populations. Systematic reviews help identify gaps in knowledge, inconsistencies in results, and areas requiring further research. By synthesizing diverse data sources, guideline developers create

a comprehensive evidence base that supports reliable and transparent recommendations. This approach also ensures that guidelines reflect current best practices grounded in robust scientific data, providing clinicians with confidence to implement personalized medicine strategies in their care delivery.

- **Grading of Recommendations:** To guide clinical decision-making effectively, many guideline organizations employ standardized grading systems, such as GRADE (Grading of Recommendations Assessment, Development and Evaluation), to assess the strength and quality of evidence underlying each recommendation. These grading frameworks consider factors like study design, risk of bias, consistency of results, and directness of evidence to classify recommendations as strong, moderate, or weak. Clear grading helps clinicians understand the certainty of the evidence and the balance of benefits and risks associated with diagnostic or therapeutic options. It also aids in prioritizing interventions with the greatest clinical impact and encourages transparency in how conclusions are drawn. By explicitly rating the quality of evidence, grading systems foster trust, facilitate informed clinical judgment, and support shared decision-making with patients.
- **Periodic Updates:** Given the rapid pace of innovation in genomics, biomarker discovery, diagnostic technologies, and targeted therapies, clinical guidelines require frequent and systematic updates to remain current and clinically relevant. Periodic revisions incorporate new scientific findings, emerging biomarkers, novel diagnostic platforms, and evolving treatment paradigms. This ongoing process ensures that healthcare providers have access to the latest evidence-based recommendations, preventing reliance on outdated practices. Updates often follow scheduled review cycles or are triggered by significant breakthroughs in research. Maintaining dynamic and up-to-date guidelines requires continuous surveillance of the literature, stakeholder engagement, and streamlined processes for revising and disseminating recommendations. This adaptability is critical to supporting the timely translation of cutting-edge science into routine patient care and optimizing personalized medicine outcomes.

11.3.3 Prominent Clinical Guidelines Bodies

- **National Comprehensive Cancer Network (NCCN):** The National Comprehensive Cancer Network (NCCN) is a leading organization that provides comprehensive, evidence-based guidelines focused on cancer care, with a strong emphasis on genomic testing and companion diagnostics. NCCN guidelines offer detailed recommendations for the use of biomarker testing to guide therapy selection across a wide range of malignancies, including lung, breast, colorectal, and hematologic cancers. These guidelines are widely respected and frequently updated to reflect the latest clinical trial results and FDA approvals. NCCN also addresses the integration of molecular diagnostics into clinical workflows, ensuring that testing is performed appropriately and interpreted accurately. Their protocols support personalized treatment plans, improve patient outcomes, and are often referenced by regulatory agencies and payers. By promoting standardization and best practices, NCCN plays a pivotal role in advancing precision oncology worldwide.

- **American Society of Clinical Oncology (ASCO):** The American Society of Clinical Oncology (ASCO) develops authoritative guidelines that focus on the use of genetic and genomic testing in cancer care, aiming to integrate precision medicine seamlessly into everyday clinical practice. ASCO's guidelines help oncologists determine when and how to use molecular diagnostics for diagnosis, prognosis, and treatment decision-making. They emphasize evidence-based recommendations for biomarker testing, companion diagnostics, and the interpretation of complex genetic data. ASCO also addresses emerging technologies and ethical considerations such as genetic counselling and patient consent. Their guidelines are designed to facilitate clinician education, improve test utilization, and optimize personalized therapeutic approaches. ASCO collaborates with other professional organizations to promote harmonization and ensure that precision medicine becomes a routine and equitable component of oncology care.
- **Clinical Pharmacogenetics Implementation Consortium (CPIC):** The Clinical Pharmacogenetics Implementation Consortium (CPIC) focuses on creating guidelines that enable clinicians to translate genetic test results into actionable prescribing decisions. CPIC guidelines provide detailed, gene-specific recommendations on drug dosing, selection, and avoidance based on patients' pharmacogenetic profiles. This helps minimize adverse drug reactions and optimize therapeutic efficacy by tailoring medications to individual genetic variability. CPIC collaborates with laboratories, clinicians, and researchers to ensure guidelines are practical, clinically relevant, and based on rigorous evidence. These guidelines cover a broad range of medications across therapeutic areas including oncology, cardiology, psychiatry, and infectious diseases. By standardizing the application of pharmacogenetics in clinical practice, CPIC supports personalized medicine efforts and improves patient safety globally.

- **European Society for Medical Oncology (ESMO):** The European Society for Medical Oncology (ESMO) provides expert recommendations on molecular testing and the use of targeted therapies in oncology, with an emphasis on harmonizing practices across Europe. ESMO guidelines address key issues such as which biomarkers to test for, optimal testing methodologies, and criteria for patient selection in various cancers. These recommendations promote consistency and quality assurance in diagnostic approaches, facilitating equitable access to precision treatments throughout European healthcare systems. ESMO also supports education and training initiatives to enhance clinician competence in molecular oncology. Their guidelines reflect evolving scientific evidence and regulatory standards, helping to bridge gaps between research, clinical practice, and policy. By fostering international collaboration, ESMO contributes significantly to advancing personalized cancer care on the continent.

11.3.4 Standardization Efforts

- **Laboratory Practices:** Standardization of laboratory practices is essential to ensure the accuracy, reliability, and reproducibility of genetic and genomic testing. This includes establishing uniform protocols for specimen collection, handling, storage, and processing, which minimize pre-analytical variability. Consistent methodologies for DNA extraction, sequencing, and biomarker detection are critical to generate dependable test results. Laboratories adopt validated assays and adhere to stringent quality assurance procedures throughout the testing workflow. Standard operating procedures (SOPs) are regularly updated to reflect technological advances and best practices. Training of laboratory personnel in these standardized techniques further reduces errors and variability. Such harmonization ensures that diagnostic results are comparable across different labs and clinical settings, fostering confidence among clinicians and patients in personalized medicine applications.
- **Reporting Formats:** The use of standardized reporting formats for genetic test results is vital for clear and effective communication among healthcare providers. Uniform terminology, interpretation criteria, and structured report layouts help clinicians accurately understand and apply genomic information in clinical decision-making. Reports typically include key elements such as detected variants, their clinical significance, test limitations, and recommended follow-up actions. Standardized guidelines, such as those from the Association for Molecular Pathology (AMP), promote consistency in variant classification and terminology. Clear, concise reports reduce misinterpretation risks and facilitate multidisciplinary discussions.

Standardization also supports integration of results into electronic health records (EHRs), enabling easy access and longitudinal patient monitoring. Ultimately, consistent reporting enhances the clinical utility of companion diagnostics and improves patient care coordination.

- **Quality Control and Accreditation:** Maintaining high standards in genomic testing laboratories requires rigorous quality control and accreditation processes. Laboratories undergo certification by recognized bodies—such as CLIA (Clinical Laboratory Improvement Amendments) in the U.S. or ISO 15189 internationally—which assess compliance with technical and operational standards. Participation in external proficiency testing programs allows labs to benchmark their performance against peers and identify areas for improvement. Ongoing quality assurance activities include regular equipment calibration, validation of assays, and review of test outcomes. Accreditation ensures that laboratories adhere to regulatory requirements and maintain consistent, high-quality testing services. This fosters trust among clinicians, patients, and regulators that diagnostic results are accurate, reproducible, and clinically valid. Quality control also supports the safe implementation of new technologies within laboratory settings.
- **Data Interoperability:** Data interoperability is a cornerstone of integrating genomic information into routine clinical practice. The development of standardized data formats, coding systems, and ontologies enables seamless sharing, aggregation, and analysis of genetic test results across diverse healthcare platforms. Integration with electronic health records (EHRs) ensures that genomic data is accessible to clinicians at the point of care, supporting timely and informed decision-making. Standardization efforts—such as the use of HL7 FHIR (Fast Healthcare Interoperability Resources) and GA4GH (Global Alliance for Genomics and Health) frameworks—facilitate consistent data exchange while protecting patient privacy and security. Interoperable systems also enable linkage with clinical databases, research registries, and decision-support tools. This connectivity enhances personalized medicine by allowing comprehensive patient data review, monitoring outcomes, and driving continuous improvement in diagnostics and therapeutics.

11.3.5 Challenges in Guideline Implementation

- **Rapid Technological Change:** The pace of innovation in genomics often outstrips the ability of guideline committees to update recommendations promptly.

- **Resource Variability:** Differences in healthcare infrastructure and expertise can limit the application of standardized guidelines in some regions.
- **Complexity of Genetic Information:** Interpretation of multi-gene panels or whole-genome sequencing data requires specialized knowledge, complicating guideline adherence.
- **Patient Diversity:** Guidelines must account for genetic variability across populations to avoid inequities in care.

11.3.6 Future Directions

- **Personalized Guidelines:** Incorporating patient-specific factors such as ancestry, comorbidities, and preferences to tailor recommendations.
- **Digital Tools:** Use of clinical decision support systems (CDSS) integrated with EHRs to provide real-time, guideline-based recommendations at the point of care.
- **Global Harmonization:** International collaboration to develop consensus guidelines that transcend regional differences and support global standards.

Clinical guidelines and standardization are foundational for the effective and ethical use of genomic information and companion diagnostics in personalized medicine. They ensure that healthcare providers have clear, evidence-based frameworks to guide testing and treatment, ultimately improving patient outcomes and fostering trust in emerging technologies.

11.4 LAB ACCREDITATION AND QUALITY CONTROL (CLIA, CAP)

Laboratory accreditation and rigorous quality control are essential to ensure the accuracy, reliability, and reproducibility of genetic and genomic testing in personalized medicine. As companion diagnostics and molecular assays become integral to clinical decision-making, maintaining high laboratory standards safeguards patient safety and supports confidence in test results.

11.4.1 Key Accreditation Bodies

Two primary organizations in the United States that regulate laboratory quality in genetic testing are:

- **Clinical Laboratory Improvement Amendments (CLIA):** Enacted by the U.S. Congress in 1988, CLIA sets federal standards for all clinical laboratory testing performed on humans (except research). CLIA certification is mandatory for labs that perform diagnostic testing and ensures consistent quality through personnel qualifications, quality assurance, proficiency testing, and proper recordkeeping.

- **College of American Pathologists (CAP):** CAP is a professional organization that provides voluntary accreditation and proficiency testing programs for clinical laboratories. CAP accreditation often exceeds CLIA requirements and is widely recognized internationally as a mark of laboratory excellence.

11.4.2 Importance of Accreditation

- **Ensures Test Accuracy:** Accredited labs follow strict protocols for specimen handling, assay validation, and result reporting, minimizing errors.
- **Protects Patient Safety:** Reliable results prevent misdiagnosis and inappropriate treatment based on faulty genetic data.
- **Facilitates Regulatory Compliance:** Accreditation is often a prerequisite for reimbursement and adherence to healthcare regulations.
- **Promotes Continuous Improvement:** Quality control programs identify and address deficiencies, leading to ongoing enhancement of laboratory performance.

11.4.3 Components of Quality Control and Assurance

- **Validation and Verification:** Laboratories must validate new tests and technologies to demonstrate analytical validity (accuracy, sensitivity, specificity) before clinical use.
- **Proficiency Testing:** Regular external proficiency testing evaluates laboratory performance by comparing results with peer labs to detect discrepancies.
- **Internal Quality Controls:** Routine checks during test runs, including controls and standards, ensure consistent assay performance.
- **Personnel Competency:** Staff qualifications, ongoing training, and competency assessments guarantee skilled execution of complex genomic tests.
- **Documentation and Recordkeeping:** Detailed logs of procedures, quality checks, and corrective actions ensure traceability and accountability.

11.4.4 Specific Challenges in Genomic Testing

- **Complex Assays:** Next-generation sequencing (NGS) and multi-gene panels require specialized validation and interpretation protocols.
- **Rapid Technological Advancements:** Labs must continually update methods and equipment, which necessitates frequent re-validation and staff training.
- **Data Management:** Secure and accurate handling of large-scale genomic data demands robust informatics infrastructure and quality checks.

11.4.5 International and Regional Standards

- **ISO 15189:** An international standard specifying requirements for quality and competence in medical laboratories, increasingly adopted globally.
- **Regional Accreditation:** Outside the U.S., laboratories may seek accreditation from organizations such as the European Molecular Genetics Quality Network (EMQN) or the Japanese Society of Clinical Genetics.

11.4.6 Impact on Personalized Medicine:

- **Trust in Test Results:** High-quality laboratory practices underpin clinical confidence in genomic diagnostics, enabling precision therapies.
- **Streamlined Clinical Integration:** Standardized quality measures facilitate incorporation of lab results into clinical workflows and decision-making.
- **Support for Research and Innovation:** Accredited labs contribute reliable data to genomic research, fostering innovation while protecting participant welfare.

Lab accreditation and robust quality control systems, exemplified by CLIA and CAP, are fundamental to the safe and effective application of genomic testing in personalized medicine. These frameworks ensure that diagnostic labs maintain high standards, which is critical for delivering accurate, trustworthy results that drive informed healthcare decisions.

11.5 IMPLEMENTATION SCIENCE IN PRECISION MEDICINE

Implementation science is the study of methods and strategies to promote the systematic uptake of research findings and evidence-based practices into routine healthcare. In the context of precision medicine, implementation science plays a crucial role in bridging the gap between genomic discoveries and their practical application in clinical settings. It focuses on understanding how to effectively integrate personalized interventions—such as genetic testing, targeted therapies, and individualized risk assessments—into healthcare systems to improve patient outcomes.

11.5.1 Challenges in Translating Precision Medicine

- **Complexity of Genomic Data:** The interpretation of vast and complex genetic information requires specialized knowledge and resources that may not be uniformly available.
- Healthcare System Readiness: Variability in infrastructure, provider expertise, and workflow integration can hinder adoption of precision medicine approaches.

- **Patient Engagement:** Ensuring patients understand and accept genomic-based recommendations is essential for successful implementation.
- **Policy and Reimbursement Barriers:** Lack of clear guidelines or financial incentives may delay the uptake of precision medicine services.

11.5.2 Focus Areas of Implementation Science

- **Assessing Context and Readiness:** Understanding the healthcare environment, including organizational culture, resources, and stakeholder attitudes, to tailor implementation strategies accordingly.
- **Developing and Testing Interventions:** Designing implementation strategies such as educational programs, decision support tools, and workflow modifications to facilitate the use of precision medicine.
- **Evaluating Outcomes:** Measuring implementation success through indicators like adoption rates, fidelity to protocols, patient outcomes, cost-effectiveness, and sustainability.
- **Addressing Barriers and Facilitators:** Identifying challenges such as clinician resistance, limited genomic literacy, or technology gaps, and leveraging facilitators like leadership support and interdisciplinary collaboration.

11.5.3 Implementation Frameworks and Models

- **Consolidated Framework for Implementation Research (CFIR):** Offers a comprehensive structure to evaluate multiple factors influencing implementation, including intervention characteristics, outer setting, inner setting, individuals involved, and the implementation process itself.
- **RE-AIM (Reach, Effectiveness, Adoption, Implementation, Maintenance):** Focuses on five critical dimensions to assess the public health impact of precision medicine interventions.
- **Knowledge-to-Action (KTA) Framework:** Guides the translation of genomic knowledge into clinical practice by mapping steps from knowledge creation to action and sustainability.

11.5.4 Role of Stakeholders

- **Clinicians:** Need training and support to interpret genetic data and incorporate precision medicine into patient care.
- **Patients:** Engagement and education help improve informed decision-making and adherence to personalized treatments.

- **Health Systems:** Must adapt infrastructure, policies, and reimbursement models to support implementation.
- **Researchers and Policymakers:** Collaborate to develop evidence-based guidelines and address regulatory and ethical issues.

11.5.6 Technological Enablers

- Integration of genomic data into electronic health records (EHRs) with decision support alerts.
- Use of telemedicine and digital tools to extend access to precision medicine services.
- Data analytics to monitor implementation progress and patient outcomes.

11.5.7 Benefits of Implementation Science in Precision Medicine

- Accelerates the translation of genomic innovations into clinical practice.
- Enhances the quality, safety, and effectiveness of personalized healthcare.
- Promotes equitable access by identifying and addressing disparities.
- Supports scalability and sustainability of precision medicine programs across diverse healthcare settings.

Implementation science is essential for realizing the full potential of precision medicine. By systematically studying and addressing the challenges of integrating genomic advances into everyday healthcare, it ensures that innovations lead to tangible health improvements, benefiting patients and healthcare systems alike.

12 Chapter

FUTURE OF PERSONALIZED MEDICINE

12.0 INTRODUCTION: AN OVERVIEW

The future of personalized medicine holds tremendous promise to revolutionize healthcare by tailoring medical treatment and prevention strategies to the unique genetic, environmental, and lifestyle factors of each individual. As advances in genomics, bioinformatics, and biotechnology continue to accelerate, personalized medicine is shifting from a niche research concept into mainstream clinical practice. This paradigm shift moves away from the traditional "one-size-fits-all" approach toward more precise, predictive, and proactive healthcare that optimizes outcomes and minimizes adverse effects. Personalized medicine leverages vast amounts of data—from whole genome sequencing and proteomics to real-time health monitoring and electronic health records—to deliver highly individualized care plans. The integration of artificial intelligence and machine learning further enhances the ability to interpret complex biological information and develop dynamic treatment algorithms. Looking ahead, the future of personalized medicine is poised to transform not only how diseases are diagnosed and treated but also how they are prevented. Predictive models using genetic and biomarker information will enable early identification of individuals at risk for chronic illnesses such as cancer, cardiovascular disease, and neurodegenerative disorders, facilitating timely interventions that can delay or even prevent disease onset. Moreover, pharmacogenomics—the study of how genes affect a person's response to drugs—will become a routine part of prescribing practices, reducing trial-and-error prescribing and enhancing drug efficacy and safety (Fig. 1).

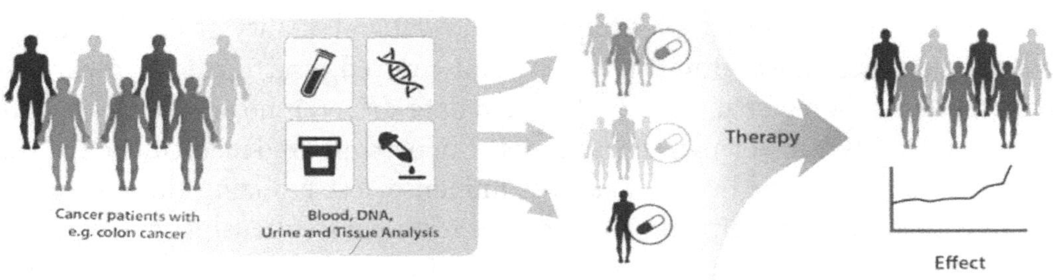

Fig. 1 Future medicine-personalised Diagnostics

The expansion of precision medicine will also be driven by advances in gene editing technologies such as CRISPR-Cas9, which offer the potential to correct genetic mutations at their source. These breakthroughs raise new possibilities for curing previously untreatable genetic disorders and for developing personalized therapies tailored to an individual's specific molecular profile. Meanwhile, the convergence of wearable devices, mobile health applications, and telemedicine will facilitate continuous health monitoring and personalized feedback, empowering patients to actively manage their health outside traditional clinical settings. Despite these exciting prospects, the future of personalized medicine also presents complex challenges that must be addressed. Issues around data privacy, security, and ownership are paramount, given the sensitive nature of genomic and health-related information. Ethical considerations surrounding equitable access, consent, and the potential for genetic discrimination require robust policy frameworks and social dialogue. Furthermore, the integration of personalized approaches into healthcare systems demands new infrastructure, workforce training, and reimbursement models to ensure sustainable implementation. Equity will be a crucial focus moving forward to prevent widening health disparities. Historically underrepresented populations in genomic research risk being left behind if inclusion efforts are not prioritized. Future initiatives must emphasize cultural competence, community engagement, and inclusive research practices to ensure that personalized medicine benefits diverse populations globally. Additionally, interdisciplinary collaboration between clinicians, researchers, data scientists, ethicists, and policymakers will be essential to navigate the technical, ethical, and social complexities of this evolving field. The global nature of genomic data and personalized medicine necessitates harmonized international regulatory frameworks and standards to facilitate data sharing, innovation, and patient safety while respecting sovereignty and cultural diversity. The establishment of dynamic consent models and transparent governance will empower individuals to control how their data is used and shared. Ultimately, the future of personalized medicine envisions a healthcare ecosystem where prevention, diagnosis, and treatment are seamlessly integrated with an individual's unique biology and life context. It is a future where precision therapies improve survival and quality of life, healthcare delivery becomes more efficient and patient-centred, and medical research is accelerated through global collaboration and data-driven innovation. As we stand at the cusp of this transformation, the promise of personalized medicine to reshape healthcare and improve human health is immense. Yet realizing these potential demands sustained commitment to innovation, ethical stewardship, and equity to ensure that the benefits of personalized medicine reach all members of society, fostering a healthier, more personalized future for everyone.

12.1 MULTI-OMICS INTEGRATION AND SYSTEMS BIOLOGY

12.1.1 Introduction to Multi-Omics

Multi-omics represents a cutting-edge approach in biomedical research that integrates multiple layers of biological data—genomics, transcriptomics, proteomics, metabolomics, epigenomics, and microbiomics—to achieve a comprehensive understanding of living systems. Each "omics" discipline offers a unique perspective: genomics reveals the fundamental DNA sequence and identifies genetic variants that may predispose to disease; transcriptomics measures gene expression, showing which genes are active under specific conditions; proteomics investigates protein abundance, modifications, and interactions; metabolomics examines small molecules and metabolites that reflect cellular metabolic states. Epigenomics adds another dimension by studying chemical modifications to DNA and histones that regulate gene activity without altering the sequence, while microbiomics explores the diverse microbial communities impacting host health. By combining these diverse datasets, researchers can trace the flow of biological information from the genome through cellular processes to phenotypic outcomes. This integrated view facilitates the identification of complex molecular mechanisms underlying diseases, moving beyond isolated findings to systems-level insights that can guide personalized diagnostics, prognostics, and therapeutic interventions.

12.1.2 Role of Systems Biology

Systems biology is an interdisciplinary field that complements multi-omics by focusing on the dynamic interactions among biological components, from genes and proteins to cells and tissues, within the context of the whole organism. It uses computational, mathematical, and statistical tools to model these interactions as networks or systems, uncovering emergent properties that cannot be understood by studying parts in isolation. Systems biology seeks to explain how molecular components collectively contribute to robustness, adaptability, and homeostasis, as well as how their dysregulation leads to disease. This holistic framework integrates heterogeneous multi-omics data, enabling the construction of predictive models that simulate biological processes over time and across conditions. By capturing the complexity of biological networks, systems biology helps identify key regulatory nodes and pathways amenable to therapeutic targeting. It also provides a quantitative basis for hypothesis generation and testing, facilitating translational research that bridges basic biology with clinical applications. In essence, systems biology turns big data into actionable knowledge for precision medicine.

12.1.3 Benefits of Multi-Omics Integration

The integration of multi-omics datasets offers transformative benefits for understanding disease biology and advancing personalized medicine. By combining genomic data with transcriptomic, proteomic, and metabolomic profiles, researchers gain a multi-dimensional view of how genetic variations influence molecular functions and contribute to pathophysiology. This layered approach helps identify robust biomarkers for early diagnosis, disease progression, and treatment response, enhancing the precision of clinical decision-making. Furthermore, multi-omics facilitates the discovery of novel therapeutic targets and elucidates molecular pathways that are disrupted in specific disease subtypes, enabling patient stratification and tailored interventions. For example, in cancer, multi-omics data can reveal tumour heterogeneity, resistance mechanisms, and metabolic alterations, guiding the development of targeted therapies. Similarly, in metabolic and autoimmune diseases, integrating metabolic and epigenetic data uncovers complex interactions driving disease progression. Ultimately, multi-omics integration bridges genotype and phenotype, improving the accuracy of risk prediction, prognostication, and personalized treatment plans.

12.1.4 Technological Advances Enabling Multi-Omics

Recent technological breakthroughs have been pivotal in enabling the rapid generation, processing, and analysis of multi-omics data at unprecedented scale and resolution. Next-generation sequencing (NGS) technologies facilitate high-throughput, cost-effective sequencing of genomes and transcriptomes, allowing comprehensive profiling of genetic and gene expression changes. Mass spectrometry advances empower sensitive and precise quantification of proteins and metabolites, essential for proteomic and metabolomic analyses. Additionally, single-cell sequencing technologies enable investigation of cellular heterogeneity and lineage relationships within complex tissues. Computational innovations, including machine learning and artificial intelligence algorithms, have become indispensable for managing the vast, heterogeneous datasets produced by multi-omics studies. These tools support data integration, pattern recognition, and predictive modelling, transforming raw data into meaningful biological insights. Cloud computing and collaborative platforms further enable sharing and joint analysis of multi-omics data across research groups, accelerating discoveries. Together, these technological advances create a robust foundation for multi-omics-driven biomedical research and clinical applications.

12.1.5 Challenges in Multi-Omics Integration

Despite its immense promise, multi-omics integration faces substantial technical and analytical challenges. Data heterogeneity is a key obstacle, as different "omics" datasets vary in scale, quality, and measurement techniques, complicating their harmonization. Batch effects and missing data can introduce bias, while the high dimensionality and complexity of interactions require advanced statistical and computational methods to extract biologically meaningful signals. Nonlinear relationships and context-dependent effects further increase analytical complexity. Developing predictive models that are both accurate and interpretable remains a challenge, particularly for clinical translation. Reproducibility is critical, necessitating validation across independent cohorts and standardized protocols. Moreover, integrating multi-omics with clinical and environmental data demands sophisticated frameworks to ensure data security and privacy compliance. Overcoming these challenges requires continuous methodological innovation, interdisciplinary collaboration, and the establishment of best practices to fully realize the clinical potential of multi-omics.

12.1.6 Clinical Applications and Case Studies

Multi-omics integration has begun to revolutionize clinical research and practice, particularly in oncology, metabolic diseases, and immunotherapy. Large-scale projects like The Cancer Genome Atlas (TCGA) exemplify the power of combining genomic, epigenomic, transcriptomic, and proteomic data to classify tumour subtypes, uncover driver mutations, and identify resistance pathways, enabling more precise and personalized cancer treatment strategies. In metabolic disorders such as diabetes, integrating metabolomic and genomic data reveals dysregulated pathways involved in insulin resistance and disease progression, informing targeted interventions. Multi-omics also enhances personalized immunotherapy by profiling tumor microenvironments and immune cell interactions, aiding in the prediction of therapy response. Beyond these areas, multi-omics supports biomarker discovery for early diagnosis, monitoring disease activity, and predicting adverse effects. These clinical applications underscore the transformative potential of multi-omics in delivering tailored, effective, and safer medical care.

12.1.7 Systems Biology Modelling for Personalized Medicine

Systems biology employs dynamic computational models that simulate biological processes over time and under varying conditions, providing a powerful tool for personalized medicine. By integrating multi-omics data with clinical and environmental variables, these models capture patient-specific molecular interactions and predict individual responses to therapies. Network-based approaches identify critical nodes and pathways as potential therapeutic targets, facilitating rational drug design. In silico simulations accelerate drug discovery by forecasting off-target effects, synergistic drug combinations, and resistance mechanisms, reducing costly trial-and-error in clinical development. Such modelling enhances clinical decision-making by providing actionable insights on disease progression and treatment optimization tailored to each patient's unique biological context. Systems biology thus bridges molecular data with practical healthcare, supporting the shift towards precision and predictive medicine.

12.1.8 Future Directions and Innovations

The future of multi-omics integration and systems biology lies in expanding the scope and resolution of biological data and enhancing computational methodologies. Emerging technologies like spatial omics will map the precise localization of molecules within tissues, providing critical insights into cellular microenvironments and tissue architecture. Single-cell omics will continue to elucidate cellular heterogeneity and lineage dynamics, deepening understanding of development and disease. Integration of multi-omics with electronic health records, lifestyle, and environmental data promises to refine personalized risk assessments and intervention strategies. Advances in artificial intelligence and deep learning will enable the creation of more sophisticated models capable of capturing the complexity of biological systems and making accurate predictions. Ethical considerations, including data privacy, consent, and equitable access, will shape implementation to ensure benefits are distributed fairly. Collectively, these innovations will drive a new era of precision medicine grounded in holistic, data-driven insights. Concise summary of multi-omics integration and systems biology is given in Table-1.

Table-1 Concise Summary of Multi-Omics Integration and Systems Biology

Area	Summary
Multi-Omics	Multi-omics integrates genomics, transcriptomics, proteomics, metabolomics, epigenomics, and microbiomics to provide a holistic view of biological systems. Each layer offers unique insights, linking genotype to phenotype for better understanding of health and disease.
Role of Systems Biology	Systems biology models biological systems as interacting networks, using computational tools to interpret complex data and understand emergent properties like robustness and disease dysregulation, complementing multi-omics integration.
Benefits of Multi-Omics Integration	Enables precise disease understanding, identification of biomarkers, therapeutic targets, and molecular pathways. Helps stratify patients by molecular subtypes for personalized treatment and prognostic predictions.
Technological Advances Enabling Multi-Omics	Advances in sequencing (NGS), mass spectrometry, and bioinformatics allow rapid generation and analysis of multi-omics data. Machine learning and computational platforms support data integration and extraction of biological insights.
Challenges in Multi-Omics Integration	Challenges include data heterogeneity, quality variability, batch effects, missing data, high dimensionality, and interpretation. Requires robust, reproducible computational models that are clinically actionable and validated across cohorts.

Area	Summary
Clinical Applications and Case Studies	Multi-omics has advanced oncology (tumour classification, drug response prediction), metabolic disease understanding, and personalized immunotherapy by profiling tumour microenvironments and immune interactions.
Systems Biology Modelling for Personalized Medicine	Uses dynamic models to simulate biological processes and predict patient-specific therapy responses. Supports identification of therapeutic targets, drug discovery, and synergistic drug combinations through network-based simulations.
Future Directions and Innovations	Future advances include spatial and single-cell omics, integration with health records and environmental data, AI-driven complex modelling, and focus on data privacy and equitable access for broader implementation.

12.2 PERSONALIZED PREVENTION AND LONGEVITY MEDICINE

12.2.1 Introduction to Personalized Prevention

Personalized prevention is an innovative healthcare paradigm that tailors' disease prevention strategies based on an individual's unique biological makeup, genetic predispositions, environmental exposures, and lifestyle factors. Moving away from traditional "one-size-fits-all" public health models, personalized prevention acknowledges that each person has distinct risk factors and vulnerabilities. This approach harnesses advances in genomic sequencing, biomarker discovery, wearable health devices, and digital health platforms to generate a detailed personal health profile. By integrating this information, healthcare providers can develop customized prevention plans targeting specific pathways that contribute to disease onset. Personalized prevention aims to shift healthcare focus from treatment to proactive risk reduction, potentially reducing the incidence and burden of chronic diseases such as heart disease, cancer, diabetes, and neurodegenerative disorders. With continuous monitoring and adaptive interventions, this model promises improved health outcomes, greater patient engagement, and optimized use of healthcare resources.

12.2.2 Genetic and Molecular Risk Profiling

A foundational element of personalized prevention is the use of genetic and molecular risk profiling to identify individuals who are predisposed to various diseases. Polygenic risk scores (PRS), which combine the effects of many genetic variants across the genome, offer a quantitative estimate of inherited susceptibility for conditions such as cardiovascular disease, breast cancer, and Alzheimer's disease. When combined with molecular biomarkers—such as circulating inflammatory proteins, hormone levels, or metabolic signatures—these profiles provide a comprehensive risk assessment. This enables clinicians to detect preclinical abnormalities or early disease states before symptoms appear. Molecular profiling supports stratification of populations into risk categories, allowing for targeted interventions like intensified screening, lifestyle modification, or prophylactic therapies. This approach moves beyond simple family history or single-gene testing, offering a more nuanced and precise prediction of disease risk and facilitating truly individualized preventive care.

12.2.3 Lifestyle and Environmental Tailoring

Personalized prevention extends beyond genetics by integrating lifestyle and environmental factors that significantly influence health outcomes. Factors such as diet, physical activity, sleep quality, stress levels, and exposure to environmental toxins like air pollution or heavy metals are critical determinants of disease risk and progression. Modern digital health technologies—including wearable fitness trackers, smartwatches, and mobile health apps—enable continuous, real-time monitoring of these parameters. These data streams allow dynamic risk assessments that capture fluctuations and trends over time. Personalized interventions can then be designed to target modifiable risk factors, such as creating customized nutrition plans to address metabolic imbalances or recommending stress reduction techniques based on physiological stress markers. This holistic approach recognizes the interplay between genetics, behaviour, and environment, empowering individuals with actionable insights and supporting sustained healthy behaviour change.

12.2.4 Role of Longevity Medicine

Longevity medicine is a growing field focused on extending both lifespan and, critically, health span—the period of life free from chronic illness and disability. This discipline seeks to delay the biological aging process and prevent or mitigate age-associated diseases through personalized strategies. Research into the molecular hallmarks of aging, including telomere shortening, cellular senescence, mitochondrial dysfunction, and epigenetic alterations, has identified potential therapeutic targets. Longevity medicine employs a combination of pharmacological agents such as senolytics, which clear senescent cells, alongside lifestyle interventions and regenerative therapies tailored to individual aging profiles. The goal is not merely to prolong life but to enhance the quality of those additional years. Personalized longevity approaches integrate biomarker assessments to monitor aging trajectories and adjust interventions dynamically, fostering resilience and maintaining physiological function well into advanced age.

12.2.5 Biomarkers of Aging and Health span

To effectively guide personalized longevity interventions, researchers have developed biomarkers that estimate biological age and health span, offering insights beyond chronological age. Epigenetic clocks, which measure DNA methylation patterns, provide a robust predictor of biological aging rates. Proteomic and metabolomic profiles reveal changes in protein expression and metabolic function that correlate with physiological decline and disease susceptibility. These biomarkers enable clinicians to monitor individual aging processes, evaluate the impact of interventions, and refine treatment plans in real time. By integrating such data, personalized medicine can identify those at higher risk of age-related functional decline or disease onset and implement preventative measures earlier. The development and validation of accurate, non-invasive biomarkers remain an active area of research critical for the clinical translation of longevity medicine.

12.2.6 Preventive Genomics in Clinical Practice

Incorporating preventive genomics into routine clinical practice represents a significant advance in personalized prevention. Genomic testing is increasingly used to identify individuals with hereditary cancer syndromes, familial hypercholesterolemia, and other inherited conditions where early detection can drastically improve outcomes. Genetic counselling is essential for interpreting complex risk information and guiding patients through preventive options, including enhanced surveillance, lifestyle changes, or prophylactic interventions. Healthcare systems are evolving to integrate precision screening programs that tailor frequency and modality based on individual risk profiles. For example, women at high genetic risk for breast cancer may begin mammographic screening earlier or consider MRI. Such risk-based approaches optimize resource allocation, reduce overdiagnosis, and improve early detection rates, marking a shift toward more efficient and effective healthcare delivery.

12.2.7 Digital Health and Remote Monitoring

The proliferation of digital health technologies significantly enhances the feasibility and effectiveness of personalized prevention. Wearable devices and sensors continuously collect physiological data such as heart rate variability, blood glucose levels, sleep patterns, and physical activity. These data feed into artificial intelligence (AI)-powered platforms that analyse trends, detect anomalies, and generate personalized health insights and alerts. Remote monitoring enables healthcare providers to track patients' health status in real time, facilitating timely interventions and reducing the need for in-person visits. This continuous feedback loop encourages patient engagement and self-management by providing immediate, actionable information. Furthermore, integrating these digital tools with electronic health records improves data continuity and supports population-level health management and research initiatives.

12.2.8 Behavioural and Psychological Considerations

Effective personalized prevention recognizes that behavioural and psychological factors profoundly influence adherence and health outcomes. Tailored communication strategies that consider individual readiness, motivation, and cultural context enhance patient engagement. Techniques such as motivational interviewing help patients explore and resolve ambivalence toward behaviour change. behavioural nudges, including reminders and incentives, promote sustained adoption of healthy habits. Additionally, addressing psychological barriers—such as anxiety, stress, or low health literacy—is crucial for successful implementation. Personalized coaching and access to mental health support services further improve outcomes by helping patients navigate challenges and maintain long-term lifestyle modifications. Ultimately, integrating behavioural science with personalized prevention creates more holistic, patient-centred care.

12.2.9 Health Equity and Access Challenges

While personalized prevention offers transformative potential, it also raises significant challenges related to equitable access. Socioeconomic disparities, limited digital literacy, and variable healthcare infrastructure may restrict availability of genomic testing, digital health tools, and personalized care for underserved populations. Without deliberate efforts, these advances risk exacerbating existing health inequalities. Addressing these barriers requires inclusive policies that subsidize access, expand digital literacy programs, and build community partnerships to engage marginalized groups. Culturally sensitive approaches and multilingual resources are essential to ensure comprehension and trust. Additionally, ethical frameworks must guide the equitable distribution of benefits from personalized prevention, ensuring that innovations reach all segments of society and contribute to reducing, rather than widening, health disparities.

12.2.10 Future Directions in Personalized Prevention and Longevity

The future of personalized prevention and longevity medicine lies in the integration of multi-omics data, real-world clinical evidence, and sophisticated artificial intelligence to develop highly precise risk prediction and intervention models. Advances in regenerative medicine—such as stem cell therapies and tissue engineering—alongside microbiome modulation and nutrigenomics will expand therapeutic options to maintain healthspan. Personalized prevention will increasingly incorporate real-time data from wearable devices and environmental sensors, allowing adaptive and proactive health management. Cross-sector collaboration among researchers, clinicians, technology developers, and policymakers will be vital to translate scientific innovations into scalable, ethical, and accessible healthcare solutions. Emphasizing patient engagement, data privacy, and health equity will ensure that the benefits of personalized prevention and longevity medicine are realized broadly across diverse populations.

12.3 CELL-BASED THERAPIES AND REGENERATIVE MEDICINE

12.3.1 Introduction to Cell-Based Therapie

Cell-based therapies are revolutionizing personalized medicine by harnessing the unique potential of living cells to repair, regenerate, or replace damaged tissues and organs, offering a fundamentally different approach compared to conventional treatments. Rather than merely alleviating symptoms, these therapies target the underlying cellular and molecular causes of disease, promoting true restoration of function. This innovative field encompasses a variety of modalities including stem cell transplantation, immune cell-based treatments such as CAR-T cell therapy, and bioengineered tissue grafts. Stem cells, with their remarkable capacity for self-renewal and differentiation into diverse cell types, serve as a critical resource for regenerating damaged tissues in conditions like spinal cord injury, Parkinson's disease, and myocardial infarction. Immune cell therapies harness the body's own immune system, engineering T-cells to recognize and destroy cancer cells more effectively, representing a major breakthrough in oncology. Additionally, advances in tissue engineering and biomaterials have enabled the creation of functional tissue constructs that can replace or support failing organs. Cell-based therapies hold immense promise for treating a wide spectrum of previously intractable diseases, including degenerative disorders, autoimmune diseases, and severe trauma. Personalized approaches are central to these therapies, as cells can be derived from the patient (autologous) or from matched donors (allogeneic), minimizing immune rejection and enhancing efficacy. The field is rapidly evolving, supported by breakthroughs in cell isolation, expansion, genetic modification, and delivery techniques. Despite their transformative potential, challenges remain, including ensuring safety, controlling cell behaviour after transplantation, and scaling production for widespread clinical use. Regulatory frameworks are adapting to these novel therapies, emphasizing rigorous clinical evaluation and long-term monitoring. As research advances, cell-based therapies are expected to become a cornerstone of precision medicine, offering tailored solutions that address individual patient needs at the most fundamental biological level, ultimately transforming healthcare paradigms.

12.3.2 Types of Cells Used in Therapy

A variety of cell types are employed in regenerative medicine, each offering distinct advantages based on their biological characteristics and therapeutic applications. Stem cells, including embryonic stem cells and adult stem cells like mesenchymal stem cells (MSCs) and hematopoietic stem cells (HSCs), are prized for their ability to self-renew and differentiate into multiple cell lineages, making them ideal for tissue regeneration. Induced pluripotent stem cells (iPSCs), reprogrammed from adult cells, provide a patient-specific source for personalized therapies without ethical concerns linked to embryonic cells. Immune cells, particularly engineered T-cells such as CAR-T cells, play a pivotal role in targeting cancers by recognizing specific antigens. Additionally, progenitor cells, which are more lineage-committed than stem cells, support tissue repair by replenishing specialized cells. Other specialized cells, like pancreatic islet cells for diabetes or cardiomyocytes for heart disease, are also explored for targeted cell replacement. Each cell type's therapeutic potential depends on factors such as ease of isolation, expansion capacity, immunogenicity, and safety profiles. Understanding these unique properties helps guide their selection and optimization for specific clinical indications.

- **Stem Cells:** Stem cells are the cornerstone of regenerative medicine due to their remarkable potential to differentiate into various cell types and self-renew. Embryonic stem cells (ESCs) are pluripotent and can give rise to virtually any cell in the body, although their use is ethically sensitive. Adult stem cells, such as mesenchymal stem cells (MSCs), are multipotent and commonly sourced from bone marrow, adipose tissue, or umbilical cord blood for use in musculoskeletal repair and immune modulation. Induced pluripotent stem cells (iPSCs), which are adult cells reprogrammed into an embryonic-like state, offer a patient-specific solution without immune rejection risks. Their use is revolutionizing disease modelling, drug testing, and personalized cell therapies. Stem cells are being actively explored for treating conditions ranging from neurodegenerative diseases and spinal cord injuries to heart failure and diabetes.
- **Immune Cells:** Immune cell-based therapies, especially Chimeric Antigen Receptor T-cell (CAR-T) therapy, have opened a new era in cancer treatment. In this approach, a patient's T cells are genetically engineered to express receptors that recognize and destroy cancer cells with high specificity. CAR-T cells have shown remarkable success in treating certain blood cancers like leukaemia and lymphoma, offering long-term remission in otherwise treatment-resistant cases. Beyond CAR-T, natural killer (NK) cells and dendritic cells are also being explored for their roles in immunotherapy. These therapies harness the natural Défense mechanisms of the immune system, reprogramming them to overcome immune evasion by tumours. Ongoing research is focused on enhancing safety, reducing side effects such as cytokine release syndrome, and extending this approach to solid tumours.

- **Progenitor and Somatic Cells:** Progenitor cells are more lineage-restricted than stem cells but still possess the capacity to proliferate and differentiate into specific cell types, making them valuable in tissue-specific therapies. Examples include neural progenitor cells for neurodegenerative conditions and cardiac progenitor cells for heart repair. Unlike pluripotent stem cells, progenitor cells are often less tumorigenic and easier to control in therapeutic applications. Somatic cells—mature, differentiated cells like pancreatic islet cells or hepatocytes—can be directly transplanted to restore lost function in diseases such as diabetes or liver failure. These cell types may be used as-is or genetically modified to enhance survival, function, or immune compatibility. Their role is expanding through innovations in cell reprogramming and tissue engineering, making them essential components in the broader landscape of cell-based regenerative therapies.

12.3.3 Mechanisms of Action

Cell-based therapies function through several dynamic and synergistic mechanisms that collectively contribute to tissue regeneration and functional restoration. One primary mechanism is cellular differentiation, wherein therapeutic cells—especially stem cells such as mesenchymal stem cells (MSCs), embryonic stem cells (ESCs), or induced pluripotent stem cells (iPSCs)—transform into specialized cell types needed to replace damaged or lost tissues, such as neurons, cardiomyocytes, or pancreatic beta cells. This allows for direct tissue reconstruction at the site of injury. Beyond this, these cells exhibit paracrine effects by secreting a broad array of growth factors, cytokines, and extracellular vesicles that do not merely support survival but actively stimulate endogenous cells to initiate repair processes, including angiogenesis, neurogenesis, and matrix remodelling. Additionally, cell therapies often play an immunomodulatory role, suppressing excessive inflammation and promoting a balanced immune environment that is conducive to healing, particularly relevant in autoimmune or chronic inflammatory diseases. In some therapies, such as CAR-T cells, immune cells are engineered to target and destroy diseased cells, such as cancerous tumours, while sparing normal tissues. Another important action is engraftment, where administered cells integrate into the host tissue, forming stable, long-term connections with native cells and extracellular matrices, thereby re-establishing physiological function. This is especially critical in conditions such as spinal cord injury or myocardial infarction, where structural and functional recovery is needed. The homing ability of some therapeutic cells enables them to migrate to injury sites, guided by chemokines and adhesion molecules, ensuring localized action. Some cells can also stimulate vascular regeneration, improving perfusion and nutrient delivery to ischemic tissues. In regenerative medicine, this multimodal functionality is what distinguishes cell therapies from pharmacological treatments. The combination of direct replacement, biochemical stimulation, immune regulation, and structural support makes these therapies uniquely suited to address complex, multifactorial conditions that involve widespread tissue damage or dysfunction.

12.3.4 Regenerative Medicine Applications

Regenerative medicine encompasses a broad spectrum of innovative strategies aimed at repairing or replacing damaged tissues and organs. Beyond cell-based therapies, it includes tissue engineering, which combines scaffolds, cells, and biologically active molecules to construct functional tissue substitutes. These engineered tissues can be used for skin grafts, cartilage repair, or even complex organs like the liver. Biomaterials, such as hydrogels and biodegradable polymers, play a crucial role by providing structural support, guiding cell differentiation, and delivering therapeutic agents. Additionally, 3D bioprinting allows for precise fabrication of tissue structures that mimic natural anatomy and microenvironments. Regenerative approaches are increasingly applied in orthopaedics, cardiovascular repair, wound healing, and organ transplantation. This field holds immense potential to transform chronic disease management and drastically improve patient quality of life.

Applications include:

- **Cardiology:** In cardiology, stem cell therapies have shown promise in regenerating heart tissue damaged by myocardial infarction (heart attack). Various types of stem cells, including mesenchymal stem cells and cardiac progenitor cells, are being explored for their ability to differentiate into cardiomyocytes and promote vascular regeneration. These cells can improve cardiac function by replacing dead tissue, enhancing perfusion, and reducing scar formation. Clinical trials have demonstrated modest improvements in ejection fraction and overall heart performance. Researchers are also investigating delivery methods, such as direct injection or scaffold implantation, to improve efficacy and engraftment. This approach aims to reduce heart failure progression and improve long-term survival in post-MI patients.
- **Neurology:** Cell-based therapies are increasingly explored for neurological disorders where conventional treatments offer limited recovery. In spinal cord injuries, transplanted neural stem cells may restore lost function by forming new neurons and glial cells. In Parkinson's disease, dopaminergic neuron replacement using fatal or induced pluripotent stem cells (iPSCs) aims to replenish depleted dopamine-producing cells. Stroke therapies involve using stem cells to reduce inflammation, stimulate angiogenesis, and replace damaged brain tissue. Preclinical and early clinical studies show encouraging outcomes in motor function and cognition. Ongoing research

focuses on ensuring safety, controlling differentiation, and achieving long-term integration in neural circuits.

- **Orthopaedics:** Regenerative medicine in orthopaedics leverages cell-seeded scaffolds to restore damaged cartilage and bone. Mesenchymal stem cells (MSCs) are commonly used due to their ability to differentiate into chondrocytes and osteoblasts, the key cellular components of cartilage and bone. These cells are often combined with biocompatible scaffolds, such as collagen or hydrogel matrices, that support tissue structure and guide regeneration. Applications include repairing osteoarthritic joints, treating fractures, and reconstructing bone defects. Autologous chondrocyte implantation and 3D-printed bone grafts are already in clinical use. The goal is to provide durable, biologically integrated repair that avoids prosthetic implants.
- **Diabetes:** In diabetes treatment, regenerative approaches aim to restore endogenous insulin production by replacing the destroyed or dysfunctional pancreatic beta cells. Pluripotent stem cells can be differentiated into insulin-producing beta-like cells in the lab and transplanted into patients. Encapsulation technologies are being developed to protect transplanted cells from immune attack without the need for immunosuppression. This strategy holds promise for Type 1 diabetes, offering a potential cure by restoring glucose regulation. Some therapies are in advanced clinical trials, showing sustained C-peptide levels and reduced insulin dependence. Combining cell replacement with immunomodulation may further enhance success rates.
- **Oncology:** Oncology has witnessed groundbreaking success through immune cell therapies, particularly chimeric antigen receptor T-cell (CAR-T) therapy. This involves engineering a patient's T cells to express receptors that recognize specific antigens on cancer cells. Once infused, these CAR-T cells selectively target and kill tumour cells with high precision. Approved CAR-T therapies have shown remarkable remission rates in haematological malignancies like leukaemia and lymphoma. Research is expanding into solid tumours, using combinations with checkpoint inhibitors and oncolytic viruses to enhance efficacy. Personalized immunotherapies are also being tailored to individual tumour profiles, ushering in a new era of precision oncology.

12.3.5 Personalization in Cell Therapies

Personalized regenerative medicine represents a transformative approach in which cell-based treatments are customized to align with the unique genetic, immunologic, and pathological features of each individual. This personalization begins with autologous therapies, where a patient's own cells are collected, modified, and reintroduced—drastically reducing the risk of immune rejection and adverse reactions compared to allogeneic sources. These cells can be expanded, reprogrammed (e.g., into iPSCs), or differentiated into specific cell types needed for tissue repair or disease correction. Genomic profiling of the patient enables clinicians to understand disease-driving mutations and cellular dysfunctions, allowing for targeted intervention. Gene editing tools, such as CRISPR-Cas9, can be employed to correct inherited genetic disorders at the cellular level before transplantation, offering a curative potential. Additionally, immune-matching algorithms help predict graft compatibility and minimize graft-versus-host disease in allogeneic therapies. In oncology, personalized CAR-T cell therapies are developed based on the patient's tumour antigen profile, improving tumour targeting and treatment response. Single-cell analysis technologies further refine patient stratification by identifying subpopulations of responsive or resistant cells. This data-driven approach optimizes safety, efficacy, and long-term integration of therapies. Ultimately, personalized cell therapies not only improve outcomes but also shift the clinical model toward proactive, individualized treatment paradigms in regenerative medicine.

12.3.6 Challenges and Risks

Despite promising results, cell-based therapies face significant challenges:

- **Safety Concerns:** Cell-based therapies, while promising, come with inherent safety risks that must be carefully managed. One major concern is immune rejection, particularly with allogeneic cells, which can lead to inflammation or graft failure. There is also a potential for tumorigenicity, especially when using pluripotent stem cells that may differentiate uncontrollably. Off-target effects during gene editing or unintended cell behaviour may result in tissue damage. Additionally, improper cell integration or migration can disrupt normal physiology. To mitigate these risks, strict preclinical testing, long-term monitoring, and patient-specific safety profiling are essential components of responsible therapy deployment.
- **Manufacturing and Standardization:** Producing cell therapies at scale presents significant manufacturing challenges. Each therapy often requires custom handling, especially for autologous products, which limits automation. Ensuring batch-to-batch consistency, viability, and purity of cells across different production sites is complex. Good Manufacturing Practice (GMP) compliance must be strictly adhered to, requiring specialized facilities and trained personnel. Cell expansion, cryopreservation, and delivery must preserve function without inducing genetic instability.

Additionally, quality control standards are still evolving, making widespread scalability a key bottleneck in commercialization.

- **Regulatory Hurdles:** Regulatory frameworks for cell-based therapies are still catching up with rapid scientific advances. Authorities like the FDA and EMA require extensive preclinical data, multi-phase clinical trials, and post-market surveillance to ensure patient safety. Because each therapy can be highly individualized, establishing uniform efficacy and safety benchmarks is challenging. Moreover, regulatory bodies must evaluate gene-edited cells, engineered tissues, and immune-modified cells, all with unique risk profiles. Collaborative efforts are needed to streamline approval pathways while maintaining rigorous standards for scientific validation and ethical compliance.
- Cost and Accessibility: Cell therapies are resource-intensive, often involving personalized cell harvesting, custom bioprocessing, and specialized clinical delivery. These factors contribute to extremely high treatment costs, sometimes exceeding hundreds of thousands of dollars per patient. Infrastructure needs, such as cell processing labs, cold-chain logistics, and trained specialists, further restrict access—especially in low- and middle-income regions. Insurance coverage is often limited or non-existent, creating barriers even in developed countries. To democratize access, innovations in cost-effective manufacturing, shared facilities, and public-private funding models are urgently needed.

12.3.7 Ethical Considerations

Cell-based therapies, while offering transformative potential, also raise significant ethical considerations that must be addressed to ensure responsible clinical application. The use of embryonic stem cells (ESCs) remains ethically contentious due to the destruction of human embryos during cell extraction, prompting debates about the moral status of embryonic life. Additionally, informed consent is crucial, especially for experimental or early-phase therapies where long-term outcomes remain uncertain. Patients must be made fully aware of potential risks, benefits, and unknowns before agreeing to treatment. Equity of access is another pressing issue, as the high cost and technological complexity of these therapies may limit their availability to privileged populations, exacerbating healthcare disparities. There are also concerns surrounding commercialization, where the drive for profit might override patient welfare or ethical transparency. Furthermore, questions around ownership of biological materials, especially in autologous therapies, and the long-term storage and use of patient-derived cells, require clear policy guidance. Ultimately, establishing robust ethical oversight, promoting transparency in research and clinical practices, and engaging diverse stakeholders—including patients, ethicists, regulators, and clinicians—are essential to ensure that cell-based therapies are developed and deployed in a socially responsible and morally sound manner.

12.3.8 Current and Emerging Innovations

The field of regenerative medicine is rapidly advancing, with cutting-edge innovations revolutionizing the development and delivery of cell-based therapies. One of the most promising breakthroughs is 3D bioprinting, which allows for the precise fabrication of complex tissue structures using bio-inks composed of living cells and supportive biomaterials. This technology holds potential for creating functional tissue grafts and, eventually, fully transplantable organs. Additionally, organoids—miniaturized, lab-grown versions of human organs—are being used for disease modelling, drug screening, and personalized medicine, offering insights into disease mechanisms and patient-specific responses. Another major trend is the integration of gene editing tools, such as CRISPR-Cas9, with cell therapy to correct genetic defects at the source before transplantation. Combination therapies are also emerging, where stem or immune cells are paired with biomaterial scaffolds or drug delivery systems to enhance stability, targeting, and therapeutic impact. Artificial intelligence (AI) is increasingly used to optimize various stages of therapy, including predicting cell behaviour, tailoring treatment protocols, and improving manufacturing efficiency. AI-driven platforms analyse large datasets from patient profiles and cell characteristics to recommend personalized therapeutic strategies. As these technologies converge, the future of regenerative medicine is moving toward highly personalized, efficient, and scalable therapeutic solutions that can address a wide range of diseases with greater precision and fewer side effects.

12.3.9 Future Prospects

The future of cell-based therapies and regenerative medicine holds transformative potential for healthcare, moving toward a paradigm where functional organ regeneration and personalized tissue replacement become standard treatment options. Scientists envision a future where patients suffering from organ failure could receive lab-grown organs derived from their own cells, eliminating the need for donor transplants and immunosuppressive therapies. Advances in stem cell biology, bioprinting, and gene editing are converging to enable the fabrication of patient-specific tissue constructs with precise structural and functional fidelity. Personalized tissue grafts, tailored to an individual's genetic and immunological profile, may significantly reduce complications like rejection and improve long-term outcomes. The integration of regenerative medicine with precision medicine platforms—including genomics, proteomics, and AI analytics—will enable highly individualized treatment strategies that adapt dynamically to disease progression and patient response. Moreover, innovations in cell manufacturing, quality control, and scalable bioprocessing are expected to lower costs and improve access. As the field advances, interdisciplinary collaboration between bioengineers, clinicians, data scientists, and regulatory agencies will be crucial to navigate ethical, logistical, and policy-related.

12.4 GLOBAL COLLABORATION AND DATA INFRASTRUCTURE

12.4.1 The Importance of Global Collaboration

Personalized medicine, with its reliance on vast amounts of biological and clinical data, thrives on international cooperation. No single institution or country possesses all the diverse datasets, expertise, or resources needed to fully realize personalized healthcare's potential. Global collaboration fosters shared knowledge, accelerates innovation, and enables the development of universally applicable precision medicine strategies.

12.4.2 Data Sharing and Integration Across Borders

To leverage the power of personalized medicine, cross-border data sharing is crucial. This includes genomic sequences, electronic health records (EHRs), clinical trial data, environmental exposures, and lifestyle information. Integrating these datasets across populations allows for improved disease risk prediction, biomarker discovery, and treatment personalization. However, seamless data sharing requires interoperable platforms, standardized formats, and common vocabularies.

12.4.3 Building Robust Data Infrastructure

A robust global data infrastructure forms the backbone of collaborative personalized medicine. The future of cell-based therapies and regenerative medicine holds transformative potential for healthcare, moving toward a paradigm where functional organ regeneration and personalized tissue replacement become standard treatment options. Scientists envision a future where patients suffering from organ failure could receive lab-grown organs derived from their own cells, eliminating the need for donor transplants and immunosuppressive therapies. Advances in stem cell biology, bioprinting, and gene editing are converging to enable the fabrication of patient-specific tissue constructs with precise structural and functional fidelity. Personalized tissue grafts, tailored to an individual's genetic and immunological profile, may significantly reduce complications like rejection and improve long-term outcomes. The integration of regenerative medicine with precision medicine platforms—including genomics, proteomics, and AI analytics—will enable highly individualized treatment strategies that adapt dynamically to disease progression and patient response. Moreover, innovations in cell manufacturing, quality control, and scalable bioprocessing are expected to lower costs and improve access. As the field advances, interdisciplinary collaboration between bioengineers, clinicians, data scientists, and regulatory agencies will be crucial to navigate ethical, logistical, and policy-related This infrastructure includes:

- High-performance computing resources for processing large datasets.
- Secure cloud-based platforms enabling remote access and collaboration.
- Advanced data storage solutions to accommodate expanding data volumes.
- Data standardization frameworks to ensure consistency and usability across datasets.

12.4.4 Privacy, Security, and Ethical Considerations

Global data sharing, particularly involving genomic and health information, raises profound privacy and security challenges that demand careful attention. Genomic data is uniquely sensitive because it contains deeply personal information that can reveal not only an individual's identity but also their predisposition to various diseases, affecting family members as well. Unauthorized access or breaches could lead to discrimination in employment, insurance, or social stigma. Moreover, the complexity of international data transfers increases risks, as varying legal frameworks and standards may leave gaps in protection. Ensuring robust encryption, secure data storage, and controlled access are vital to safeguarding this information. Ethical concerns also arise around informed consent, as individuals must fully understand how their data will be used and shared globally. Transparency and accountability from organizations handling such data are essential to maintain trust. Additionally, there is a risk of data misuse or exploitation by commercial entities, emphasizing the need for clear governance policies. Ultimately, balancing the benefits of global data sharing for medical research with stringent privacy and ethical safeguards is critical to protect individuals' rights while advancing science. Protecting individual rights while enabling research requires:

- Strict adherence to data protection laws (e.g., GDPR).
- Use of de-identification and anonymization techniques.
- Implementation of consent models that accommodate broad and dynamic permissions.
- Deployment of cybersecurity measures to prevent unauthorized access or breaches.

12.4.5 Role of International Consortia and Networks

Several international consortia exemplify the power of collaboration:

- The Global Alliance for Genomics and Health (GA4GH) works to develop standards and policies for responsible data sharing.

- The International Cancer Genome Consortium (ICGC) aggregates cancer genomic data from multiple countries.
- The Human Cell Atlas project maps all human cell types through worldwide cooperation.

These networks foster data harmonization, resource sharing, and joint research initiatives.

12.4.6 Challenges in Global Collaboration

Despite benefits, multiple challenges exist:

- **Legal and regulatory differences complicate data sharing agreements:** Data sharing across borders is often hindered by diverse legal frameworks and regulatory requirements. Each country or region may have its own privacy laws, data protection standards, and compliance mandates that must be navigated carefully. This complexity can delay or even prevent the establishment of agreements necessary for smooth data exchange. Additionally, differing interpretations of consent and ownership rights can create uncertainty for organizations involved. As a result, legal teams must invest significant effort to ensure agreements are both compliant and mutually acceptable.
- **Variable technological capabilities across regions lead to disparities in data contribution and use:** Not all regions have equal access to advanced technologies, which creates gaps in how data is collected, processed, and shared. Some areas may lack robust digital infrastructure, modern data management tools, or skilled personnel to handle complex datasets. This technological divide results in uneven data contributions, where regions with more resources dominate the shared pools. Consequently, the utility and accuracy of aggregated data can be skewed, limiting the overall benefits. Addressing these disparities requires targeted investments and capacity-building initiatives to foster equitable participation.
- **Cultural and language barriers may affect collaboration dynamics:** Collaboration between international partners can be complicated by differences in language and cultural norms. Misunderstandings can arise from varying communication styles, idiomatic expressions, and expectations around hierarchy or decision-making. These barriers might slow down negotiations, reduce efficiency, or even cause conflicts within teams. Furthermore, cultural perceptions of data privacy and sharing can influence willingness to collaborate openly. To foster effective cooperation, teams must prioritize cross-cultural training and use clear, inclusive communication methods.

- **Trust issues, particularly in sharing sensitive patient data internationally:** Trust is a fundamental challenge when sharing sensitive health data across borders, especially patient information. Concerns about data misuse, unauthorized access, or breaches can make organizations hesitant to share valuable datasets. Differences in cybersecurity practices and enforcement of privacy protections exacerbate these fears. Without strong trust frameworks and transparency, collaborations risk breakdowns or overly restrictive data sharing policies. Building trust requires clear agreements, robust security measures, and ongoing dialogue to reassure all parties of data integrity and ethical use.

12.4.7 Technological Innovations Facilitating Collaboration

Emerging technologies support global data infrastructure:

- **Blockchain offers decentralized, tamper-proof data management enhancing trust and transparency:** Blockchain technology introduces a decentralized framework where data is stored across multiple nodes rather than a single central authority. This structure inherently reduces the risk of data tampering or unauthorized alterations, as every transaction is cryptographically secured and recorded in an immutable ledger. Because every participant has access to the same transparent record, trust between parties is significantly increased, even among those who do not fully trust each other. This transparency also facilitates auditing and accountability, making it easier to trace data provenance and changes over time. In sectors like healthcare or finance, where data integrity is paramount, blockchain can play a transformative role. Moreover, smart contracts automate data sharing agreements by enforcing predefined rules without intermediaries. Despite challenges such as scalability and energy consumption, ongoing innovations continue to improve blockchain's practicality for secure data management.
- **Federated learning enables AI model training across distributed datasets without moving data, preserving privacy:** Federated learning represents a groundbreaking approach where AI models are trained locally on decentralized data sources, eliminating the need to centralize sensitive datasets. Instead of aggregating raw data, only model updates or gradients are shared and aggregated centrally, significantly reducing privacy risks. This technique allows organizations to collaboratively build powerful AI models without exposing individual-level data, which is especially crucial in fields like healthcare and finance with strict data protection regulations. Federated learning also mitigates concerns over data ownership and legal compliance by keeping data within its original jurisdiction. By preserving

data privacy while leveraging distributed datasets, federated learning helps overcome data silos and fosters innovation through cooperative intelligence. However, challenges such as communication overhead and model convergence require continued research to optimize performance. Ultimately, federated learning offers a privacy-preserving balance between data utility and security.

- **Cloud platforms with advanced encryption ensure secure and scalable data access:** Modern cloud computing platforms provide a flexible infrastructure for storing and processing vast amounts of data with high availability and scalability. To address security concerns, these platforms integrate advanced encryption methods both at rest and in transit, ensuring that sensitive data remains protected from unauthorized access or breaches. Encryption keys can be managed by the users themselves, adding an additional layer of control over data security. Furthermore, cloud providers offer compliance certifications and adhere to international security standards, helping organizations meet regulatory requirements more easily. The scalability of cloud resources enables dynamic allocation of computing power, allowing organizations to handle fluctuating workloads efficiently. Beyond storage, cloud platforms often include built-in tools for data analytics, machine learning, and access management. This combination of security and scalability makes cloud platforms indispensable for modern data ecosystems, facilitating collaboration without compromising privacy.
- **Application programming interfaces (APIs) allow interoperability between diverse data systems:** APIs serve as critical connectors that enable different software systems, applications, and databases to communicate and exchange data seamlessly. By providing standardized methods and protocols for data access, APIs break down silos created by proprietary systems or incompatible formats. This interoperability is essential for integrating heterogeneous data sources across organizations, industries, or geographic regions. APIs can be designed to support varying levels of data access, ensuring that sensitive information is shared securely and in compliance with governance policies. They also facilitate automation by enabling real-time data updates and interaction between applications, enhancing efficiency. Moreover, APIs support modular system architectures, allowing components to evolve independently without disrupting the overall ecosystem. In healthcare, finance, and other data-intensive sectors, APIs are foundational to building connected, scalable platforms that drive innovation and collaboration. With the rise of RESTful and GraphQL APIs, developers have powerful tools to build flexible and user-friendly data interfaces.

12.4.8 Impact on Research and Healthcare Delivery

Global collaboration in research and healthcare delivery has profoundly transformed the landscape of personalized medicine and public health. By pooling genomic and clinical datasets from diverse populations worldwide, it significantly reduces the biases that often arise from studies limited to homogeneous groups. This enhanced diversity improves the generalizability and applicability of research findings, ensuring that medical innovations are effective across different ethnicities, genetic backgrounds, and environmental contexts. Large-scale international studies become feasible, allowing researchers to identify rare genetic variants and complex disease patterns that would be impossible to detect in smaller cohorts.

Such collaboration has proven especially crucial during global health crises, such as the COVID-19 pandemic, where rapid sharing of viral genomic data accelerated the understanding of virus evolution, transmission, and vaccine development. This real-time data exchange enabled coordinated international responses and informed public health strategies that saved countless lives. Beyond emergency contexts, global data sharing fosters continuous innovation in diagnosing, treating, and preventing diseases by integrating insights from multiple healthcare systems and research institutions.

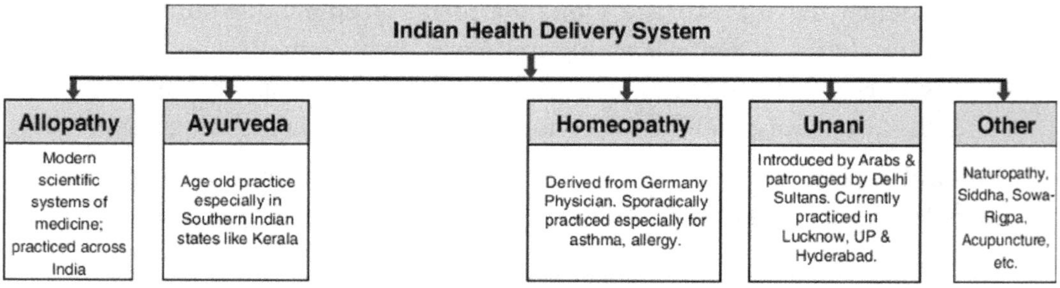

Fig. 2 Indian healthcare delivery system

Importantly, this global approach promotes health equity by extending the benefits of cutting-edge medical research to underserved and resource-limited regions. By democratizing access to genomic technologies and clinical knowledge, it helps bridge disparities in healthcare quality and outcomes. Collaborative platforms also support capacity building, training local researchers and clinicians to participate actively in global science and healthcare improvement. Moreover, integrating diverse datasets encourages the development of more inclusive AI and machine learning models that can predict disease risk, treatment response, and prognosis with greater accuracy for all populations. This advances the promise of truly personalized medicine, tailored to individuals' unique genetic and clinical profiles. In sum, global collaboration not only accelerates scientific discovery but also transforms healthcare delivery by making it more responsive, equitable, and effective worldwide. It fosters a new era of shared knowledge and collective action, where the benefits of research breakthroughs are accessible to everyone, irrespective of geography or socioeconomic status (Fig.- 2).

12.4.9 Future Directions

Sustaining and enhancing global collaboration in research and healthcare demands a multifaceted approach. First, harmonized international policies must be established to promote ethical and transparent data sharing while respecting privacy and regulatory differences. Significant investments are needed to build and upgrade infrastructure, especially in low-resource settings, to ensure equitable participation and data contribution. Alongside this, the ongoing development of technical standards and secure data platforms is crucial to maintain interoperability and safeguard sensitive information. Strengthening partnerships across academia, industry, governments, and patient communities will foster trust, innovation, and shared responsibility. By aligning these efforts, the global community can unlock the full potential of collaborative research, driving advances that benefit populations worldwide and paving the way for more inclusive, effective healthcare solutions. Sustaining and enhancing global collaboration requires:

- Harmonized international policies promoting ethical data sharing.
- Investments in infrastructure for low-resource settings.
- Continued development of technical standards and secure platforms.
- Strengthening partnerships between academia, industry, governments, and patient communities.

Global collaboration and a robust data infrastructure are indispensable for the future of personalized medicine. By uniting diverse expertise and resources worldwide, these efforts promise to unlock the full potential of precision healthcare, benefiting patients universally through more accurate diagnoses, targeted therapies, and preventive strategies.

12.5 TOWARD UNIVERSAL, INCLUSIVE PRECISION HEALTH

12.5.1 The Vision of Precision Health for All

The vision of precision health for all represents a transformative shift in how healthcare is conceived and delivered, moving beyond the traditional one-size-fits-all approach toward individualized care that integrates genetic, environmental, and lifestyle factors unique to each person. Precision health aspires to harness cutting-edge technologies, such as genomics, digital health tools, and big data analytics, to predict, prevent, and treat diseases more effectively and proactively. However, this vision extends far beyond technological innovation; it is fundamentally about equity and inclusion. To realize precision health for all, it is imperative to ensure that these medical advances reach every individual, regardless of socioeconomic status, ethnicity, geographic location, or other social determinants that have historically limited access to high-quality healthcare. Achieving universal access requires addressing deep-rooted disparities in healthcare infrastructure, education, and resource allocation. Marginalized and underserved populations often face barriers such as lack of insurance, limited access to specialized care, and insufficient representation in research studies, all of which can perpetuate health inequities. Precision health must actively work to dismantle these obstacles by designing inclusive research protocols that encompass diverse populations, investing in healthcare infrastructure in low-resource settings, and developing culturally sensitive health interventions. Moreover, policy frameworks need to support equitable access through affordable and accessible diagnostic tools, therapies, and personalized prevention strategies (Fig. 3).

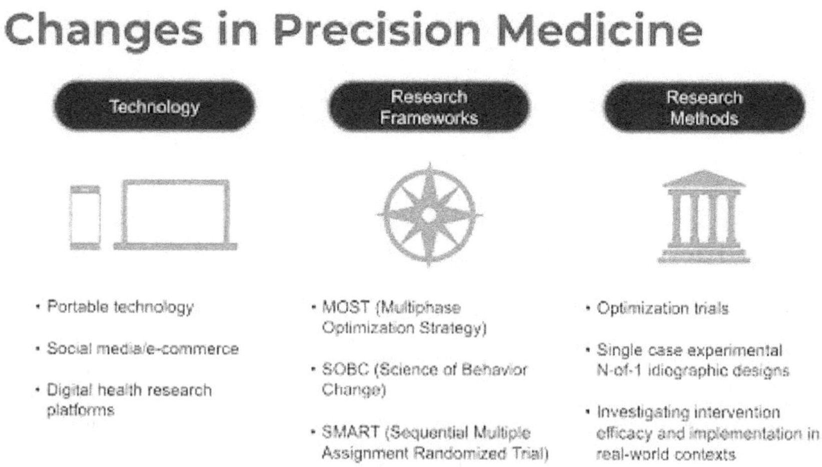

Fig. 3 Opportunities for social and behavioural sciences to drive precision health

This vision also embraces the social determinants of health, recognizing that genetics alone do not determine health outcomes. Factors like housing, nutrition, education, and environmental exposures play critical roles and must be integrated into precision health models to truly personalize care. Community engagement and patient empowerment are essential components, ensuring that individuals from all backgrounds can participate in decision-making and have their unique needs addressed. Ultimately, precision health for all aims to build healthcare systems that are not only technologically advanced but also just and inclusive, bridging gaps between different populations and fostering global health equity. By centring equity and diversity, this vision promises to transform health outcomes worldwide, enabling a future where everyone can benefit from the promise of precision medicine—improving quality of life and longevity on a truly global scale.

12.5.2 Addressing Health Disparities in Precision Medicine

Current precision medicine initiatives face significant challenges due to the underrepresentation of minority, indigenous, and underserved populations in genomic databases and clinical research. This lack of diversity creates gaps in knowledge, which limits the accuracy and effectiveness of personalized treatments and interventions for these groups. Without inclusive data, precision medicine risks perpetuating or even worsening existing health disparities, as medical decisions and innovations may be primarily based on genetic information derived from predominantly European or other well-represented ancestries. To overcome these challenges, deliberate and sustained efforts are necessary to actively recruit diverse participants in clinical trials and genomic studies. This recruitment must be accompanied by outreach and education programs that build trust within historically marginalized communities, addressing concerns around data privacy, misuse, and ethical considerations. Additionally, improving equitable access to genetic testing and counselling services is crucial, as many underserved populations face barriers related to cost, geography, and healthcare infrastructure. Culturally sensitive healthcare delivery models that respect and incorporate community values and traditions further enhance engagement and adherence to personalized care plans. By fostering inclusivity and representation, precision medicine can become a truly transformative tool that benefits all populations, helping to close the gap in health outcomes and promote equity in medical innovation.

12.5.3 Socioeconomic and Geographic Barriers

Economic constraints and geographic isolation remain major obstacles to accessing precision health services, disproportionately affecting rural and low-income populations. The high costs associated with genetic testing, specialized treatments, and counselling can place precision medicine out of reach for many individuals. Additionally, healthcare infrastructure in underserved or remote areas often lacks the necessary resources, including trained personnel and advanced technology, to support these services effectively. Digital literacy and access to reliable internet connectivity are also critical factors that limit patients' ability to engage with telemedicine and digital health tools integral to precision health. Addressing these challenges requires comprehensive policy reforms to provide subsidies and insurance coverage for precision health interventions. Investments in healthcare infrastructure must prioritize rural and economically disadvantaged communities, ensuring they are equipped with the tools and expertise needed. Moreover, community-based outreach and education programs can enhance awareness and digital skills, fostering greater acceptance and utilization of precision health. By bridging these socioeconomic and geographic gaps, precision health can become more inclusive, ensuring that advances benefit all populations regardless of their location or income.

12.5.4 Cultural Competence and Community Engagement

Promoting inclusion in precision health requires more than just scientific and technological innovation; it necessitates deep cultural competence and meaningful community engagement. Precision health programs must recognize and respect the diverse cultural values, beliefs, and preferences that influence how different populations perceive health, illness, and medical interventions. Many communities hold unique worldviews about genetics, hereditary conditions, and data privacy that can shape their willingness to participate in research or adopt new healthcare practices. Without careful attention to these perspectives, well-intentioned initiatives risk alienating or misunderstanding the very populations they aim to serve. Engaging communities early and throughout the entire research and healthcare delivery process is essential to build trust, foster mutual respect, and ensure that programs are relevant and responsive to local needs. This includes involving community leaders, patient advocates, and cultural experts in the design of studies, outreach strategies, and educational materials. Such collaboration helps address concerns about confidentiality, potential stigma, and misuse of genetic information, which can be particularly sensitive in marginalized or historically exploited populations. Tailored communication strategies are vital for conveying complex scientific concepts in culturally meaningful and accessible ways. This may involve using local languages, culturally familiar metaphors, or trusted communication channels to ensure understanding and acceptance. Culturally competent care goes beyond language to include sensitivity to customs, health beliefs, and decision-making processes that differ across communities. Healthcare providers trained in cultural competence can better support patients in navigating precision health options, improving adherence and outcomes. Moreover, community engagement empowers individuals by giving them a voice in how precision health services are developed and delivered. This participatory approach fosters a sense of ownership and accountability, which is crucial for sustained collaboration and success. It also helps identify barriers and facilitators unique to each community, guiding more effective and equitable interventions. Ultimately, integrating cultural competence and community engagement into precision health not only enhances inclusion but also enriches the science itself. By honouring diverse perspectives and experiences, precision health becomes more ethical, effective, and equitable—laying the foundation for healthcare that truly serves all people, everywhere.

12.5.5 Integration with Public Health Initiatives

The vision of universal precision health extends beyond individual clinical care to encompass population-level public health strategies, creating a more holistic and effective healthcare ecosystem. By integrating personalized genetic, environmental, and lifestyle data with traditional public health surveillance, precision health enables more accurate identification of at-risk populations and early detection of emerging health threats. This fusion allows for tailored prevention and intervention programs that are specifically designed to address the unique needs and susceptibilities of diverse communities. For example, genomic insights can guide vaccination campaigns, screening programs, and lifestyle recommendations, optimizing their impact and cost-effectiveness. Precision public health leverages advanced data analytics and bioinformatics to analyse large-scale datasets, identifying patterns that inform targeted resource allocation and health policies. This approach enhances the ability of public health systems to respond rapidly to outbreaks, chronic disease burdens, and environmental health challenges by focusing efforts where they are most needed. Moreover, it supports the development of equitable strategies that consider social determinants of health, reducing disparities and promoting health justice on a systemic level. Integrating precision health with public health initiatives requires strong collaboration among healthcare providers, researchers, policymakers, and community stakeholders. It also demands robust infrastructure for data sharing, privacy protection, and ethical governance to maintain public trust. By aligning personalized medicine with population health goals, universal precision health promises to improve outcomes not only for individuals but for entire communities, making healthcare more predictive, preventive, and inclusive. Ultimately, this integrated approach strengthens health systems globally and moves us closer to achieving sustainable, equitable health for all.

12.5.6 Ethical and Legal Frameworks for Inclusion

Creating truly inclusive precision health requires the development and enforcement of robust ethical and legal frameworks that prioritize justice, equity, and the protection of patient rights. These frameworks must address the unique challenges posed by the collection, storage, and use of sensitive genetic and health data, ensuring that individuals and communities are safeguarded against discrimination and exploitation. Policies need to be designed to protect data privacy rigorously, incorporating state-of-the-art security measures and clear consent processes that empower patients with control over how their information is shared and used. Transparent and participatory governance models are essential, involving stakeholders—including patients, researchers, ethicists, and policymakers—in decision-making processes to foster trust and accountability. Legal protections must extend beyond privacy to guarantee equitable access to precision health technologies and interventions, preventing socioeconomic status, ethnicity, or geography from becoming barriers to care. Specific laws should prohibit the misuse of genetic information in contexts such as insurance underwriting, employment, or law enforcement, which could lead to stigmatization or unfair treatment. These protections help create a safe environment where individuals feel confident to participate in research and healthcare programs without fear of repercussions. Furthermore, ethical guidelines should emphasize cultural sensitivity and respect for diverse values and beliefs, ensuring that inclusion efforts are both meaningful and respectful. By embedding equity and patient rights at the core of precision health policies, societies can work toward eliminating disparities and ensuring that the benefits of genomic and personalized medicine are accessible to all. These frameworks are not static but must evolve alongside technological advances and emerging societal challenges, maintaining a balance between innovation and human dignity. Ultimately, strong ethical and legal foundations are indispensable for building inclusive, trustworthy, and sustainable precision health systems that serve the global community fairly and responsibly.

12.5.7 Technological Innovations to Bridge Gaps

Technological innovations hold immense promise for bridging gaps and fostering inclusion in precision health, especially for remote and underserved populations. Mobile health (mHealth) applications enable individuals to monitor their health, receive personalized guidance, and connect with healthcare providers regardless of geographic barriers. Telemedicine platforms expand access to specialists and genetic counselling, overcoming challenges posed by limited local healthcare infrastructure. Artificial intelligence (AI) and machine learning tools enhance diagnostic accuracy and treatment personalization by analysing vast datasets quickly, making precision health more efficient and scalable. Advances in low-cost genomic sequencing technologies are revolutionizing access by dramatically reducing the cost and complexity of genetic testing. When combined with scalable cloud-based data platforms, these innovations democratize precision medicine by allowing a wider range of institutions and communities to participate in and benefit from genomic research and clinical applications. Such platforms also facilitate secure data sharing and collaboration, which are critical for advancing global health equity. However, technological progress alone is not enough. Digital inclusion initiatives—such as improving internet connectivity, enhancing digital literacy, and providing culturally appropriate technology training—are essential to ensure that innovations do not inadvertently widen existing disparities. Without addressing these social and infrastructural barriers, the most vulnerable populations risk being left behind as precision health advances. Therefore, a dual focus on cutting-edge technology and inclusive implementation strategies is crucial to realize the full potential of precision health for all. By doing so, we can build a future where personalized medicine is accessible, affordable, and effective across diverse global communities.

12.5.8 Global Collaboration for Equity

Global collaboration is a cornerstone for achieving equity in universal precision health, as it enables the sharing of critical resources, expertise, and data across national boundaries. International partnerships foster the creation of diverse and representative genomic databases that reflect the genetic variability of populations worldwide, addressing a major limitation in current precision medicine efforts. These collaborations also promote the development of standardized protocols and ethical guidelines that ensure care delivery is both effective and equitable, regardless of geographic or socioeconomic context. By pooling knowledge and infrastructure, collaborative networks accelerate scientific discovery and reduce duplication of efforts, ultimately speeding the translation of research into practical healthcare solutions. Moreover, global initiatives play a vital role in building capacity within low- and middle-income countries, where healthcare systems often lack the technology, training, and funding needed to implement precision health. Through training programs, technology transfer, and funding support, these efforts empower local researchers and clinicians to lead precision health initiatives tailored to their populations. This fosters self-sufficiency and sustainability, reducing reliance on external aid over time. Collaborative platforms also encourage data sharing with robust privacy protections, enabling inclusive research while respecting local regulations and cultural values. Such global partnerships help bridge the divide between affluent and resource-limited regions, promoting health equity on a truly international scale. By working together, countries can ensure that the benefits of precision health innovations are accessible to all, driving improvements in health outcomes worldwide and advancing a more just and inclusive future for medicine.

12.5.9 Measuring and Monitoring Inclusion

To ensure meaningful progress toward inclusive precision health, establishing clear metrics and robust monitoring systems is essential. These tools enable the systematic evaluation of equity in access to precision health services, clinical outcomes, and research participation across diverse populations. By collecting and analysing disaggregated data—such as by ethnicity, socioeconomic status, geography, and gender—health systems can identify disparities and uncover underserved groups that require targeted support. Data-driven assessments provide critical insights that inform policy decisions, resource allocation, and program design, ensuring that interventions are responsive to actual needs rather than assumptions. Furthermore, transparency in reporting these metrics fosters accountability among stakeholders, including healthcare providers, researchers, and policymakers. Incorporating community feedback and patient-reported outcomes into monitoring frameworks enriches understanding of barriers and facilitators to inclusion from the perspective of those most affected. This participatory approach ensures that measures of success reflect not only quantitative indicators but also qualitative experiences, enhancing the relevance and effectiveness of precision health programs. Accountability mechanisms, such as public dashboards, performance incentives, and regular audits, promote continuous improvement and reinforce commitments to equity. Moreover, international benchmarking and collaboration enable the sharing of best practices and drive global standards for inclusive precision health. Ultimately, ongoing measurement and monitoring create a feedback loop that supports adaptive strategies, helping to close equity gaps and realize the full potential of precision health for all populations.

12.5.10 Realizing the Promise of Precision Health for All

The future of precision health truly depends on its ability to be universal and inclusive, reaching all individuals regardless of their background, socioeconomic status, or geographic location. To realize this promise, it is essential to actively address existing disparities that limit access to cutting-edge technologies, genetic testing, and personalized treatments. Engaging communities through culturally sensitive education, transparent communication, and collaborative decision-making fosters trust and empowers individuals to participate fully in their healthcare journey. Equitable access to precision health services requires thoughtful policy reforms, investment in infrastructure, and dedicated efforts to build capacity in underserved regions. This inclusive approach not only enhances the effectiveness of personalized medicine but also ensures that its benefits are shared fairly across diverse populations. Achieving this vision demands coordinated and sustained efforts from multiple stakeholders, including healthcare providers, researchers, policymakers, industry leaders, and patient advocacy groups. Collaboration among these sectors can drive innovation while prioritizing ethics, equity, and social justice. It also requires continuous monitoring and adaptation to emerging challenges, such as technological disparities or evolving societal needs. By embracing a holistic, equity-centred model, precision health can transform healthcare delivery—improving disease prevention, diagnosis, and treatment outcomes worldwide. Ultimately, fulfilling the promise of precision health for all is a shared responsibility and an achievable goal, one that holds the potential to elevate global health standards and improve the lives of millions, regardless of their circumstances.

REFERENCES

Adams J. Pharmacogenomics and personalized medicine. Nature Education, 2008;1(1):194.

Agrawal, R.; Prabakaran, S. Big data in digital healthcare: Lessons learnt and recommendations for general practice. Heredity 2020, 124, 525–534.

Agyeman AA, Ofori-Asenso R. Perspective: Does personalized medicine hold the future for medicine? J Pharm Bioallied Sci. 2015;7:239-244.

Alemayehu, D.; Berger, M.L. Big Data: Transforming drug development and health policy decision making. Health Serv. Outcomes Res. Methodol. 2016, 16, 92–102

Alexander, C.A.; Wang, L. Big data analytics in heart attack prediction. J. Nurs. Care 2017, 6, 2167–2168.

Álvarez-Machancoses, Ó.; De Andrés-Galiana, E.J.; Fernández-Martínez, J.L.; Kloczkowski, A. Robust prediction of single and multiple point protein mutations stability changes. Biomolecules 2019, 10, 67.]

Álvarez-Machancoses, Ó.; deAndrés-Galiana, E.; Fernández-Martínez, J.L.; Kloczkowski, A. In The Utilization of Different Classifiers to Perform Drug Repositioning in Inclusion Body Myositis Supports the Concept of Biological Invariance. In Proceedings of the International Conference on Artificial Intelligence and Soft Computing, ICAISC 2020, Zakopane, Poland, 12–14 October 2020; Springer: Berlin/Heidelberg, Germany; pp. 589–598.

Álvarez-Machancoses, Ó.; Fernández-Martínez, J.L. Using artificial intelligence methods to speed up drug discovery. Expert Opin. Drug Discov. 2019, 14, 769–777.

Angermueller, C.; Clark, S.J.; Lee, H.J.; Macaulay, I.C.; Teng, M.J.; Hu, T.X.; Krueger, F.; Smallwood, S.A.; Ponting, C.P.; Voet, T. Parallel single-cell sequencing links transcriptional and epigenetic heterogeneity. Nat. Methods 2016, 13, 229–232.

Apweiler, R.; Beissbarth, T.; Berthold, M.R.; Blüthgen, N.; Burmeister, Y.; Dammann, O.; Deutsch, A.; Feuerhake, F.; Franke, A.; Hasenauer, J. Whither systems medicine? Exp. Mol. Med. 2018, 50, e453.

Arrieta, A.B.; Díaz-Rodríguez, N.; Del Ser, J.; Bennetot, A.; Tabik, S.; Barbado, A.; García, S.; Gil-López, S.; Molina, D.; Benjamins, R. Explainable Artificial

Intelligence (XAI): Concepts, taxonomies, opportunities and challenges toward responsible AI. Inf. Fusion 2020, 58, 82–115.

Ashley, E.A. Towards precision medicine. Nat. Rev. Genet. 2016, 17, 507–522.

Association of the British Pharmaceutical Industry. The stratification of disease for personalized medicines. http://www.abpi.org.uk/our-work/library/medical-disease/Pages/personalised-medicines.aspx. Accessed April 16, 2009.

Auffray, C.; Balling, R.; Barroso, I.; Bencze, L.; Benson, M.; Bergeron, J.; Bernal-Delgado, E.; Blomberg, N.; Bock, C.; Conesa, A. Making sense of big data in health research: Towards an EU action plan. Genome Med. 2016, 8, 1–13.

Bates, D.W.; Saria, S.; Ohno-Machado, L.; Shah, A.; Escobar, G. Big data in health care: Using analytics to identify and manage high-risk and high-cost patients. Health Aff. 2014, 33, 1123–1131.

Beckmann, J.S.; Lew, D. Reconciling evidence-based medicine and precision medicine in the era of big data: Challenges and opportunities. Genome Med. 2016, 8, 1–11.

Bejnordi, B.E.; Veta, M.; Van Diest, P.J.; Van Ginneken, B.; Karssemeijer, N.; Litjens, G.; Van Der Laak, J.A.; Hermsen, M.; Manson, Q.F.; Balkenhol, M. Diagnostic assessment of deep learning algorithms for detection of lymph node metastases in women with breast cancer. JAMA 2017, 318, 2199–2210.]

Bell GC, Caudle KE, Whirl-Carrillo M. Clinical pharmacogenetics implementation consortium (CPIC) guideline for CYP2D6 genotype and use of ondansetron and tropisetron. Clin Pharmacol Ther. 2017;102:213-218.

Bellazzi, R.; Ferrazzi, F.; Sacchi, L. Predictive data mining in clinical medicine: A focus on selected methods and applications. WIREs Data Min. Knowl. Discov. 2011, 1, 416–430.

Belle, A.; Thiagarajan, R.; Soroushmehr, S.; Navidi, F.; Beard, D.A.; Najarian, K. Big data analytics in healthcare. BioMed Res. Int. 2015, 2015, 370194.

Bibault, J.-E. Real-life clinical data mining: Generating hypotheses for evidence-based medicine. Ann. Transl. Med. 2020, 8, 69.]

Bijl MJ, Visser LE, Hofman A. Influence of the CYP2D6*4 polymorphism on dose, switching and discontinuation of antidepressants. Br J Clin Pharmacol. 2008;65:558-564.

Biswas M, Ershadian M, Shobana J. Associations of HLA genetic variants with carbamazepine-induced cutaneous adverse drug reactions: an updated meta-analysis. Clin Transl Sci. 2022;15:1887-1905.

Bochner F, Hooper WD, Eadie MJ, Tyrer JH. Decreased capacity to metabolize diphenylhydantoin in a patient with hypersensitivity to warfarin. Aust N Z J Med. 1975;5:462-466.

Bonder, M.J.; Kasela, S.; Kals, M.; Tamm, R.; Lokk, K.; Barragan, I.; Buurman, W.A.; Deelen, P.; Greve, J.-W.; Ivanov, M. Genetic and epigenetic regulation of gene expression in fetal and adult human livers. BMC Genom. 2014, 15, 860.

Bosco, G.L.; Rizzo, R.; Fiannaca, A.; La Rosa, M.; Urso, A. A deep learning model for epigenomic studies. In Proceedings of the 2016 12th International Conference on Signal-Image Technology & Internet-Based Systems (SITIS), Naples, Italy, 28 November–1 December 2016; Institute of Electrical and Electronics Engineers (IEEE): New York, NY, USA; pp. 688–692.

Bozina N, Vrkic KM, Simicevic L. Use of pharmacogenomics in elderly patients treated for cardiovascular diseases. Croat Med J. 2020;61:147-158.

Brown, B. HIPAA Beyond HIPAA: ONCHIT, ONC, AHIC, HITSP, and CCHIT. J. Health Care Compliance 2008, 10, 41–44.

Budai B, Prekopp P, Noszek L. GSTM1 null and GSTT1 null: predictors of cisplatin-caused acute ototoxicity measured by DPOAEs. J Mol Med (Berl). 2020;98:963-971.

Cacabelos R, Cacabelos N, Carril JC. The role of pharmacogenomics in adverse drug reactions. Expert Rev Clin Pharmacol. 2019;12:407-442.

Cahan, E.M.; Hernandez-Boussard, T.; Thadaney-Israni, S.; Rubin, D.L. Putting the data before the algorithm in big data addressing personalized healthcare. NPJ Digit. Med. 2019, 2, 1–6.

Caliebe A, Tekola-Ayele F, Darst BF. Including diverse and admixed populations in genetic epidemiology research. Genet Epidemiol. 2022;46:347-371.

Camacho, D.M.; Collins, K.M.; Powers, R.K.; Costello, J.C.; Collins, J.J. Next-generation machine learning for biological networks. Cell 2018, 173, 1581–1592.

Cardoso, F.; van't Veer, L.J.; Bogaerts, J.; Slaets, L.; Viale, G.; Delaloge, S.; Pierga, J.-Y.; Brain, E.; Causeret, S.; DeLorenzi, M. 70-gene signature as an aid to treatment decisions in early-stage breast cancer. N. Engl. J. Med. 2016, 375, 717–729.

Carlson B, KRAS testing: optimizing cancer therapy. Biotechnol Healthcare. 2009;6(5):7-9.

Castellani C, Assael BM. Cystic fibrosis: a clinical view. Cell Mol Life Sci. 2016;74:129-140.

Caudle KE, Thorn CF, Klein TE. Clinical Pharmacogenetics Implementation Consortium guidelines for dihydropyrimidine dehydrogenase genotype and fluoropyrimidine dosing. Clin Pharmacol Ther. 2013;94:640-645.

Cernea, A.; Fernández-Martínez, J.L.; de Andrés-Galiana, E.J.; Fernández-Muñiz, Z.; Bermejo-Millo, J.C.; González-Blanco, L.; Solano, J.J.; Abizanda, P.; Coto-Montes, A.; Caballero, B. Prognostic networks for unraveling the biological mechanisms of Sarcopenia. Mech. Ageing Dev. 2019, 182, 111129.

Cernea, A.; Fernández-Martínez, J.L.; deAndrés-Galiana, E.J.; Fernández-Ovies, F.J.; Alvarez-Machancoses, O.; Fernández-Muñiz, Z.; Saligan, L.N.; Sonis, S.T. Robust pathway sampling in phenotype prediction. Application to triple negative breast cancer. BMC Bioinform. 2020, 21, 1–13.

Chan SW, Hu M, Ko SS. CYP2C19 genotype has a major influence on labetalol pharmacokinetics in healthy male Chinese subjects. Eur J Clin Pharmacol. 2013;69:799-806.

Chan, I.S.; Ginsburg, G.S. Personalized medicine: Progress and promise. Annu. Rev. Genom. Hum. Genet. 2011, 12, 217–244.

Chang M, Soderberg MM, Scordo MG, Tybring G, Dahl ML. CYP2C19*17 affects R-warfarin plasma clearance and warfarin INR/dose ratio in patients on stable warfarin maintenance therapy. Eur J Clin Pharmacol. 2015;71:433-439.

Cheng Y, Wang G, Zhang W. Effect of CYP2C9 and SLCO1B1 polymorphisms on the pharmacokinetics and pharmacodynamics of nateglinide in healthy Chinese male volunteers. Eur J Clin Pharmacol. 2013;69:407-413.

Ciccacci C, Latini A, Politi C. Impact of glutathione transferases genes polymorphisms in nevirapine adverse reactions: a possible role for GSTM1 in SJS/TEN susceptibility. Eur J Clin Pharmacol. 2017;73:1253-1259.

Cifuentes, C.; Romero, E.; Godoy, J. Design and implementation of a telepediatric primary-level and low-cost system to reduce unnecessary patient transfers. Telemed. e-Health 2017, 23, 521–526.

Cirillo, D.; Valencia, A. Big data analytics for personalized medicine. Curr. Opin. Biotechnol. 2019, 58, 161–167.

Classen DC, Pestotnik SL, Evans SR, et al. Adverse drug events in hospitalized patients: excess length of stay, extra costs, and attributable mortality. JAMA. 1997;277(4):301-306.

Collin, C.B.; Gebhardt, T.; Golebiewski, M.; Karaderi, T.; Hillemanns, M.; Khan, F.M.; Salehzadeh-Yazdi, A.; Kirschner, M.; Krobitsch, S.; Consortium, E.-S.P. Computational Models for Clinical Applications in Personalized Medicine—Guidelines and Recommendations for Data Integration and Model Validation. J. Pers. Med. 2022, 12, 166.

Crews KR, Gaedigk A, Dunnenberger HM. Clinical Pharmacogenetics Implementation Consortium (CPIC) guidelines for codeine therapy in the context of cytochrome P450 2D6 (CYP2D6) genotype. Clin Pharmacol Ther. 2012;91:321-326.

Cutter, G.R.; Liu, Y. Personalized medicine: The return of the house call? Neurol. Clin. Pract. 2012, 2, 343–351.]

Daly AK, Donaldson PT, Bhatnagar P. HLA-B*5701 genotype is a major determinant of drug-induced liver injury due to flucloxacillin. Nat Genet. 2009;41:816-819.

Danziger, J.; Ángel Armengol de la Hoz, M.; Li, W.; Komorowski, M.; Deliberato, R.O.; Rush, B.N.; Mukamal, K.J.; Celi, L.; Badawi, O. Temporal trends in critical care outcomes in US minority-serving hospitals. Am. J. Respir. Crit. Care Med. 2020, 201, 681–687.

Dash, S.; Shakyawar, S.K.; Sharma, M.; Kaushik, S. Big data in healthcare: Management, analysis and future prospects. J. Big Data 2019, 6, 54.

Davaalkham J, Hayashida T, Tsuchiya K. Allele and genotype frequencies of cytochrome P450 2B6 gene in a Mongolian population. Drug Metab Dispos. 2009;37:1991-1993.

Dean L, Victoria MP, Stuart AS. Abacavir therapy and HLA-B*57:01 genotype. In: Medical Genetics Summaries [Internet]. Bethesda (MD): National Center for Biotechnology Information (US); 2012. Updated 2018.

Dean L. Metoprolol Therapy and CYP2D6 Genotype. 2017, Apr 4. In: Pratt VM, Scott SA, Pirmohamed M, eds. Medical Genetics Summaries. Bethesda (MD): National Center for Biotechnology Information (US); 2012-. Available from: https://www.ncbi.nlm.nih.gov/books/ NBK100663.

deAndrés-Galiana, E.J.; Bea, G.; Fernández-Martínez, J.L.; Saligan, L.N. Analysis of defective pathways and drug repositioning in Multiple Sclerosis via machine learning approaches. Comput. Biol. Med. 2019, 115, 103492.

deAndrés-Galiana, E.J.; Fernández-Martínez, J.L.; Luaces, O.; del Coz, J.J.; Fernández, R.; Solano, J.; Nogués, E.A.; Zanabilli, Y.; Alonso, J.M.; Payer, A.R. On the prediction of Hodgkin lymphoma treatment response. Clin. Transl. Oncol. 2015, 17, 612–619.

deAndrés-Galiana, E.J.; Fernández-Martínez, J.L.; Sonis, S.T. Design of biomedical robots for phenotype prediction problems. J. Comput. Biol. 2016, 23, 678–692.

Dendukuri N, Khetani K, McIsaac M, Brophy J. Testing for HER2-positive breast cancer: a systematic review and cost-effectiveness analysis. CMAJ. 2007;176:1429-1434.

Diebold, F.X.; Cheng, X.; Diebold, S.; Foster, D.; Halperin, M.; Lohr, S.; Mashey, J.; Nickolas, T.; Pai, M.; Pospiech, M. A Personal Perspective on the Origin (s) and

Development of "Big Data": The Phenomenon, the Term, and the Discipline*. CiteSeer 2012.

Dimiduk, D.M.; Holm, E.A.; Niezgoda, S.R. Perspectives on the impact of machine learning, deep learning, and artificial intelligence on materials, processes, and structures engineering. Integr. Mater. Manuf. Innov. 2018, 7, 157–172.

Dimitrov, D.V. Medical internet of things and big data in healthcare. Healthc. Inform. Res. 2016, 22, 156–163.

Duggal P, Ladd-Acosta C, Ray D, Beaty TH. The evolving field of genetic epidemiology: from familial aggregation to genomic sequencing. Am J Epidemiol. 2019;188:2069-2077.

Edginton, A.N.; Willmann, S. Physiology-based simulations of a pathological condition. Clin. Pharmacokinet. 2008, 47, 743–752.

Eduati, F.; Jaaks, P.; Wappler, J.; Cramer, T.; Merten, C.A.; Garnett, M.J.; Saez-Rodriguez, J. Patient-specific logic models of signaling pathways from screenings on cancer biopsies to prioritize personalized combination therapies. Mol. Syst. Biol. 2020, 16, e8664.

Elens L, Capron A, van Schaik RH. Impact of CYP3A4*22 allele on tacrolimus pharmacokinetics in early period after renal transplantation: toward updated genotype-based dosage guidelines. Ther Drug Monit. 2013;35:608-616.

El-Jaick KB, Ribeiro-Alves M, Soares MVG. Homozygotes NAT2*5B slow acetylators are highly associated with hepatotoxicity induced by anti-tuberculosis drugs. Mem Inst Oswaldo Cruz. 2022;117

Endicott S, Haas DM. The current state of therapeutic drug trials in pregnancy. Clin Pharmacol Ther. 2012;92:149-150.

Epstein RS, Moyer TP, Aubert RE, et al. Warfarin genotyping reduces hospitalization rates. Results from the MM-WES. J Amer Col Cardiol. 2010;55(25):2804-2812.

Erban, A.; Fehrle, I.; Martinez-Seidel, F.; Brigante, F.; Más, A.L.; Baroni, V.; Wunderlin, D.; Kopka, J. Discovery of food identity markers by metabolomics and machine learning technology. Sci. Rep. 2019, 9, 9697.

Espinal-Enríquez, J.; Mejía-Pedroza, R.; Hernández-Lemus, E. Computational approaches in precision medicine. In Progress and Challenges in Precision Medicine; Elsevier: Amsterdam, The Netherlands, 2017; pp. 233–250.

Evans WE, Relling MV. Pharmacogenomics: translating functional genomics into rational therapeutics. Science. 1999;15:487-491.

Fan, J.; Han, F.; Liu, H. Challenges of big data analysis. Natl. Sci. Rev. 2014, 1, 293–314.

Fang P, Zheng X, He J. Functional characterization of wild-type and 24 CYP2D6 allelic variants on gefitinib metabolism in vitro. Drug Des Devel Ther. 2017;11:1283-1290.

Farlex. Perlegen Sciences to Analyze Genetics of Common Diseases in Postmenopausal Women; Collaboration with Women's Health Initiative Funded by the National Institutes of Health. 2005. Last accessed on 2015 Jun 02. Available from: http://www.businesswire.com/news/home/20050630005199/en/Perlegen-Sciences-Analyze-Genetics-Common-Diseases-Postmenopausal#VW2J50ZJUdU.

FDA. Resources Related to Pharmacogenomics. U.S. Food and Drug Administration. 2005. https://www.fda.gov/drugs/science-and-research-drugs/table-pharmacogenomic-biomarkers-drug-labeling.

Fernandez Martinez, J.L.; Fernandez Muniz, M.Z.; Tompkins, M.J. On the topography of the cost functional in linear and nonlinear inverse problems. Geophysics 2012, 77, W1–W15.

Fernández-Martínez, J.L.; de Andrés-Galiana, E.J.; Fernández-Ovies, F.J.; Cernea, A.; Kloczkowski, A. Robust sampling of defective pathways in multiple myeloma. Int. J. Mol. Sci. 2019, 20, 4681.

Fernández-Martínez, J.L.; Fernández-Muñiz, Z.; Cernea, A.; Pallero, J.; DeAndrés-Galiana, E.J.; Pedruelo-González, L.M.; Álvarez, O.; Fernández-Ovies, F.J. How to deal with uncertainty in inverse and classification problems. In Advances in Modeling and Interpretation in Near Surface Geophysics; Springer: Berlin/Heidelberg, Germany, 2020; pp. 401–414.

Fernández-Martínez, J.L.; Fernández-Muñiz, Z.; Pallero, J.; Pedruelo-González, L.M. From Bayes to Tarantola: New insights to understand uncertainty in inverse problems. J. Appl. Geophys. 2013, 98, 62–72.

Fernández-Martínez, J.L.; Pallero, J.; Fernández-Muñiz, Z.; Pedruelo-González, L.M. The effect of noise and Tikhonov's regularization in inverse problems. Part I: The linear case. J. Appl. Geophys. 2014, 108, 176–185.

Fernández-Martínez, J.L.; Pallero, J.; Fernández-Muñiz, Z.; Pedruelo-González, L.M. The effect of noise and Tikhonov's regularization in inverse problems. Part II: The nonlinear case. J. Appl. Geophys. 2014, 108, 186–193.

Figueiras A, Estany-Gestal A, Aguirre C. CYP2C9 variants as a risk modifier of NSAID-related gastrointestinal bleeding: a case-control study. Pharmacogenet Genomics. 2016;26:66-73.

Finan C, Gaulton A, Kruger FA. The druggable genome and support for target identification and validation in drug development. Sci Transl Med. 2017;9:1166.

Finkelstein J, Friedman C, Hripcsak G, Cabrera M.Potential utility of precision medicine for older adults with polypharmacy: a case series study. Pharmgenomics Pers Med. 2016;15(9):31–45. doi: 10.2147/PGPM.S101474.

Folchetti, L.G.D.; da Silva, I.T.; de Almeida-Pititto, B.; Ferreira, S.R.G. Nutritionists' Health Study cohort: A web-based approach of life events, habits and health outcomes. BMJ Open 2016, 6, e012081.

Fontana RJ, Li YJ, Phillips E. Allopurinol hepatotoxicity is associated with human leukocyte antigen Class I alleles. Liver Int. 2021;41:1884-1893.

Fröhlich, H.; Balling, R.; Beerenwinkel, N.; Kohlbacher, O.; Kumar, S.; Lengauer, T.; Maathuis, M.H.; Moreau, Y.; Murphy, S.A.; Przytycka, T.M. From hype to reality: Data science enabling personalized medicine. BMC Med. 2018, 16, 1–15.

Fujita, K.A.; Ostaszewski, M.; Matsuoka, Y.; Ghosh, S.; Glaab, E.; Trefois, C.; Crespo, I.; Perumal, T.M.; Jurkowski, W.; Antony, P. Integrating pathways of Parkinson's disease in a molecular interaction map. Mol. Neurobiol. 2014, 49, 88–102.

Furda, R.; Gregus, M. Impediments in healthcare digital transformation. Int. J. Appl. Res. Public Health Manag. (IJARPHM) 2019, 4, 21–34.

Gandomi, A.; Haider, M. Beyond the hype: Big data concepts, methods, and analytics. Int. J. Inf. Manag. 2015, 35, 137–144.

Gao C, Wang Y, Tian W, Zhu Y, Xue F. The therapeutic significance of aromatase inhibitors in endometrial carcinoma. Gynecol Oncol. 2014;134:190-195.

Gediya, L.K.; Njar, V.C. Promise and challenges in drug discovery and development of hybrid anticancer drugs. Expert Opin. Drug Discov. 2009, 4, 1099–1111.

Gelb, M.H. Drug discovery for malaria: A very challenging and timely endeavor. Curr. Opin. Chem. Biol. 2007, 11, 440–445.

Giacomini KM, Balimane PV, Cho SK. International Transporter Consortium commentary on clinically important transporter polymorphisms. Clin Pharmacol Ther. 2013;94:23-26.

Ginsburg, G.S.; Willard, H.F. Genomic and personalized medicine: Foundations and applications. Transl. Res. 2009, 154, 277–287.

Grant DM, Mörike K, Eichelbaum M, Meyer UA. Acetylation pharmacogenetics. The slow acetylator phenotype is caused by decreased or absent arylamine N-acetyltransferase in human liver. J Clin Invest. 1990;85:968-972.

Greene, N.; Fisk, L.; Naven, R.T.; Note, R.R.; Patel, M.L.; Pelletier, D.J. Developing structure- activity relationships for the prediction of hepatotoxicity. Chem. Res. Toxicol. 2010, 23, 1215–1222.

Guha, R. On exploring structure–activity relationships. Silico Models Drug Discov. 2013, 81–94.

Haas DM. Pharmacogenetics and individualizing drug treatment during pregnancy. Pharmacogenomics. 2014;15:69-78.

Hagrman D, Goodisman J, Souid AK. Kinetic study on the reactions of platinum drugs with glutathione. J Pharmacol Exp Ther. 2004;308:658-666.

Hagstrom SA, Ying GS, Pauer GJT. Pharmacogenetics for genes associated with age-related macular degeneration in the Comparison of AMD Treatments Trials (CATT). Ophthalmology. 2013;120:593-599.

Hamey, F.K.; Göttgens, B. Machine learning predicts putative hematopoietic stem cells within large single-cell transcriptomics data sets. Exp. Hematol. 2019, 78, 11–20.

Hartenfeller, M.; Schneider, G. De novo drug design. Chem. Inform. Comput. Chem. Biol. 2010, 299–323

Hassan, M.; Raza, H.; Abbasi, M.A.; Moustafa, A.A.; Seo, S.-Y. The exploration of novel Alzheimer's therapeutic agents from the pool of FDA approved medicines using drug repositioning, enzyme inhibition and kinetic mechanism approaches. Biomed. Pharmacother. 2019, 109, 2513–2526.

Hastings, J.F.; O'Donnell, Y.E.; Fey, D.; Croucher, D.R. Applications of personalised signalling network models in precision oncology. Pharmacol. Ther. 2020, 212, 107555.

Hayes JD, Pulford DJ. The glutathione S-transferase supergene family: regulation of GST and the contribution of the isoenzymes to cancer chemoprotection and drug resistance. Crit Rev Biochem Mol Biol. 1995;30:445-600.

Higgins G. "The role of pharmacogenomics (PGx) in drug discovery" in Drug Discovery: Practices, Processes, and Perspectives, eds. Li JJ, Corey EJ.

Hirvensalo P, Tornio A, Neuvonen M. Enantiospecific pharmacogenomics of fluvastatin. Clin Pharmacol Ther. 2019;106:668-680.

Hodgson K, Tansey K, Dernovsekiimj MZ. Genetic differences in cytochrome P450 enzymes and antidepressant treatment response. J Psychopharmacol. 2014;28:133-141.

Hood, L. Systems biology and p4 medicine: Past, present, and future. Rambam Maimonides Med. J. 2013, 4.

Howe LA. Pharmacogenomics and management of cardiovascular disease. JNP. 2009;34:28-35.

Hulsen, T.; Jamuar, S.; Moody, A.; Karnes, J.; Varga, O.; Hedensted, S.; Spreafico, R.; Hafler, D.; McKinney, E. From big data to precision medicine. Front. Med. 2019, 6, 34.

Iriart, J.A.B. Precision medicine/personalized medicine: A critical analysis of movements in the transformation of biomedicine in the early 21st century. Cadernos. Cad. De Saúde Publica 2019, 35.]

Iyer L, Das S, Janisch L. UGT1A1*28 polymorphism as a determinant of irinotecan disposition and toxicity. Pharmacogenomics J. 2002;2:43-47.

Jain KK. Textbook of Personalised Medicine. Netherlands: Springer Science + Business Media; 2009.

Jakka S, Rossbach M. An economic perspective on personalized medicine. Hugo J. 2013;7:1.

Janga, S.C.; Edupuganti, M.M.R. Systems and network-based approaches for personalized medicine. Curr. Synth. Syst. Biol. 2014, 2.

Jimenez-Sanchez, G. Genomics innovation: Transforming healthcare, business, and the global economy. Genome 2015, 58, 511–517.

Johnson JA, Bootman JL. Drug-related morbidity and mortality. A cost-of-illness model. Arch Intern Med. 1995;155(18)1949-1956.

Jordan, M.I.; Mitchell, T.M. Machine learning: Trends, perspectives, and prospects. Science 2015, 349, 255–260.

Kasowski M, Grubert F, Heffelfinger C. Variation in transcription factor binding among humans. Science. 2010;328:232-235.

Khennou, F.; Khamlichi, Y.I.; Chaoui, N.E.H. Improving the use of big data analytics within electronic health records: A case study based OpenEHR. Procedia Comput. Sci. 2018, 127, 60–68

Khrunin AV, Filippova IN, Aliev AM. GSTM1 copy number variation in the context of single nucleotide polymorphisms in the human GSTM cluster. Mol Cytogenet. 2016;19:30.

Kim SD, Lee JH, Hur EH. Influence of GST gene polymorphisms on the clearance of intravenous busulfan in adult patients undergoing hematopoietic cell transplantation. Biol Blood Marrow Transplant. 2011;17:1222-1230.

Kitano, H.; Funahashi, A.; Matsuoka, Y.; Oda, K. Using process diagrams for the graphical representation of biological networks. Nat. Biotechnol. 2005, 23, 961–966.

Kolch, W.; Fey, D. Personalized computational models as biomarkers. J. Pers. Med. 2017, 7, 9.

Kubinyi H. Nature Reviews, Drug Discovery. 2003;2:665-668.

Kuperstein, I.; Bonnet, E.; Nguyen, H.-A.; Cohen, D.; Viara, E.; Grieco, L.; Fourquet, S.; Calzone, L.; Russo, C.; Kondratova, M. Atlas of Cancer Signalling Network: A systems biology resource for integrative analysis of cancer data with Google Maps. Oncogenesis 2015, 4, e160.

Labrinidis, A.; Jagadish, H.V. Challenges and opportunities with big data. Proc. VLDB Endow. 2012, 5, 2032–2033.

Lamb, J.; Crawford, E.D.; Peck, D.; Modell, J.W.; Blat, I.C.; Wrobel, M.J.; Lerner, J.; Brunet, J.-P.; Subramanian, A.; Ross, K.N. The Connectivity Map: Using gene-expression signatures to connect small molecules, genes, and disease. Science 2006, 313, 1929–1935.

Laurence LB, Björn CK, Randa H. Goodman & Gilman's: The Pharmacological Basis of Therapeutics, 13e. McGraw-Hill Education LLC.; 2018.

Lavanderos MA, Cayun JP, Roco A. Association study among candidate genetic polymorphisms and chemotherapy-related severe toxicity in testicular cancer patients. Front Pharmacol. 2019;10:206.

Lavrač, N. Machine learning for data mining in medicine. In Proceedings of the Joint European Conference on Artificial Intelligence in Medicine and Medical Decision Making, Aalborg, Denmark, 20–24 June 1999; Springer: Aalborg, Denmark; pp. 47–62.

Leape LL, Brennan TA, et al. NEJM. The nature of adverse events in hospitalized patients—results of the Harvard Medical Practice Study II. 1991;324(6)377-384.

Lee MR, Huang HL, Lin SW. Isoniazid concentration and NAT2 genotype predict risk of systemic drug reactions during 3HP for LTBI. J Clin Med. 2019;8:812.

Lee, B.S.; McIntyre, R.S.; Gentle, J.E.; Park, N.S.; Chiriboga, D.A.; Lee, Y.; Singh, S.; McPherson, M.A. A computational algorithm for personalized medicine in schizophrenia. Schizophr. Res. 2018, 192, 131–136.

Leff, D.; Yang, G. Big data for precision medicine. Engineering 2015, 1, 277–279.

Lek, M.; Karczewski, K.; Minikel, E.; Samocha, K.; Banks, E.; Fennell, T.; O'Donnell-Luria, A.; Ware, J.; Hill, A.; Cummings, B.; et al. Analysis of protein-coding genetic variation in 60,706 humans. Nature 2016, 536, 285–291.

Li J, Zhang L, Zhou H, Stoneking M, Tang K. Global patterns of genetic diversity and signals of natural selection for human ADME genes. Hum Mol Genet. 2011;20:528-540.

Liao Q, Chen DJ, Zhang F. Effect of CYP3A4*18B polymorphisms and interactions with OPRM1 A118G on postoperative fentanyl requirements in patients undergoing radical gastrectomy. Mol Med Rep. 2013;7:901-908.

Libbrecht, M.W.; Noble, W.S. Machine learning applications in genetics and genomics. Nat. Rev. Genet. 2015, 16, 321–332.

Light DW. New prescription drugs: a major health risk with few offsetting advantages. Harvard University. Edmond J. Safra Center for Ethics. June 27, 2014. Liou, S.-Y.; Stringer, F.; Hirayama, M. The impact of pharmacogenomics research on drug development. Drug Metab. Pharmacokinet. 2012, 27, 2–8.

Lucena MI, Molokhia M, Shen Y. Susceptibility to amoxicillin-clavulanate-induced liver injury is influenced by multiple HLA class I and II alleles. Gastroenterology. 2011;141:338-347.

Lui G, Bouazza N, Denoyelle F. Association between genetic polymorphisms and platinum-induced ototoxicity in children. Oncotarget. 2018;9:30883-30893.

Luz, C.F.; Vollmer, M.; Decruyenaere, J.; Nijsten, M.W.; Glasner, C.; Sinha, B. Machine learning in infection management using routine electronic health records: Tools, techniques, and reporting of future technologies. Clin. Microbiol. Infect. 2020, 26, 1291–1299.

Luzzatto L, Nannelli C, Notaro R. Glucose-6-phosphate dehydrogenase deficiency. Hematol Oncol Clin North Am. 2016;30:373-393.

Lv J, Liu F, Feng N. CYP3A4 gene polymorphism is correlated with individual consumption of sufentanil. Acta Anaesthesiol Scand. 2018;62:1367-1373.

MacLean, M.; Miles, C. Swift action needed to close the skills gap in bioinformatics. Nature 1999, 401, 10.

Madani, A.; Ong, J.R.; Tibrewal, A.; Mofrad, M.R. Deep echocardiography: Data-efficient supervised and semi-supervised deep learning towards automated diagnosis of cardiac disease. NPJ Digit. Med. 2018, 1, 1–11.

Malik-Sheriff, R.S.; Glont, M.; Nguyen, T.V.; Tiwari, K.; Roberts, M.G.; Xavier, A.; Vu, M.T.; Men, J.; Maire, M.; Kananathan, S. BioModels—15 years of sharing computational models in life science. Nucleic Acids Res. 2020, 48, D407–D415.

Mamoshina, P.; Vieira, A.; Putin, E.; Zhavoronkov, A. Applications of deep learning in biomedicine. Mol. Pharm. 2016, 13, 1445–1454.

Marchio, C.; Balmativola, D.; Castiglione, R.; Annaratone, L.; Sapino, A. Predictive diagnostic pathology in the target therapy era in breast cancer. Curr. Drug Targets 2017, 18, 4–12.

Mardinoglu, A.; Agren, R.; Kampf, C.; Asplund, A.; Nookaew, I.; Jacobson, P.; Walley, A.J.; Froguel, P.; Carlsson, L.M.; Uhlen, M. Integration of clinical data with a genome-scale metabolic model of the human adipocyte. Mol. Syst. Biol. 2013, 9, 649.

Martin-Sanchez, F.; Verspoor, K. Big data in medicine is driving big changes. Yearb. Med. Inform. 2014, 23, 14–20.

Masoudi-Nejad, A.; Wang, E. Cancer Modeling and Network Biology: Accelerating toward Personalized Medicine. Semin. Cancer Biol. 2015, 30, 1–3.

Mathew, P.S.; Pillai, A.S. Big Data solutions in Healthcare: Problems and perspectives. In Proceedings of the International Conference on Innovations in Information, Embedded and Communication Systems (ICIIECS), Coimbatore, India, 19–20 March 2015; pp. 1–6.]

Mazzei, M.J.; Noble, D. Big Data and Strategy: Theoretical Foundations and New Opportunities. In Strategy and Behaviors in the Digital Economy; IntechOpen: London, UK, 2019.

McCarthy AD, Kennedy JL, Middleton LT. Pharmacogenetics in drug development. Philos Trans R Soc Lond B Biol Sci. 2005;29:1579-1588.

McDonagh EM, Thorn CF, Bautista JM. PharmGKB summary: very important pharmacogene information for G6PD. Pharmacogenet Genomics. 2012;22:219-228.

McGuire AL, Burke W. An unwelcome side effect of direct-to-consumer personal genome testing: raiding the medical commons. JAMA. 2008;300:2669-2671.

McIlwain CC, Townsend DM, Tew KD. Glutathione S-transferase polymorphisms: cancer incidence and therapy. Oncogene. 2006;25:1639-1648.

Meyer, U.A. Pharmacogenetics–five decades of therapeutic lessons from genetic diversity. Nat. Rev. Genet. 2004, 5, 669–676.

Mifsud J, Maliepaard M. "Bringing the magic bullet closer to reality" in Preventive and Predictive Genetics: Towards Personalised Medicine, eds. Grech G, Grossman I.

Miller AM, Garfield S, Woodman RC. Patient and provider readiness for personalized medicine. Pers Med Oncol. 2016;5:158-167.

Minucci A, Moradkhani K, Hwang MJ. Glucose-6-phosphate dehydrogenase (G6PD) mutations database: review of the old and update of the new mutations. Blood Cells Mol Dis. 2012;48:154-165.

Monshi MM, Faulkner L, Gibson A. Human leukocyte antigen (HLA)-B*57:01-restricted activation of drug-specific T cells provides the immunological basis for flucloxacillin-induced liver injury. Hepatology. 2013;57:727-739.

Morrison, T.M.; Pathmanathan, P.; Adwan, M.; Margerrison, E. Advancing regulatory science with computational modeling for medical devices at the FDA's office of science and engineering laboratories. Front. Med. 2018, 5, 241.

Murdoch, T.B.; Detsky, A.S. The inevitable application of big data to health care. JAMA 2013, 309, 1351–1352.

Musuamba, F.T.; Skottheim Rusten, I.; Lesage, R.; Russo, G.; Bursi, R.; Emili, L.; Wangorsch, G.; Manolis, E.; Karlsson, K.E.; Kulesza, A. Scientific and regulatory evaluation of mechanistic in silico drug and disease models in drug development: Building model credibility. CPT Pharmacomet. Syst. Pharmacol. 2021, 10, 804–825.

Naqvi, M.R.; Jaffar, M.A.; Aslam, M.; Shahzad, S.K.; Iqbal, M.W.; Farooq, A. Importance of big data in precision and personalized medicine. In Proceedings of the 2020 International Congress on Human-Computer Interaction, Optimization and Robotic Applications (HORA), Ankara, Turkey, 30 July 2020; pp. 1–6.

Narita, A.; Ueki, M.; Tamiya, G. Artificial intelligence powered statistical genetics in biobanks. J. Hum. Genet. 2021, 66, 61–65.

Nelson MR, Tipney H, Painter JL. The support of human genetic evidence for approved drug indications. Nat Genet. 2015;47:856-860.

NHGRI. Genome-Wide Association Studies. 2013. Last accessed on 2013 Aug 09. Available from: http://www.genome.gov/20019523.

Niu, N.; Liu, T.; Cairns, J.; Ly, R.C.; Tan, X.; Deng, M.; Fridley, B.L.; Kalari, K.R.; Abo, R.P.; Jenkins, G. Metformin pharmacogenomics: A genome-wide association study to identify genetic and epigenetic biomarkers involved in metformin anticancer response using human lymphoblastoid cell lines. Hum. Mol. Genet. 2016, 25, 4819–4834.

Nowell SA, Ahn J, Rae JM. Association of genetic variation in tamoxifen-metabolizing enzymes with overall survival and recurrence of disease in breast cancer patients. Breast Cancer Res Treat. 2005;91:249-258.

O'Mara TA, Batra J, Glubb D. Editorial: Establishing genetic pleiotropy to identify common pharmacological agents for common diseases. Front Pharmacol. 2019;10:1038.

Oates JT, Lopez D. Pharmacogenetics: an important part of drug development with a focus on its application. Int J Biomed Investig. 2018;1:111.

Obstetric-Fetal Pharmacology Research Units Network. http://opru.rti.org.

Ogg MS, Brennan P, Meade T, Humphries SE. CYP2C9*3 allelic variant and bleeding complications. Lancet. 1999;354:1124.

Oh JH, Choi MG, Dong MS. Low-dose intravenous pantoprazole for optimal inhibition of gastric acid in Korean patients. J Gastroenterol Hepatol. 2007;22:1429-1434.

Olagunju A, Schipani A, Siccardi M. CYP3A4*22 (c.522-191 C>T; rs35599367) is associated with lopinavir pharmacokinetics in HIV-positive adults. Pharmacogenet Genomics. 2014;24:459-463.

Ozen AY, Duman DG. Pancreatic involvement in cystic fibrosis. Minerva Med. 2016;107:427-436.

Pastorino, R.; De Vito, C.; Migliara, G.; Glocker, K.; Binenbaum, I.; Ricciardi, W.; Boccia, S. Benefits and challenges of Big Data in healthcare: An overview of the European initiatives. Eur. J. Public Health 2019, 29 (Suppl. S3), 23–27.

Patil, H.K.; Seshadri, R. Big data security and privacy issues in healthcare. In Proceedings of the 2014 IEEE International Congress on Big Data, Washington, DC, USA, 27–30 October 2014; pp. 762–765.

Patil, P.; Chaudhari, P.; Sahu, M.; Duragkar, N. Review article on gene therapy. Int. J. Genet. 2012, 4, 74.

Pérez-Urizar, J.; Granados-Soto, V.; Flores-Murrieta, F.J.; Castañeda-Hernández, G. Pharmacokinetic-pharmacodynamic modeling: Why? Arch. Med. Res. 2000, 31, 539–545.

Personal Genome Project. Volunteers from the General Public Working Together with Researchers to Advance Personal Genomics. 2013. Last accessed on 2013 Aug 09. Available from: http://www. personalgenomes.org.

Personalized Medicine Coalition. The basics, 2016. Available from: www. personalizedmedicinecoalition.org.

Pincinato EC, Costa EFD, Lopes-Aguiar L. GSTM1, GSTT1 and GSTP1 Ile105Val polymorphisms in outcomes of head and neck squamous cell carcinoma patients treated with cisplatin chemoradiation. Sci Rep. 2019;9:9312.

Pison, C.; Consortium, C. THE CASyM ROADMAP Implementation of Systems Medicine across

Podlesny, N.J.; Kayem, A.V.; Meinel, C. Towards identifying de-anonymisation risks in distributed health data silos. In Proceedings of the International Conference on Database and Expert Systems Applications, Linz, Austria, 26–29 August 2019; Springer: Berlin/Heidelberg, Germany; pp. 33–43.

Policy brief. Testing for G-6-PD Deficiency for Safe Use of Primaquine in Radical Cure of P. vivax and P. ovale. 2016. Available online at: https://www.who.int/malaria/publications/atoz/g6pd-testing-PQ-radical-cure-vivax/en.

Raghupathi, W.; Raghupathi, V. Big data analytics in healthcare: Promise and potential. Health Inf. Sci. Syst. 2014, 2, 3.

Rahman, J.A. Knowledge Based Trade, Technical Change and Location Environment: The Case of Small and Medium Sized Enterprises Engaged in Advanced Producer Software Services in the South East Region. Ph.D. Thesis, University College London, London, UK, 2005.

Ramírez J, Ratain MJ, Innocenti F. Uridine 5′-diphospho-glucuronosyltransferase genetic polymorphisms and response to cancer chemotherapy. Future Oncol. 2010;6:563-585.

Rauschert, S.; Raubenheimer, K.; Melton, P.; Huang, R. Machine learning and clinical epigenetics: A review of challenges for diagnosis and classification. Clin. Epigenet. 2020, 12, 1–11.

Razzak, M.I.; Imran, M.; Xu, G. Big data analytics for preventive medicine. Neural Comput. Appl. 2020, 32, 4417–4451.

Realizing the promise of personalized medicine. Available from: www.hbr.org.

Rebbeck T. Molecular epidemiology of the human glutathione S-transferase genotypes GSTM1 and GSTT1 in cancer susceptibility. Cancer Epidemiol Biomarkers Prev. 1997;6:733-743.

Reinbolt, R.E.; Sonis, S.; Timmers, C.D.; Fernández-Martínez, J.L.; Cernea, A.; de Andrés-Galiana, E.J.; Hashemi, S.; Miller, K.; Pilarski, R.; Lustberg, M.B. Genomic risk prediction of aromatase inhibitor-related arthralgia in patients with breast cancer using a novel machine-learning algorithm. Cancer Med. 2018, 7, 240–253.

Relling MV, Gardner EE, Sandborn WJ. Clinical Pharmacogenetics Implementation Consortium guidelines for thiopurine methyltransferase genotype and thiopurine dosing. Clin Pharmacol Ther. 2011;89:387-391.

Relling MV, Klein TE. CPIC: Clinical pharmacogenetics implementation consortium of the pharmacogenomics research network. Clin Pharmacol Ther. 2011;89(3):464-467.

Ritchie, M.D.; Holzinger, E.R.; Li, R.; Pendergrass, S.A.; Kim, D. Methods of integrating data to uncover genotype–phenotype interactions. Nat. Rev. Genet. 2015, 16, 85–97.

Roses AD. Pharmacogenetics in drug discovery and development: A translational perspective. Nat Rev Drug Discov. 2008;7(10):807-817.

Ross S, Anand SS, Joseph P, Pare G. Promises, and challenges of pharmacogenetics: an overview of study design, methodological and statistical issues. JRSM Cardiovasc Dis. 2012;1:1-13.

Russmann S, Jetter A, Kullak-Ublick GA. Pharmacogenetics of drug-induced liver injury. Hepatology. 2010;52:748-761.

Sadee W, Dai Z. Pharmacogenetics/genomics and personalized medicine. Hum Mol Genet. 2005;14:207-214.

Sahana S, Bhoyar RC, Sivadas A. Pharmacogenomic landscape of Indian population using whole genomes. Clin Transl Sci. 2022;15:866-877.

Samardzic J, Bozina N, Skoric B. CYP2C19*2 genotype influence in acute coronary syndrome patients undergoing serial clopidogrel dose tailoring based on platelet function testing: analysis from randomized controlled trial NCT02096419. Int J Cardiol. 2015;186:282-285.

Sawers L, Ferguson MJ, Ihrig BR. Glutathione S-transferase P1 (GSTP1) directly influences platinum drug chemosensitivity in ovarian tumour cell lines. Br J Cancer. 2014;111:1150-1158.

Schaefer, G.O.; Tai, E.S.; Sun, S. Precision medicine and big data. Asian Bioeth. Rev. 2019, 11, 275–288.

Schneider, G. Automating drug discovery. Nat. Rev. Drug Discov. 2018, 17, 97–113.

Scott SA, Sangkuhl K, Gardner EE. Clinical Pharmacogenetics Implementation Consortium guidelines for cytochrome P450-2C19 (CYP2C19) genotype and clopidogrel therapy. Clin Pharmacol Ther. 2011;90:328-332.

Scott SA. Personalizing medicine with clinical pharmacogenetics. Genet Med. 2011;13:987-995.

Seripa D, Latina P, Fontana A. Role of CYP2D6 polymorphisms in the outcome of postoperative pain treatment. Pain Med. 2015;16:2012-2023.

Seth P, Lunetta KL, Bell DW. Phenol sulfotransferases: hormonal regulation, polymorphism, and age of onset of breast cancer. Cancer Res. 2000;60:6859-6863.

Shams ME, Arneth B, Hiemke C. CYP2D6 polymorphism and clinical effect of the antidepressant venlafaxine. J Clin Pharm Ther. 2006;31:493-502.

Shen, Y.; Zhang, Y. Transmission protocol for secure big data in two-hop wireless networks with cooperative jamming. Inf. Sci. 2014, 281, 201–210.

Shin J. Clinical pharmacogenomics of warfarin and clopidogrel. J Pharm Pract. 2012;25:428-438.

Shirai N, Furuta T, Xiao F. Comparison of lansoprazole and famotidine for gastric acid inhibition during the daytime and night-time in different CYP2C19 genotype groups. Aliment Pharmacol Ther. 2002;16:837-846.

Shull, F. The true cost of mobility? IEEE Softw. 2014, 31, 5–9.

Smith G, Stanley LA, Sim E, Strange RC, Wolf CR. Metabolic polymorphisms and cancer susceptibility. Cancer Surv. 1995;25:27-65.

Sreter KB, Barisic B, Popovic-Grle S. Pharmacogenomics and tailored polypharmacy: an 80-year-old lady with rosuvastatin-associated rhabdomyolysis and maprotiline-related Ogilvie's syndrome. Int J Clin Pharmacol Ther. 2017;55(5):442-448.

Stempler, S.; Yizhak, K.; Ruppin, E. Integrating transcriptomics with metabolic modeling predicts biomarkers and drug targets for Alzheimer's disease. PLoS ONE 2014, 9, e105383.

Stephens, Z.D.; Lee, S.Y.; Faghri, F.; Campbell, R.H.; Zhai, C.; Efron, M.J.; Iyer, R.; Schatz, M.C.; Sinha, S.; Robinson, G.E. Big data: Astronomical or genomical? PLoS Biol. 2015, 13, e1002195.

Strang, K.D.; Sun, Z. Hidden big data analytics issues in the healthcare industry. Health Inform. J. 2020, 26, 981–998.

Sy SK, de Kock L, Diacon AH. N-acetyltransferase genotypes and the pharmacokinetics and tolerability of para-aminosalicylic acid in patients with drug-resistant pulmonary tuberculosis. Antimicrob Agents Chemother. 2015;59:4129-4138.

Sykiotis GP, Kalliolians GD, Papavassiliou AG. Pharmacogenetic principles in the Hippocratic writings. J Clin Pharmacol. 2005;45(11):1218–1220.

Teng JW, Yang ZM, Li J, Xu B. Predictive role of Glutathione S-transferases (GSTs) on the prognosis of osteosarcoma patients treated with chemotherapy. Pak J Med Sci. 2013;29:1182-1186.

Testa B, Pedretti A, Vistoli G. Reactions and enzymes in the metabolism of drugs and other xenobiotics. Drug Discov Today. 2012;17:549-560.

The 1000 Genomes Project Consortium. A map of human genome variation from population-scale sequencing. Nature. 2010;467:1061-1073.

The Global Alliance for Genomics and Health. A federated ecosystem for sharing genomic, clinical data. Science 2016, 352, 1278–1280.

Thiele, I.; Palsson, B.Ø. A protocol for generating a high-quality genome-scale metabolic reconstruction. Nat. Protoc. 2010, 5, 93–121.

Tuena, C.; Semonella, M.; Fernández-Álvarez, J.; Colombo, D.; Cipresso, P. Predictive precision medicine: Towards the computational challenge. In P5 eHealth: An Agenda for the Health Technologies of the Future; Springer: Cham, Switzerland, 2020; pp. 71–86.

Tukey RH, Strassburg CP, Mackenzie PI. Pharmacogenomics of human UDP-glucuronosyltransferases and irinotecan toxicity. Mol Pharmacol. 2002;62:446-450.

Tukey RH, Strassburg CP. Human UDP-glucuronosyltransferases: metabolism, expression, and disease. Annu Rev Pharmacol Toxicol. 2000;40:581-616.

Udyavar, A.R.; Wooten, D.J.; Hoeksema, M.; Bansal, M.; Califano, A.; Estrada, L.; Schnell, S.; Irish, J.M.; Massion, P.P.; Quaranta, V. Novel hybrid phenotype revealed in small cell lung cancer by a transcription factor network model that can explain tumor heterogeneity. Cancer Res. 2017, 77, 1063–1074.

Uhlen, M.; Zhang, C.; Lee, S.; Sjöstedt, E.; Fagerberg, L.; Bidkhori, G.; Benfeitas, R.; Arif, M.; Liu, Z.; Edfors, F. A pathology atlas of the human cancer transcriptome. Science 2017, 357, e2507.

Ulyantsev, V.I.; Kazakov, S.V.; Dubinkina, V.B.; Tyakht, A.V.; Alexeev, D.G. MetaFast: Fast reference-free graph-based comparison of shotgun metagenomic data. Bioinformatics 2016, 32, 2760–2767.

Vaithinathan AG, Asokan V. Public health and precision medicine share a goal. J Evid Based Med. 2017;10:76-80.

van Loenen, B.; Kulk, S.; Ploeger, H. Data protection legislation: A very hungry caterpillar: The case of mapping data in the European Union. Gov. Inf. Q. 2016, 33, 338–345.

Van't Veer, L.J.; Dai, H.; Van De Vijver, M.J.; He, Y.D.; Hart, A.A.; Mao, M.; Peterse, H.L.; Van Der Kooy, K.; Marton, M.J.; Witteveen, A.T. Gene expression profiling predicts clinical outcome of breast cancer. Nature 2002, 415, 530–536.

Viale, G.; De Snoo, F.; Slaets, L.; Bogaerts, J.; Van't Veer, L.; Rutgers, E.; Piccart-Gebhart, M.; Stork-Sloots, L.; Glas, A.; Russo, L. Immunohistochemical versus molecular (BluePrint and MammaPrint) subtyping of breast carcinoma. Outcome results from the EORTC 10041/BIG 3-04 MINDACT trial. Breast Cancer Res. Treat. 2018, 167, 123–131.

Vizirianakis IS. Challenges in current drug delivery from the potential application of pharmacogenomics and personalized medicine in clinical practice. Curr Drug Deliv. 2004;1:73-80.

Vreuls CP, Olde Damink SW, Koek GH. Glutathione S-transferase M1-null genotype as risk factor for SOS in oxaliplatin-treated patients with metastatic colorectal cancer. Br J Cancer. 2013;108:676-680.

Vu T, Claret FX. Trastuzumab: updated mechanisms of action and resistance in breast cancer. Front Oncol. 2012;2:1-6.

Wang X, Lai Y, Luo Y. Relationship between clopidogrel-related polymorphisms and variable platelet reactivity at 1 year: a cohort study from Han Chinese. J Res Med Sci. 2016;7:111.

Wang, H.; Jiang, X.; Kambourakis, G. Special issue on Security, Privacy and Trust in network-based Big Data. Inf. Sci.—Inform. Comput. Sci. Intell. Syst. Appl. Int. J. 2015, 318, 48–50.

Wang, L. Heterogeneous data and big data analytics. Autom. Control. Inf. Sci. 2017, 3, 8–15.

Wang, R.-S.; Saadatpour, A.; Albert, R. Boolean modeling in systems biology: An overview of methodology and applications. Phys. Biol. 2012, 9, 055001.

Wang, Y.; Kung, L.; Byrd, T.A. Big data analytics: Understanding its capabilities and potential benefits for healthcare organizations. Technol. Forecast. Soc. Chang. 2018, 126, 3–13

Wenger, A.M.; Guturu, H.; Bernstein, J.A.; Bejerano, G. Systematic reanalysis of clinical exome data yields additional diagnoses: Implications for providers. Genet. Med. 2017, 19, 209–214.

Wielki, J. Implementation of the big data concept in organizations-possibilities, impediments and challenges. In Proceedings of the 2013 Federated Conference on Computer Science and Information Systems, Kraków, Poland, 8–11 September 2013; pp. 985–989.

Wilke RA, Ramsey LB, Johnson SG. The clinical pharmacogenomics implementation consortium: CPIC guideline for SLCO1B1 and simvastatin-induced myopathy. Clin Pharmacol Ther. 2012;92:112-127.

Windsor RE, Strauss SJ, Kallis C, Wood NE, Whelan JS. Germline genetic polymorphisms may influence chemotherapy response and disease outcome in osteosarcoma: a pilot study. Cancer. 2012;118:1856-1867.

Wooden, B.; Goossens, N.; Hoshida, Y.; Friedman, S.L. Using big data to discover diagnostics and therapeutics for gastrointestinal and liver diseases. Gastroenterology 2017, 152, 53–67.e3.

Wright, C.F.; McRae, J.F.; Clayton, S.; Gallone, G.; Aitken, S.; FitzGerald, T.W.; Jones, P.; Prigmore, E.; Rajan, D.; Lord, J. Making new genetic diagnoses with old data: Iterative reanalysis and reporting from genome-wide data in 1133 families with developmental disorders. Genet. Med. 2018, 20, 1216–1223.

Wu, P.-Y.; Cheng, C.-W.; Kaddi, C.D.; Venugopalan, J.; Hoffman, R.; Wang, M.D. Omic and electronic health record big data analytics for precision medicine. IEEE Trans. Biomed. Eng. 2016, 64, 263–273.

Xin HW, Liu HM, Li YQ. Association of CYP3A418B and CYP3A53 polymorphism with cyclosporine-related liver injury in Chinese renal transplant recipients. Int J Clin Pharmacol Ther. 2014;52:497-503.

Xu JM, Wang Y, Ge FJ. Severe irinotecan-induced toxicity in a patient with UGT1A1 28 and UGT1A1 6 polymorphisms. World J Gastroenterol. 2013;19:3899-3903.

Yee J, Heo Y, Kim H. Association between the CYP2C9 genotype and hypoglycemia among patients with type 2 diabetes receiving sulfonylurea treatment: a meta-analysis. Clin Ther. 2021;43:836-843.

Zhang A, Sun H, Wang P, Han Y, Wang X. Future perspectives of personalized medicine in traditional Chinese medicine: a systems biology approach. Complement Ther Med. 2011;20:93-99.

Zhang BL, Sun T, Zhang BN. Polymorphisms of GSTP1 is associated with differences of chemotherapy response and toxicity in breast cancer. Chin Med J (Engl). 2011;124:199-204.

Zhang J, Wu Y, Hu X. GSTT1, GSTP1, and GSTM1 genetic variants are associated with survival in previously untreated metastatic breast cancer. Oncotarget. 2017;8:105905-105914.

Zhang, H. Overview of sequence data formats. In Statistical Genomics; Springer: Berlin/Heidelberg, Germany, 2016; pp. 3–17.

Zhou SF, Wang LL, Di YM. Substrates and inhibitors of human multidrug resistance associated proteins and the implications in drug development. Curr Med Chem. 2008;15:1981-2039.

Zhou Y, Lauschke VM. Population pharmacogenomics: an update on ethnogeographic differences and opportunities for precision public health. Hum Genet. 2022;141:1113-1136.

Zikopoulos, P.; Eaton, C. Understanding Big Data: Analytics for Enterprise Class Hadoop and Streaming Data; McGraw-Hill Osborne Media: New York, NY, USA, 2011.

Zoon CK, Starker EQ, Wilson AM, Emmert-Buck MR, Libutti SK, Tangrea MA. Current molecular diagnostics of breast cancer and the potential incorporation of microRNA. Expert Rev Mol Diagn. 2009;9:455-467.

Index

www.ingramcontent.com/pod-product-compliance
Lightning Source LLC
LaVergne TN
LVHW081941200926
848484LV00009B/2487
* 9 7 8 1 7 8 7 1 5 6 1 5 9 *